OSCE
and Clinical Skills Handbook

OSCE

and Clinical Skills Handbook

SECOND EDITION

KATRINA F. HURLEY, MD, FRCPC, MHI

Assistant Professor, Emergency Medicine
Dalhousie University
Halifax, Nova Scotia, Canada

ELSEVIER
SAUNDERS

OSCE AND CLINICAL SKILLS HANDBOOK   ISBN: 978-1-926648-15-6
Copyright © 2011 Elsevier Canada, a division of Reed Elsevier Canada, Ltd.

Notice

Medicine is an ever-changing field. Standard safety precautions must be followed, but as new research and clinical experience broaden our knowledge, changes in treatment and drug therapy may become necessary or appropriate. Every effort has been made to ensure that the drug dosage schedules are accurate and in accord with standards accepted at the time of printing. However, it is important to mention that the doses used in this publication do not necessarily conform to manufacturer's recommendations. Readers are advised to check the most current product information provided by the manufacturer of each drug to be administered to verify the recommended dose, the method and duration of administration, and contraindications. It is the responsibility of the licensed prescriber, relying on knowledge of the patient and experience, to determine the dosages and best treatment for each patient. Neither the publishers nor the editors assume any liability for any injury and/or damage to persons or property arising from this publication.

The Publisher

Library and Archives Canada Cataloguing in Publication
Hurley, Katrina F., 1976-
   OSCE and clinical skills handbook / Katrina F. Hurley.—2nd ed.
ISBN: 978-1-926648-15-6
   1. Clinical medicine—Examinations—Study guides. 2. Clinical competence—Examinations, questions, etc. 3. Medical history taking—Examinations, questions, etc. 4. Physical diagnosis—Examinations, questions, etc. I. Title.
   RC71.H87 2011   616.0076   C2010-905447-4

Vice President, Publishing: Ann Millar
Managing Developmental Editor: Martina van de Velde
Publishing Services Manager: Jeff Patterson
Project Manager: Mary Stueck
Copy Editor: Anne Ostroff
Cover Design: Karen Pauls
Interior Design: Karen Pauls
Typesetting and Assembly: Graphic World India

Elsevier Canada
905 King Street West, 4th Floor, Toronto, ON, Canada M6K 3G9
Phone: 1-866-896-3331
Fax: 1-866-359-9534

To my by'e and our little monsters.

"In spite of pain and injustice, life is good.
Under the badness, goodness lives;
and if good doesn't exist, we will make it exist; and we will save the world
although it might not want us to."

Rafael Barrett
Great writer, journalist, and Spanish mathematician

CONTENTS

CONTRIBUTORS

Peter Green, MD, FRCPC

Program Director, Division of Dermatology
Associate Professor of Dermatology
Dalhousie University
Halifax, Nova Scotia, Canada
CHAPTER 7: DERMATOLOGY

Rose P. Mengual, ACP, MD

Emergency Medicine Resident
Dalhousie University
Halifax, Nova Scotia, Canada
Royal College of Physicians and Surgeons of Canada
CHAPTER 5: NERVOUS SYSTEM

James Chan, MD, MEd, FRCPC

Associate Program Director, Internal Medicine Program
Division of General Internal Medicine
University of Ottawa
Ottawa, Ontario, Canada

Chris King-Talley, RN, MSN, FNP-BC

Senior Instructor
Family Nurse Practitioner
University of Calgary
Calgary, Alberta, Canada

Nancy McNaughton, MEd, PhD

Associate Director, Standardized Patient Program
Fellow, Wilson Center for Research in Education
Faculty of Medicine
University of Toronto
Toronto, Ontario, Canada

Amil Shah, MDCM, FACP, FRCPC

Clinical Competency Assessment Director
Undergraduate MD Program
Faculty of Medicine
University of British Columbia
Vancouver, British Columbia, Canada

Diana Tabak, MEd(S)

Lecturer, Family and Community Medicine
Associate Director, Standardized Patient Program
University of Toronto
Toronto, Ontario, Canada

PREFACE

STATEMENT OF PURPOSE

The *OSCE and Clinical Skills Handbook* is designed as a study aid for medical students preparing for Objective Structured Clinical Examinations (OSCEs). In my own experience as a student at Memorial University of Newfoundland, I found OSCE preparation difficult because of the broad range of materials available and the lack of a centralized study aid that reflected the style of the examination. For this reason, I saw an opportunity to develop a book that not only summarized important history and physical examination skills in a centralized way, but also supplied the information through the use of patient presentations or examination scenarios. The format is designed to facilitate both individual and group study.

The clinical examination was devised by medical pioneers who used these techniques as diagnostic tests: for example, tactile fremitus, percussion, and auscultation to detect pneumonia. The physical examination has endured the test of time, and one instrument, the stethoscope, has come to be viewed as a symbol of the profession as a whole. Technology has advanced the field of medicine substantially in the past century, leading some authorities to question the value of the clinical examination in modern medicine. Prudent use of clinical examination can guide the application of diagnostic and treatment technologies.

Your feedback and ideas are welcome; contact me at kfhurley@dal.ca.

DISCLAIMER

By no means is this book all-inclusive; although it contains a multitude of scenarios that may not be presented in your OSCE, it fails to include every *possible* question. The *OSCE and Clinical Skills Handbook,* 2nd edition, has not been officially endorsed by medical schools, the Medical Council of Canada, or the United States Medical Licensing Examination (USMLE).

The scope of this book is limited primarily to basic clinical medicine and contains only a cursory review of anatomy that would be considered the minimum requirement needed to learn the core clinical competencies. Furthermore, physiology, therapy, and current management are beyond the scope of this book, and students are encouraged to consult appropriate textbooks (such as those included in the Resource List) and online evidence-based resources as needed.

Communication and interviewing skills are considered core clinical competencies in medicine, and their importance cannot be overemphasized. The subtleties of interpersonal, cross-cultural, and interprofessional communication skills are not addressed in this handbook. Students are assumed to have attained these core skills in their teaching curriculums early in their training. Consult appropriate references in the Resource List to review this information.

ACKNOWLEDGMENTS

Many thanks to the students who have contributed feedback and new ideas that have helped to improve this book during its development, namely, those at Memorial University of Newfoundland, who were the first to read the book, many drafts ago.

It was the positive responses from these students that convinced me to carry on in this endeavor.

Special thanks to the staff at Elsevier who made this publication possible, especially Ann Millar, Martina van de Velde, and Anne Ostroff. I am thankful for the substantial contributions of Drs. Rose Mengual and Peter Green, who wrote the Nervous System and Dermatology chapters, respectively. Without these contributions, this project could not have been completed. I am also grateful for the expert advice provided by Dr. Graham Bullock for the Musculoskeletal System chapter; Dr. Lara Hazelton for the Psychiatry chapter; Drs. Katalin Koller and Paige Moorhouse for the Geriatrics chapter; and Drs. Lynette Reid, Merril Pauls, and John Campbell for their feedback and suggestions for the Ethics chapter.

Finally, I wish to thank my husband, who continues to support my authorship and academic pursuits. With three young children, this sort of support is no longer an abstract concept . . . those of you who are parents will understand what I mean!

RESOURCE LIST

ANATOMY AND PHYSIOLOGY

Blumenfeld H. *Neuroanatomy through Clinical Cases.* 2nd ed. Sunderland, Mass.: Sinauer Associates; 2010.

Hall JE. *Guyton and Hall Textbook of Medical Physiology.* 12th ed. Philadelphia: Elsevier; 2010.

Moore KL, Dalley AF, Agur AMR. *Clinically Oriented Anatomy.* 6th ed. Philadelphia: Lippincott Williams & Wilkins; 2009.

Netter FH. *Atlas of Human Anatomy.* 5th ed. St. Louis: Elsevier; 2010.

COMMUNICATION

Buckman R. *How to Break Bad News: A Guide for Health Care Professionals.* Baltimore: Hopkins Fulfillment Service; 1992.

Gordon T, Edwards WS. *Making the Patient Your Partner: Communication Skills for Doctors and Other Caregivers.* Westport, Conn.: Auburn House; 1997.

Silverman J, Kurtz S, Draper J. *Skills for Communicating with Patients.* 2nd ed. Abingdon, UK: Radcliffe Medical Press; 2005.

DEFINITIONS AND TERMINOLOGY

Dorland's Illustrated Medical Dictionary. 31st ed. Philadelphia: Elsevier; 2007.

Stedman's Medical Dictionary. 28th ed. Philadelphia: Lippincott Williams & Wilkins; 2005.

OSCE

Byrne G, Hill J, Dornan T, et al. *Core Clinical Skills for OSCEs in Surgery.* Edinburgh: Churchill Livingstone; 2007.

Dornan T, O'Neill PA. *Core Clinical Skills for OSCEs in Medicine.* 2nd ed. Edinburgh: Churchill Livingstone; 2006.

Jugovic PJ, Bitar R, McAdam LC. *Fundamental Clinical Situations: A Practical OSCE Study Guide.* 4th ed. Toronto, ON: WB Saunders; 2003.

Singer PA, Robb AK. *Ethics OSCE Project,* Toronto, 1994, Centre for Bioethics and Department of Medicine, University of Toronto; http://wings.buffalo.edu/bioethics/osce.html

MedEdPORTAL is a program of the Association of American Medical Colleges (http://services. aamc.org/30/mededportal/servlet/segment/mededportal/information/). The "Featured Collection" on Standardized Patients is very useful.

CLINICAL SKILLS

Bickley LS. *Bates' Guide to Physical Examination and History Taking.* 10th ed. Philadelphia: Lippincott Williams & Wilkins; 2008.

Douglas G, Nicol F, Robertson C. *MacLeod's Clinical Examination.* 12th ed. Edinburgh: Churchill Livingstone; 2009.

Gill D, O'Brien N. *Paediatric Clinical Examination Made Easy.* 5th ed. Edinburgh: Churchill Livingstone; 2006.

Jarvis C. *Physical Examination and Health Assessment.* 5th ed. Philadelphia: Elsevier; 2007.

LeBlond RF, Brown D, DeGowin R. *DeGowin's Diagnostic Examination.* 9th ed. New York: McGraw-Hill Professional; 2008.

Marks JG, Miller JJ. *Lookingbill and Marks' Principles of Dermatology.* 4th ed. Philadelphia: Elsevier; 2006.

Seidel HM, Ball JW, Dains JE, et al. *Mosby's Guide to Physical Examination.* 7th ed. St. Louis: Mosby; 2010.

Singer PA. *Bioethics at the Bedside: A Clinician's Guide.* Ottawa, ON: Canadian Medical Association; 1999.

Swartz MH. *Textbook of Physical Diagnosis: History and Examination.* 6th ed. Philadelphia: Elsevier; 2009.

Weller R, Hunter JAA, Savin J, et al. *Clinical Dermatology.* 4th ed. New York: Wiley-Blackwell; 2008.

Zimmerman M. *Interview Guide for Evaluating DSM-IV Psychiatric Disorders and the Mental Status Examination.* East Greenwich, RI: Psych Products Press; 1994.

INTRODUCTION

WHAT IS AN OSCE?

The Objective Structured Clinical Examination (OSCE) is a tool widely used for measuring clinical competence. The OSCE was first described by Harden and colleagues at the University of Dundee in 1975.[1] It was developed to improve the evaluation of medical students' clinical skills, such as communication. The first OSCE consisted of a number of timed stations through which students rotated and evaluators used itemized checklists with "controlled grading criteria." The authors found the results to be easily reproducible.

Since that time, the OSCE has been adopted by many medical schools in North America and Europe, by the Medical Council of Canada (Qualifying Examination Part II; see http://www.mcc.ca/en/exams/qe2/), and by the United States Medical Licensing Examination (Step 2; see http://www.usmle.org/Examinations/step2/step2.html). Of 126 schools accredited by the Liaison Committee on Medical Education (LCME) in 2002 to 2003, 82 used a comprehensive clerkship-level OSCE.[2] Furthermore, numerous residency programs and several specialty examination boards are also using OSCE-type examinations with "standardized patients" (from whom the student obtains the history or performs the examination). OSCEs have been extensively studied in undergraduate and postgraduate medical settings and have also been used in other professional education domains such as nursing and dentistry.[3,4]

The advantage of this tool has been its ability to test the many dimensions of clinical competence: history taking, physical examination, interpersonal and communication skills, professionalism, technical skills, problem solving, decision making, management, and documentation.[5]

The reliability or the reproducibility of OSCE scores over time is "acceptable."[6] A wide range of reliabilities have been reported over the years for the OSCEs, citing influences such as standardization of patients, number, range and length of stations;

[1]Harden RM, Stevenson M, Downie WW, et al. Assessment of clinical competence using objective structured examination. *BMJ.* 1975;1:447-451.

[2]Barzansky B, Etzel SI. Educational programs in US medical schools, 2002–2003. *JAMA.* 2003;290:1190-1196.

[3]Mitchell ML, Henderson A, Groves M, et al. The Objective Structured Clinical Examination (OSCE): optimising its value in the undergraduate nursing curriculum. *Nurse Educ Today.* 2009;29:398-404.

[4]Cannick GF, Horowitz AM, Garr DR, et al. Use of the OSCE to evaluate brief communication skills training for dental students. *J Dent Educ.* 2007;71:1203-1209.

[5]Casey PM, Goepfert AR, Espey EL, et al. To the point: reviews in medical education—the Objective Structured Clinical Examination. *Am J Obstet Gynecol.* 2009;200:25-34.

[6]Turner JL, Dankoski ME. Objective structured clinical exams: a critical review. *Fam Med.* 2008;40: 574-578.

and student fatigue and anxiety.[7-12] Construct validity can be ensured through the process of blueprinting, whereby the complexity, scope, outcomes, and expectations are defined.[13] OSCEs have also been validated using the construct of experience: that is, more senior trainees should perform better than more junior trainees.[14]

OSCEs can be expected to vary from setting to setting in terms of specific scenarios, standardized patients, grading criteria, time allowed for each scenario, and outcomes. Although I have attempted to eliminate my own biases, the evolution of this book reflects my own experiences with OSCEs at Memorial University of Newfoundland and Dalhousie University.

HOW IS AN OSCE GRADED?

Traditionally, a trainee's performance has been evaluated through the use of a standardized clinical scenario and a structured binary checklist. The "observer" completing the checklist may be an examiner (who witnesses the examination), the standardized patient, or a combination of both. Some checklist items are considered "critical actions": that is, actions that are considered essential or core for ensuring patient safety and an optimal outcome.[15] In some examinations, failure to complete critical actions may be grounds for remediation or for failing the station.

Some OSCEs are evaluated through the use of a global rating scale. This type of scale may reflect, for example, communication skills, professionalism, cohesiveness, and responsiveness to the patient's needs or feelings.[16] A global rating scale can be used independently of, or as a supplement to, a checklist.

For the specific objectives and format of the Medical Council of Canada Qualifying examination, see the council's Website (www.mcc.ca). For specific information on the United States Medical Licensing Examination, see www.usmle.org.

---

[7]van der Vleuten CPM, Swanson DB. Assessment of clinical skills with standardized patients: state of the art. *Teach Learn Med.* 1990;2(2):58-76.

[8]Cohen R, Reznick RK, Taylor BR, et al. Reliability and validity of the Objective Structured Clinical Examination in assessing surgical residents. *Am J Surg.* 1990;160:302-305.

[9]Matsell DG, Wolfish NM, Hsu E. Reliability and validity of the Objective Structured Clinical Examination in paediatrics. *Med Educ.* 1991;25:293-299.

[10]Newble DI, Sawnson DB. Psychometric characteristics of the Objective Structured Clinical Examination. *Med Educ.* 1988;22:325-334.

[11]Petrusa ER, Blackwell TA, Ainsworth MA. Reliability and validity of the Objective Structured Clinical Examination for assessing the clinical performance of residents. *Arch Intern Med.* 1990;150:573-577.

[12]Roberts J, Norman G. Reliability and learning from the Objective Structured Clinical Examination. *Med Educ.* 1990;24:219-233.

[13]Roberts C, Newble D, Jolly B, et al. Assuring the quality of high-stakes undergraduate assessments of clinical competence. *Med Teach.* 2006;28:535-543.

[14]Merrick HW, Nowacek GA, Boyer J, et al. Ability of the Objective Structured Clinical Examination to differentiate surgical residents, medical students, and physician assistant students. *J Surg Res.* 2002;106:319-322.

[15]Payne NJ, Bradley EB, Heald EB, et al. Sharpening the eye of the OSCE with critical action analysis. *Acad Med.* 2008;83:900-905.

[16]Hodges B, McIlroy JH. Analytic global OSCE ratings are sensitive to level of training. *Med Educ.* 2003;37:1012-1016.

HOW SHOULD I PREPARE FOR AN OSCE?

The OSCE is viewed by students as a high-stakes examination and provokes significant anxiety.[17] Female students, in particular, report more anxiety and lower confidence than do their male counterparts.[18]

It is thus not surprising that students spend a significant amount of time studying and preparing for their OSCEs. Students often collaborate in their preparations, taking the time to practice with one another.[19] "Good performance" appears to be linked to learning styles. Well-organized study methods and learning styles characterized by desire to achieve and an orientation toward learning for meaning (rather than surface learning or rote learning) appear to be positively associated with better OSCE performance.[20]

Some research findings have suggested that students change their behavior in accordance with how the OSCE is graded.[21] For example, students expecting to be evaluated with a structured checklist ask highly focused questions, whereas students expecting to be evaluated with a global rating scale ask more open-ended questions.[22]

There is evidence that, paradoxically, expert clinicians may perform more poorly than trainees on checklist-scored OSCEs. Experts may use heuristic methods and more focused assessments, overlooking some of the thoroughness rewarded by checklists.[22,23]

Although prior academic performance may be the best predictor of success, OSCE performance is a "product of complex relationships between skills and knowledge, mediated by perceptions of anxiety, self-confidence and preparedness."[24,25]

KEY TIPS FOR SUCCESS IN THE OSCE

PRIOR TO THE EXAMINATION

Find out about the format of the examination, including the number, length, and scope of stations, and the assessment method (checklist versus global rating; scoring by an examiner, a standardized patient, or a combination of the two, if possible. High-stakes

---

[17]Brand HS, Schoonheim-Klein M. Is the OSCE more stressful? Examination anxiety and its consequences in different assessment methods in dental education. *Eur J Dent Educ.* 2009;13:147-153.

[18]Blanch DC, Hall JA, Roter DL, et al. Medical student gender and issues of confidence. *Patient Educ Couns.* 2008;72:374-281.

[19]Rudland J, Wilkinson T, Smith-Han K, et al. "You can do it late at night or in the morning. You can do it at home, I did it with my flatmate." The educational impact of an OSCE. *Med Teach.* 2008;30:206-211.

[20]Martin IG, Stark P, Jolly B. Benefiting from clinical experience: the influence of learning style and clinical experience on performance in an undergraduate Objective Structured Clinical Examination. *Med Educ.* 2000;34:530-534.

[21]McIlroy JH, Hodges B, McNaughton N, et al. The effect of candidates' perceptions of the evaluation method on reliability of checklist and global rating scores in an Objective Structured Clinical Examination. *Acad Med.* 2002;77:725-728.

[22]Hodges B, Regehr G, McNaughton N, et al. Checklists do not capture increasing levels of expertise. *Acad Med.* 1999;74:1129-1134.

[23]Hodges B, McNaughton N, Regehr G, et al. The challenge of creating new OSCE measures to capture the characteristics of expertise. *Med Educ.* 2002;36:742-748.

[24]Mavis BE. Does studying for an Objective Structured Clinical Examination make a difference? *Med Educ.* 2000;34:808-812.

[25]Mavis B. Self-efficacy and OSCE performance among second year medical students. *Adv Health Sci Educ Theory Pract.* 2001;6(2):93-102.

examinations such as those administered by the Medical Council of Canada have detailed objectives that are published online. Understanding the format and expected content of the examination will help you tailor your studying and group practice exercises. Knowing what to expect may also help reduce anxiety about the process.

DURING THE EXAMINATION

In OSCEs, as in clinical practice, you can expect to encounter new problems. It may not be possible to prepare yourself for every question that *could* be asked on your OSCE. More important than knowing the content of each question is to face each question with a method or strategy. When you encounter a question that you have not studied or when you begin to draw a blank, you can rely on a framework such as **ChLORIDE FPP** to delineate a history, **VITAMINS C** to sort through differential diagnoses, and **IPPA** to approach physical examination.

Thus, when in doubt, take a systematic approach:

Character	**V**ascular	**I**nspection
Location	**I**nfectious	**P**alpation
Onset	**T**raumatic	**P**ercussion
Radiation	**A**utoimmune/allergic	**A**uscultation
Intensity	**M**etabolic	
Duration	**I**diopathic/iatrogenic	
Events associated	**N**eoplastic	
Frequency	**S**ubstance abuse and psychiatric	
Palliative factors	**C**ongenital	
Provocative factors		

TIPS TO IMPROVE PERFORMANCE

- Read the instructions to candidate carefully.
- Suspend disbelief; treat the standardized patient the way you would treat a real patient.
- Ignore the presence of the examiner; do not be distracted by what the examiner is doing with the checklist or scoring sheet.
- Be sure to introduce yourself to the patient and find out the patient's name or confirm the patient's identity.
- Wash your hands.
- Develop a rapport with the patient, just as you would with a real patient.
- Be conscientious about the patient's comfort during the physical examination.
- Ensure that you drape the patient properly.
- Explain aloud what you are doing in your examination of the patient. State what you are looking for and your findings (both for the patient and for the examiner).
- If you make a mistake, move on! If you perform badly on a station, you need to put that out of your mind and focus on what is being asked of you right now. Remember that the examiner and the standardized patient in subsequent stations do not know about your performance on other stations. Each station marks a fresh start.

HOW TO USE THIS BOOK

A list of abbreviations is provided at the end of the introduction. All abbreviations used in this book can be found in this alphabetized list.

This book is organized in scenarios that are suitable to a variety of learning levels, from the most basic physical examination skills, such as examining the liver, to questions whose answers require a multisystem approach, such as assessing a patient with a complaint of "chest pain."

Chapters 1 to 6 and 8 to 14 reflect core competencies in clinical medicine. Chapter 7, *Dermatology*, provides a fundamental approach to the examination and description of some common skin problems. Dermatology is considered a subspecialty area and is thus not a core area of study in most undergraduate clinical clerkships. The problem-based scenarios in this chapter are examples of what you may commonly encounter in a primary care or emergency department setting and are not intended to be all-inclusive; it is hoped that a background of some common problems will be helpful in guiding you to formulate a differential diagnosis and approach to other skin conditions not covered here.

Chapters 1 to 11 are divided into sections on **Anatomy, Glossary of Signs and Symptoms, Essential Skills,** and **Advanced Skills.** Each chapter also contains **Sample Checklists** that are worthy of review by learners at all levels. In general, junior-level students should focus on the Essential Skills, whereas more senior trainees should extend their focus to Advanced Skills.

Although the majority of the book is arranged in a systems-based manner, Chapters 11, 12, and 13 reflect specific populations (women, children, and elderly patients, respectively). In general, the Essential Skills and Advanced Skills presented in Chapters 1 to 10 can be applied to these specific populations (at times, in a modified way).

Chapter 14, *Ethics*, differs from the other chapters with regard to format; an ethical scenario is presented, followed by a discussion of the principal learning points for the case and a performance summary of what the student should accomplish in the course of a compassionate conversation with the patient.

The Sample Checklists that appear in each chapter are an example of the performance assessment sheets that an OSCE examiner might use to grade your demonstrated skill-set at each timed station. These lists serve as a means of testing yourself or group members in preparation for the OSCE.

Approach the material as a guide only. You need not perform the physical examination tasks or approach the history in the order presented in this handbook; the content is meant to be illustrative rather than prescriptive. However, you should take an organized approach, developing a consistent method that you can apply in each encounter with a patient. It is difficult to construct clinical encounters on paper. A real-life encounter would allow for the patient to respond to your queries, which would shape your thoughts and alter your subsequent questions. Do not treat the scenarios in this book as a list of questions that should be memorized; the goal is to present a framework. You need to apply the framework and *customize* it to the patient presenting in your OSCE.

DECIPHERING THE EVIDENCE FOR THE CLINICAL EXAMINATION

The clinical examination was devised by medical pioneers who used these techniques as diagnostic tests. Viewed as representative of healing professions as a whole, the clinical examination has endured the test of time and provides an opportunity to deepen patient relationships and add a "human touch."[26]

Technology has advanced the field of medicine substantially over the past century, leading some authorities to question the value of the clinical examination in modern medicine. In general, high-quality evidence that tests the usefulness of the clinical examination is sparse. However, informed use of clinical examination can guide the application of diagnostic and treatment technologies.

Where possible, I have outlined evidence to support or refute features of the clinical examination. "Good" evidence on the diagnostic use of clinical examination would include a blind comparison with an independent "gold standard" irrespective of examination results; an appropriate spectrum of patients; a description of the setting and the patient population; and a description of the examination technique, detailed enough to be accurately replicated. The endpoint would be a measure of the examination's precision or reliability and its accuracy. Precision is often measured in terms of interrater reliability. The κ statistic is one measure of precision that establishes whether the observer agreement is beyond chance (Table 1).

Accuracy is the correctness of the test in diagnosing (or not diagnosing) disease when it is actually present (or absent). *Precision* is a prerequisite for accuracy, but a test that is very precise may still be rather inaccurate: for example, the use of eye color as a predictor of multiple gestation. Determination of eye color would probably have high intraobserver and interobserver agreement (precision). However, in comparison with the "gold standard" of ultrasonography, the use of eye color for determining the presence of multiple gestations yields poor accuracy.

Accuracy can be measured in terms of sensitivity or specificity, or it can be measured with likelihood ratios. The likelihood ratio combines sensitivity and specificity. You can use the likelihood ratio, pretest probability, and a Fagan nomogram to arrive at an estimate of the posttest probability (Table 2 and Figures 1 and 2). *Pretest probability* is the probability that a particular disease is present before a diagnostic test such as the physical examination is used. In most cases, this can be equated to the prevalence of disease in a given population, which can be stratified by age and sex when applicable.

A *positive likelihood ratio* is used to "rule in" disease—that is, it reflects the likelihood that disease is present when the test result is positive—whereas a *negative likelihood ratio* is used to "rule out" disease when the test result is negative or the clinical finding is absent. Where possible in this book, I have presented the positive and negative likelihood ratios for features of the clinical examination.

To explore this topic further, consult an evidence-based resource such as the book by McGee.[26a]

---

[26]Bickley LS. *Bates' Guide to Physical Examination and History Taking.* 8th ed. Philadelphia: Lippincott, Williams & Wilkins; 2003.

[26a]McGee S. *Evidence-Based Physical Diagnosis.* 2nd ed. Philadelphia: Elsevier; 2007.

Table 1 Interpretation of κ Values

κ	Conventional Levels
≤0	Poor agreement (less than chance)
0.01–0.2	Slight agreement
0.21–0.4	Fair agreement
0.41–0.6	Moderate agreement
0.61–0.8	Substantial agreement
0.81–1.0	Almost perfect agreement

Viera AJ, Garrett JM. Understanding interobserver agreement: The kappa statistic. *Fam Med.* 2005;37:360-363.

Table 2 Interpretation of Likelihood Ratios (LRs)

LR	Effect
>10 \<0.1	High
5–10 0.1–0.2	Moderate
2–5 0.2–0.5	Small
1–2 0.5–1	Rarely useful

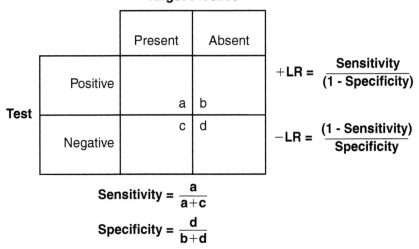

Figure 1 Calculating likelihood ratios. −LR, Negative likelihood ratio; +LR, positive likelihood ratio.

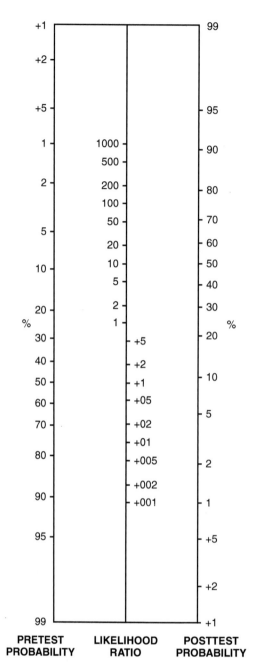

Figure 2 The Fagan nomogram, used to estimate the posttest probability of disease. To use the Fagan nomogram, draw a line from the pretest probability on the left to the likelihood ratio in the middle, and extrapolate the line to the posttest probability on the right.

Medicine is often considered *the* paradigm of professionalism. A physician must fulfill the role of a healer and a professional simultaneously. The role of healer dates back to ancient times, whereas the role of professional arose in the Middle Ages as a means of organizing health care delivery. The "profession" has the privilege of self-regulation and self-policing. Physicians were consequently granted prestige and status within the community, according to the assumption that altruism and moral behavior would be adopted by people practicing medicine. Such prestige and status are still accorded to physicians today, and so they have an obligation to maintain a code of professional conduct.

Cruess and associates[27] published a working definition of professionalism as follows:

> Profession: An occupation whose core element is work based upon the mastery of a complex body of knowledge and skills. It is a vocation in which knowledge of some department of science or learning or the practice of an art founded upon it is used in the service of others. Its members are governed by codes of ethics and profess a commitment to competence, integrity and morality, altruism, and the promotion of the public good within their domain. These commitments form the basis of a social contract between a profession and society, which in return grants the profession a monopoly over the use of its knowledge base, the right to considerable autonomy in practice and the privilege of self-regulation. Professions and their members are accountable to those served and to society. (p. 74)

The concept of professionalism has gained considerable support since 2000; it has received nearly universal acceptance as a core competency in North America and beyond. Some domains that may be considered include work ethic; response to feedback; and conduct, including dress, appearance, and language.[28] However, putting professionalism into practical, observable terms has proved challenging. For example, faculty struggle with context-specific definitions of professionalism (e.g., variations based on specialty, geography, gender, culture, media) that may conflict with one another.[29]

Educators aim to instill in students the attitudes and behaviors expected of the profession as a whole. The challenge has been devising a means of evaluating the outcomes of these efforts in a standardized manner. Evaluations often focus on observable behaviors. Unfortunately, people do not always act or behave in accordance with their held attitudes and values,[30] so it is difficult to reduce the subtle and complex construct of professionalism to a simple, single-dimensional scale; thus, professionalism is hard to

---

[27]Cruess SR, Johnston S, Cruess RL. "Profession": a working definition for medical educators. *Teach Learn Med.* 2004;16:74-76.

[28]Ginsburg S, McIlroy J, Oulanova O, et al. Toward authentic clinical evaluation: pitfalls in the pursuit of competency. *Acad Med.* 2010;85:780-786.

[29]Bryden P, Ginsburg S, Kurabi B, et al. Professing professionalism: are we our own worst enemy? Faculty members' experiences of teaching and evaluating professionalism in medical education at one school. *Acad Med.* 2010;85:1025-1034.

[30]Rees CE, Knight LV. The trouble with assessing students' professionalism: theoretical insights from sociocognitive psychology. *Acad Med.* 2007;82:46-50.

evaluate reliably in an OSCE setting.[31] Despite these limitations, observable dimensions of professionalism are likely to continue to appear on OSCEs until more acceptable tools are developed.

COMMUNICATION

Entire courses in medical curricula have been developed on the topic of communication. The following series of key pointers is intended to refresh your memory[32]:

- Setting up the interview: It is best to conduct patient interviews in a quiet, nonthreatening setting. Avoid using physical barriers, such as sitting behind a desk. It is not always possible to arrange this type of setting (e.g., in the emergency department); in those situations, do your best to maintain patient privacy by drawing the curtains and speaking as quietly as possible (if the patient does not have a hearing deficit).
- Beginning the interview: Begin by establishing the identity of the patient. Make eye contact with the patient, and introduce yourself. Determine how the patient would like to be addressed.
- Nonverbal cues: Throughout the interview, it is important to avoid appearing rushed, because this will probably interfere with the patient's desire to disclose information. Maintain eye contact when possible. Remain nonjudgmental. You should also observe the patient's nonverbal cues; observations about how things are said and what is *not* said may be as important and informative as the content of the patient's words.
- Open-ended questions: It is optimal to start with an open-ended question such as "What brought you in here today?" Do not interrupt the patient's account of his or her chief complaint. Physicians interrupt patients during their opening statement in 69% of encounters after a mean of only 18 to 23 seconds.[33,34] It is helpful to prompt the patient for more information: "Tell me more about that."
  - Directed questions may be used later to clarify specific points in the history.
  - Be an active listener. Take the time to ensure that you have heard the patient's story correctly by summarizing from time to time: "So, what you are saying is. . . . Is there anything else?"
  - **FIFE:** Many interviewers find the FIFE mnemonic helpful for remembering to elicit the patient's **f**eelings, **i**deas, **f**ears, and **e**xpectations about his or her complaint or illness. This information can be very revealing.[35]
  - Closing remarks: Draw the encounter to a close by summarizing any findings. Outline the next steps in delineating and managing the patient's complaint and a broader action plan. Provide an opportunity for the patient to ask questions.

CROSS-CULTURAL COMMUNICATION

Lack of understanding of cultural issues can lead to impaired physician-patient communication and negative health outcomes. In our multicultural environment, it is important for physicians to take time to understand patients' beliefs and their effects on perceptions of health and illness.

[31]Ginsburg S, Regehr G, Mylopoulos M. From behaviours to attributions: further concerns regarding the evaluation of professionalism. *Med Educ.* 2009;43:414-425.

[32]Teutsch C. Patient-doctor communication. *Med Clin North Am.* 2003;87:1115-1145.

[33]Beckman HB, Frankel RM. The effect of physician behavior on the collection of data. *Ann Intern Med.* 1984;101:692-696.

[34]Marvel MK, Epstein RM, Flowers K, et al. Soliciting the patient's agenda. Have we improved? *JAMA.* 1999;281:283-287.

[35]Silverman J, Kurtz S, Draper J. How to discover the patient's perspective (pp. 93-97). In *Skills for Communicating with Patients.* 2nd ed. Abingdon, UK: Radcliffe Medical Press; 2005.

The **LEARN** mnemonic provides a framework for physicians[36]:
- **L**isten with sympathy and understanding to the patient's perception of the problem.
- **E**xplain your perceptions of the problem.
- **A**cknowledge and discuss the differences and similarities.
- **M**ake recommendations for next steps in investigation and management of the problem.
- **N**egotiate with the patient in the context of cultural and religious beliefs to arrive at an acceptable action plan.

Alternatively, you can use the **ETHNIC(S)** mnemonic:[37,38]

Explanation: Find out the patient's explanation of their symptoms, illness, or condition. If the patient cannot offer an explanation, find out what concerns the patient most about it.

Treatment: Find out what kinds of treatments (prescription and nonprescription) the patient has tried for this symptom, illness, or condition thus far.

Healers: Find out whom the patient has consulted about this symptom, illness, or condition thus far (e.g., physicians, friends, alternative medicine practitioners).

Negotiate: Find options that will be mutually acceptable to you and your patient (i.e., that incorporates the patient's beliefs).

Intervention: Determine an intervention with your patient.

Collaboration: Collaborate with the patient, family members, other members of the health care team, healers, and community resources.

Spirituality: Clarify the role that spirituality and faith play in the ways the patient copes with his or her symptoms, illness, or condition.

BREAKING BAD NEWS

The definition of "bad news" depends on the individual and varies somewhat from patient to patient. Death and dying are generally considered to be the main topics in this area, but chronic pain or a psychiatric illness, for example, may engender a comparable degree of turmoil and difficulty. The encounter in which such news is delivered may affect the patient's satisfaction with his or her care, any future coping mechanisms, and the level of hopefulness. Whereas physicians' stress peaks during the clinical encounter, patients' stress peaks afterward.[39]

The main goals of this type of patient encounter are to gather information from the patient, deliver the "bad news," provide patient support, and collaborate with the patient in developing a plan. The **SPIKES** protocol, as outlined by Baile and colleagues,[40] is presented as follows:
- **S**etting up the interview: Mentally rehearse the interview. Arrange for a private space for the encounter, and involve significant others. Sit down, because you do not wish to appear rushed. Maintain eye contact when possible.
- Assess the patient's **p**erceptions: Find out how the patient perceives his or her current situation: "What have you been told about your condition so far?"
- Obtain the patient's **i**nvitation: Find out at what level the patient wishes to have information disclosed (e.g., details versus the big picture). The optimal time for disclosure is when particular investigations are ordered.

---

[36]Berlin EA, Fowkes WC Jr. A teaching framework for cross-cultural health care. Application in family practice. *West J Med.* 1983;139:934-938.

[37]Kobylarz FA, Heath JM, Like RC. The ETHNIC(S) mnemonic: a clinical tool for ethnogeriatric education. *J Am Geriatr Soc.* 2002;50:1582-1589.

[38]Levin SJ, Like RC, Gottlieb JE. ETHNIC: a framework for culturally competent clinical practice. In Appendix: Useful clinical interviewing mnemonics. *Patient Care.* 2000;34:188-189.

[39]Ptacek JT, Eberhardt TL. Breaking bad news: a review of the literature. *JAMA.* 1996;276:496-502.

[40]Baile WF, Buckman R, Lenzi R, et al. SPIKES—a six-step protocol for delivering bad news: application to the patient with cancer. *Oncologist,* 2000;5:302-311.

- Pass along **k**nowledge to the patient: Precede the bad news with a "warning shot" so as not to take the patient off guard: "I have bad news to tell you." Avoid medical jargon and talk to the patient at a level that he or she can understand. Check that the patient understands the information, when possible.
- Address the patient's **e**motions: Offer support by identifying the patient's emotions and the reason for them. Be empathic.
- **S**trategy and **s**ummary: It is important to outline a plan of next steps for the patient, including another planned encounter. Having a plan provides some security for the patient and the patient's family. Written information and a planned second encounter to further discuss their concerns are vital, because patients are unlikely to retain most of the information disclosed after the "bad news."

Robert Buckman[41] elaborated strategies for breaking bad news.

---

[41]Buckman R. *How to Break Bad News: A Guide for Health Care Professionals*, Baltimore: Hopkins Fulfillment Service; 1992.

Introduce yourself to the patient: "Hello. My name is Joe/Jane Doe, and I am a medical student."

Wash your hands.

- **Identifying data (ID):** Verify the patient's name, age or date of birth, sex, race, place of birth, marital status, religion, and other personal data. Ask yourself whether the historian is reliable. Inquire about the source of the referral (e.g., self, family doctor).
- **Chief concern:** One or more symptoms or concerns for which the patient is seeking care or advice. Use the patient's own words when possible.
- **History of present illness (HPI):** This history clarifies the chief concern; it is a chronologic account of how each symptom developed and related events **(ChLORIDE FPP).** Ask when the patient last felt "well."
  - **Ch**aracter: "What is [the symptom] like?"
  - **L**ocation: "Where is it?"
  - **O**nset: "When did it start?"
  - **R**adiation: "Does it go anywhere else?"
  - **I**ntensity: "How bad is it (scale of 1 to 10, with 1 being mild and 10 being the worst)?"
  - **D**uration: "How long does it last? How has it changed or progressed since it started?"
  - **E**vents associated: "What were you doing or where were you when the symptom began?"
  - **F**requency: "Has this happened before? If so, how often does it happen?"
  - **P**alliative factors: "What makes it better?"
  - **P**rovocative factors: "What makes it worse?"
- Remember to
  - Develop a rapport with the patient.
  - Ascertain the patient's thoughts and feelings about his or her illness or symptom.
  - Clarify the patient's concerns that led to seeking medical attention.
  - Find out how the illness or symptom has affected the patient's life.
- **Past medical history (PMH)/past surgical history (PSH):** In chronologic order, past illnesses (including psychiatric illnesses and childhood illnesses), past hospitalizations, current medical illnesses, injuries, and medical or surgical interventions and anesthetics
- **Medications (MEDS):** All current medications (including prescription, over-the-counter, and alternative medicines); may include relevant past medications
- **Allergies:** Allergies to drugs (prescription, over-the-counter, and alternative medicines) and environmental allergens, such as latex
- **Social history (SH):** Smoking; use of alcohol (EtOH); use of street drugs; diet; sleep patterns; exercise and leisure activities; hazards and safety issues; employment; relationship with family, peers, and partner; sexual history
- **Immunizations:** Especially important in children, persons with infectious diseases, and travelers
- **Family history (FH):** Age, health, and cause of death of each member of the patient's immediate family (parents, siblings, and children)
- **Review of systems (ROS):** Ask about common symptoms in each major body system. Be sure to address the patient (as always) in language consistent with his or

her level of understanding. ROS pertinent to the chief concern should be included in the HPI.

- **General:** Ask about current state of health (includes past medical problems relevant to the current state of health).
- **Cardiovascular system (CVS):** Ask about chest pain, pressure, or tightness; palpitations; orthopnea; paroxysmal nocturnal dyspnea (PND); shortness of breath; pedal edema; claudication; varicose veins; history of rheumatic fever; heart murmur; hypertension; hyperlipidemia; and mitral valve prolapse.
- **Respiratory system (Resp):** Ask about cough, sputum, hemoptysis, dyspnea, pleuritic chest pain, wheezing, asthma, chronic obstructive pulmonary disease (COPD), recurrent respiratory infections, occupational exposures (e.g., asbestos, radiation), results of most recent chest radiograph (CXR), tuberculosis, pulmonary embolism, and sleep patterns (snoring, sleep apnea).
- **Gastrointestinal system (GI):** Ask about weight gain or loss, results of previous endoscopy and digital rectal examination (DRE), nausea or vomiting, diarrhea, constipation, hematemesis, hematochezia, melena, change in stool caliber, hemorrhoids, hepatitis, peptic ulcer disease (PUD), gastroesophageal reflux (GER) or "heartburn," dysphagia, difficulty chewing, excessive belching or flatus, abdominal pain, appetite, and diet.
- **Genitourinary system (GU):** Ask about dysuria, hematuria, nocturia, urinary frequency, polyuria, decreased force of urination, hesitancy, urgency, incontinence, nephrolithiasis, urinary tract infection (UTI), and pyelonephritis.
  - ◆ **Female:** Ages at menarche and at menopause; regularity of menstrual cycle; presence of premenstrual symptoms; date of last menstrual period (LMP); presence of dysmenorrhea, postmenopausal bleeding, vaginal discharge, labial sores or lesions, sexually transmitted infections (STIs), sexual dysfunction, and endometriosis; birth control method; presence of breast lumps and nipple discharge; gravida, para, and abortus status; presence of dyspareunia; date of last Pap smear; history of abnormal Pap smear results; past mammography results
  - ◆ **Male:** Presence of hernias, testicular masses or pain, penile discharge, penile sores or lesions, prostatitis, sexual dysfunction, and STIs; prostate-specific antigen (PSA) level; results of DRE of the prostate
- **Neurologic system (Neuro):** Ask about headache, diplopia, blurred vision, eye pain or redness, cataracts, glaucoma, visual field losses, hearing loss, tinnitus, vertigo, dizziness, syncope, seizures, paresthesias, weakness or paralysis, tremor, pain, ataxia, falls, and head injury.
- **Musculoskeletal system (MSK):** Ask about arthritis, joint stiffness or swelling, myalgias, gout, and back pain.
- **Skin:** Ask about rashes, changing moles, birthmarks, dryness, pruritus, lumps, pigmentation change, hair loss, hirsutism, and nail changes.
- **Hematologic (Heme):** Ask about blood type, anemia, easy bruising or bleeding, prior transfusions and reactions, lymph node enlargement, constitutional symptoms (pain, fatigue, fever, chills, night sweats), and thromboembolic disease.
- **Endocrine system (Endo):** Ask about polyuria, polydipsia, polyphagia, cold or heat intolerance, diabetes mellitus, thyroid disease, goiter, tremors, osteoporosis, galactorrhea, hirsutism, purple striae, central obesity, and amenorrhea.
- **Head, eyes, ears, nose, and throat (HEENT):** Ask about sinusitis, postnasal drip, nasal polyps, epistaxis, condition of teeth and gums, ulcers or growths in the oral cavity, sore throat, change in voice, hoarseness, glasses, contact lenses, and use of dentures.
- **Mental health:** Ask about depression, agitation, panic or anxiety, memory disturbance, confusion, personality disorders, hallucinations, delusions, mania, and substance abuse.

DOCUMENTATION

In general, documentation should be as complete as possible at all times. From the perspective of persons reading and reviewing your documentation of the patient's history and physical examination, *if it is not documented, it did not happen.* Document not only positive findings but also pertinent negative findings. It is important to be consistent in your approach to charting; you will be less likely to omit information if you approach it systematically. When time permits, document in the same format as the medical history just outlined, documenting the physical examination in a systems-based format.

Writing a **SOAP** note is a useful way to quickly summarize a patient encounter:

Subjective: Write the history in the patient's own words.

Objective: Write your physical examination findings and laboratory investigations.

Assessment: Write your provisional diagnosis and differential diagnosis.

Plan: Outline your plan to delineate or confirm the diagnosis and to manage the patient's problems. It is useful to organize the plan with a *problem list.* Develop the problem list by starting with the patient's chief concern, positive symptoms identified in the ROS, and active medical conditions.

For example, a SOAP note for Mark Bartholomew (see Appendix A) is outlined as follows:

S: Mark Bartholomew is a 24-year-old male student who presents to the Emergency Department with fatigue, muscle aches, abdominal discomfort, and jaundice. He is previously healthy, with no history of hepatobiliary disease. He is sexually active and uses condoms regularly. He drinks alcohol on the weekends (24 beers) and denies use of IV [intravenous] drugs. He denies any new medications or intentional ingestions. He recently took part in a cross-country adventure race in Nevada (4 weeks ago), where he had some diarrhea that resolved spontaneously. His stools are now normal, although his urine is slightly darker than usual. He does not know of any sick contacts. He is not immunized against viral hepatitis.

O: Vital signs are within normal limits. The patient is in no apparent distress and looks his stated age. He appears faintly jaundiced. No scleral icterus and no further extrahepatic stigmata of liver dysfunction are noted. Bowel sounds are present. He notes epigastric and right upper quadrant tenderness with deep palpation. There is no guarding and no evidence of hepatosplenomegaly. The results of the cardiorespiratory examination are unremarkable.

A: Possible infectious hepatitis
- DD$_X$: VITAMINS C (jaundice)
  - **I**nfectious: Viral hepatitis
  - **A**utoimmune/**a**llergic: Autoimmune hepatitis
  - **M**etabolic: Hemolysis
  - **I**diopathic/**i**atrogenic: Biliary obstruction (stone or stricture)
  - **S**ubstance abuse and psychiatric: Alcoholic or toxic hepatitis
  - **C**ongenital/genetic: Gilbert syndrome

P: Supportive care
- Patient should take enteric precautions (for at least 1 week after jaundice), including hand washing.
- Contact local public health agency for advice on management of reportable illnesses such as infectious hepatitis.
- Investigations should include complete blood cell count; measurements of urea level, creatinine level, electrolytes, glucose level, liver enzymes, and bilirubin level (direct and indirect); coagulation profile; and hepatitis A, B, and C serologic studies.

ABBREVIATIONS

A_2: aortic component of second heart sound
AAA: abdominal aortic aneurysm
ABCs: airway, breathing, and circulation
ABI: ankle-brachial index
ACE: angiotensin-converting enzyme
ACL: anterior cruciate ligament
ACTH: adrenocorticotropic hormone
AIDS: acquired immune deficiency syndrome
AMI: acute myocardial infarction
AP: anteroposterior
Apgar: appearance, pulse, grimace, activity, respiratory
AR: aortic regurgitation
AS: aortic stenosis
ASA: acetylsalicylic acid
ASIS: anterior superior iliac spine
AV: atrioventricular
AVPU: alert, verbal, pain, and unresponsive (scale)
BCC: basal cell carcinoma
BCG: bacille bilié de Calmette-Guérin (tuberculosis vaccine)
BM: bowel movement
BMI: body mass index
BP: blood pressure
CAD: coronary artery disease
CAGE (questionnaire): cut down, annoyed by criticism, guilty about drinking, eye-opener
CAH: congenital adrenal hyperplasia
CBC: complete blood cell count
CHF: congestive heart failure
CI: confidence interval
CNS: central nervous system
COPD: chronic obstructive pulmonary disease
COX-2: cyclooxygenase-2
CPR: cardiopulmonary resuscitation
CT: computed tomographic
CVA: costovertebral angle
CVD: cardiovascular disease
CVS: cardiovascular system
CXR: chest radiograph (x-ray)
DDAVP: desmopressin
DDH: developmental dysplasia of the hip
DDST: Denver Developmental Screening Test
DD_X: differential diagnosis

DEET: diethyltoluamide
DIC: disseminated intravascular coagulation
DIP: distal interphalangeal (joint)
DKA: diabetic ketoacidosis
DM: diabetes mellitus
DRE: digital rectal examination
DTaP: diphtheria, tetanus, and acellular pertussis (vaccine)
DVT: deep venous thrombosis
ECG: electrocardiogram
ED: emergency department
EDC: estimated date of confinement
Endo: endocrine system
EtOH: alcohol
FABERE (maneuver): flexion, abduction, external rotation, and extension
FEV_1: forced expiratory volume in first second
FH: family history
FVC: forced vital capacity
GCS: Glasgow Coma Scale
GER: gastroesophageal reflux
GI: gastrointestinal
GU: genitourinary
Gyne: gynecologic
HbA_{1c}: hemoglobin A_{1c}
HBV: hepatitis B virus
HEENT: head, eyes, ears, nose, and throat
Heme: hematologic
Hep B: hepatitis B vaccine
Hib: *Haemophilus influenzae* type b conjugate vaccine
HIV: human immunodeficiency virus
HPI: history of present illness
HPV: human papillomavirus
HR: heart rate
Hz: hertz
IBD: inflammatory bowel disease
IBS: irritable bowel syndrome
ICP: intracranial pressure
ICS: intercostal space
ID: identifying data
IHD: ischemic heart disease
INR: international normalized ratio
IP: interphalangeal (joint)
IPV: inactivated polio vaccine

IV: intravenous
IVC: inferior vena cava
JVD: jugular venous distension
JVP: jugular venous pressure
LCME: Liaison Committee on Medical Education
LDL: low-density lipoprotein
LEEP: loop electrocautery excision procedure
LLL: left lower lobe (lung)
LLQ: left lower quadrant (abdomen)
LMP: last menstrual period
−LR: negative likelihood ratio
+LR: positive likelihood ratio
LSCS: lower segment cesarean section
LUL: left upper lobe (lung)
LUQ: left upper quadrant (abdomen)
LV: left ventricle
LVH: left ventricular hypertrophy
MAL: midaxillary line
MCL: midclavicular line
MCP: metacarpophalangeal (joint)
MCV: mean corpuscular volume
MEDS: medication
MEN: multiple endocrine neoplasia
MI: myocardial infarction
mm: millimeter
mm Hg: millimeters of mercury
MMR: measles, mumps, and rubella (vaccine)
MMSE: Mini-Mental State Examination
MR: mitral regurgitation
MS: mitral stenosis
MSK: musculoskeletal
MTP: metatarsophalangeal (joint)
MVP: mitral valve prolapse
Neuro: neurologic
NSAID: nonsteroidal anti-inflammatory drug
NSVD: normal spontaneous vaginal delivery
Obs: obstetric
OCD: obsessive-compulsive disorder
OSCE: Objective Structured Clinical Examination
OTC: over-the-counter (medications)
P_2: pulmonary component of second heart sound
$Paco_2$: partial pressure of arterial carbon dioxide
PAD: peripheral arterial disease
Pap smear: Papanicolaou test
PCL: posterior cruciate ligament
PCOS: polycystic ovarian syndrome
PE: pulmonary embolism

PID: pelvic inflammatory disease
PIP: proximal interphalangeal (joint)
PMH: past medical history
PMS: premenstrual syndrome
PND: paroxysmal nocturnal dyspnea
PSA: prostate-specific antigen
PSH: past surgical history
PTHrp: parathyroid hormone–related protein
PTSD: posttraumatic stress disorder
PUD: peptic ulcer disease
PVC: premature ventricular contraction
RBC: red blood cell
Resp: respiratory
RLL: right lower lobe (lung)
RLQ: right lower quadrant (abdomen)
RML: right middle lobe (lung)
ROM: range of motion
ROS: review of systems
RR: respiratory rate
RUL: right upper lobe (lung)
RUQ: right upper quadrant (abdomen)
S_1: first heart sound
S_2: second heart sound
S_3: third heart sound
S_4: fourth heart sound
SCC: squamous cell carcinoma
SCM: sternocleidomastoid muscle
SH: social history
SIADH: syndrome of inappropriate antidiuretic hormone
SOBOE: shortness of breath on exertion
SSRI: selective serotonin reuptake inhibitors
SSSS: staphylococcal scalded skin syndrome
STI: sexually transmitted infection
SVC: superior vena cava
TB: tuberculosis
Td: tetanus and diphtheria vaccine
TIA: transient ischemic attack
TIMI: Thrombolysis In Myocardial Infarction
TORCH: toxoplasmosis, other agents, rubella, cytomegalovirus, and herpes simplex virus (association)
TPN: total parenteral nutrition
TURP: transurethral resection of the prostate
URTI: upper respiratory tract infection
USMLE: United States Medical Licensing Examination
UTI: urinary tract infection
WHO: World Health Organization

MNEMONICS

ABCDE (for assessment of skin lesions for malignancy): asymmetry, border (irregularity), color (variegated), diameter, and elevation or enlargement

BEANN (for complications of diabetes): bugs (infections), eyes, arteries, nephropathy, nerves

ChLORIDE FPP: character, location, onset, radiation, intensity, duration, events associated, frequency, palliative factors, provocative factors

COWS: cold opposite, warm same (normal response to caloric stimulation)

Dduv (for informed consent): decision-making capacity, disclosure, understanding, voluntariness

DRIP (for differential diagnosis of urinary incontinence): drugs, delirium; restricted mobility, retention; infection, impaction; polydipsia

ETHNICS (for cross-cultural communication): explanation (patient's explanation of symptoms, illness, or condition), treatment, healers (whom patient has consulted), negotiate (options), intervention, collaboration (with patient, family members, health care providers, community resources), spirituality

FIFE: feelings, ideas, fears, and expectations

ImPAIRED (for mania): impulsivity, pressured speech, activity (increased), insomnia, racing thoughts, esteem inflation, and distractibility

IPPA: inspection, palpation, percussion, auscultation

LEARN (for cross-cultural communication): listen (to patient's perception of problem), explain (your perception of problem), acknowledge (differences and similarities of perceptions), recommendations (for next steps in investigation and management of problem), negotiate

MAD FOCS (for psychosis): memory deficits, activity, distortions, feelings, orientation, cognition, some other findings

POLICE (for differentiating jugular venous pulsation from carotid pulsation): palpability, occlusion, location, inspiration (effect of), contour, erect position (effect of)

SAD PERSONS (scale): age; depression; previous suicide attempts; EtOH (alcohol); rational thinking loss; separated, divorced, or widowed; organized plan (for suicide); no social support; stated future intent (to commit suicide)

SEADS (for musculoskeletal assessment): swelling; erythema, ecchymosis; atrophy; deformity; skin changes

SIGE CAPS (for depression): sleeplessness, interest (loss of), guilt, energy (decreased), concentrate (inability to), appetite (loss of), psychomotor retardation or agitation, suicidal ideation

SOAP (note): subjective (patient's version of history), objective (findings of physical examination and laboratory investigations), assessment (provisional and differential diagnoses), plan (treatment)

SPACED (for consideration in respiratory assessment): smoking, shortness of breath on expiration, sputum production; pain, pigeons; asthma; cough, chest radiograph; exercise tolerance, environmental/occupational exposure; dyspnea

TEST CA (for musculoskeletal assessment): tenderness, effusion, swelling, temperature, crepitus, atrophy

VITAMINS C (for generating a differential diagnosis): vascular, infectious, traumatic, autoimmune/allergic, metabolic, idiopathic/iatrogenic, neoplastic, substance abuse/psychiatric, congenital/genetic

Cardiovascular System

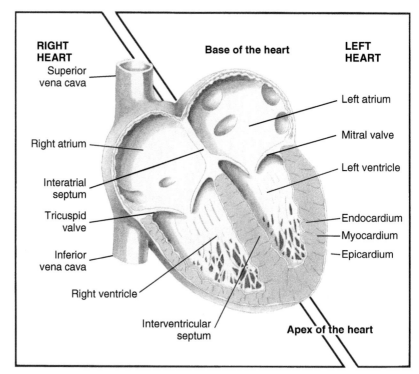

Figure 1-1 Gross anatomy of the heart. (From Wilkins RL, Sheldon RL, Krider SJ. *Clinical Assessment in Respiratory Care.* 4th ed. St. Louis: Mosby; 2000 [p. 192, Figure 9-1].)

ANATOMY

- The heart is enclosed in a thin sac of parietal pericardium. A small amount of pericardial fluid lubricates the space between the heart and the pericardium.
- The heart comprises four chambers (Figure 1-1).

Surface Anatomy (Figure 1-2)
- The **right atrium** forms the right border of the heart and is usually not identifiable on physical examination.
- The **right ventricle** occupies most of the anterior cardiac surface, narrowing superiorly to meet the pulmonary artery at the level of the third left costal cartilage.
- The **left atrium** lies mostly posterior and cannot be examined directly.
- The **left ventricle** lies to the left of and behind the right ventricle, forming the left border of the heart. The tip of the left ventricle produces the **apical impulse,** a systolic beat usually found in the fifth intercostal space (ICS).

Figure 1-2 Surface anatomy of the heart. ICS, intercostal space; MCL, midclavicular line. (Adapted from Swartz M. *Textbook of Physical Diagnosis: History and Examination.* 6th ed. Philadelphia: Elsevier; 2010 [p. 396, Figure 14-4].)

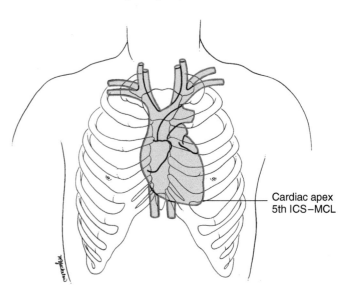

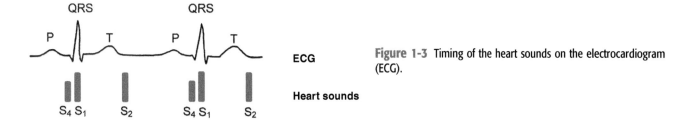

Figure 1-3 Timing of the heart sounds on the electrocardiogram (ECG).

Review of Heart Sounds

- Heart sounds are produced by the sudden deceleration of blood flow when the heart valves close and their timing relates to events within the cardiac cycle (Figure 1-3).
- The cardiac cycle is initiated by the conduction of an impulse generated by the **sinoatrial (SA) node** in the right atrium. This impulse propagates through the atria to the **atrioventricular (AV) node.** The impulse then continues to be propagated through the bundle of His, the right and left bundle branches, and the Purkinje fibers (Figure 1-4).
- At the onset of systole, contraction of the ventricles increases interventricular pressure, causing closure of the mitral and tricuspid valves and opening of the aortic and pulmonic valves. The closure of the mitral and tricuspid valves is heard as the **first heart sound (S_1).**
- As diastole begins, the ventricles relax and interventricular pressure decreases, allowing the aortic and pulmonic valves to close, producing the **second heart sound (S_2).**
- A period of rapid ventricular filling follows and may be marked by a **third heart sound (S_3).**
- Although not often heard in normal adults, a **fourth heart sound (S_4)** marks atrial contraction and immediately precedes S_1 of the next beat.
- Pressures in the right side of the heart are significantly lower than pressures in the left side of the heart. Thus, right-sided events usually occur slightly later than left-sided events; this phenomenon contributes to the splitting of heart sounds.
  - Normal inspiratory splitting of S_2 is the separation of S_2 into A_2 and P_2, which correspond to the closure of the aortic and pulmonic valves, respectively. Splitting of S_2 on both inspiration and expiration (persistent splitting) is suggestive of an abnormality.
  - S_1 also has two components: an earlier mitral sound and a later tricuspid sound. Splitting of S_1 does not vary with respiration, and it is best heard at the lower left sternal border. Wide splitting of S_1 is abnormal, arising from delayed closure of the tricuspid valve as in complete right bundle branch block or atrial septal defect with significant left-to-right shunting.

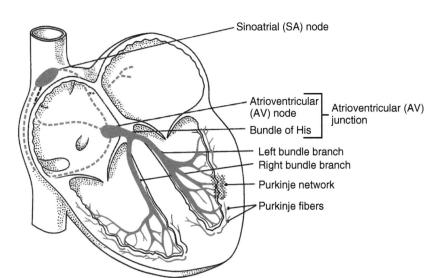

Figure 1-4 Intrinsic electrical conduction in the heart. (From Wilkins RL, Sheldon RL, Krider SJ. *Clinical Assessment in Respiratory Care.* 4th ed. St. Louis: Mosby; 2000 [p. 193, Figure 9-2].)

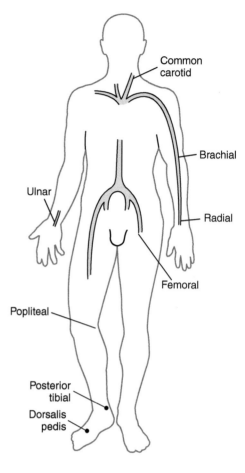

Figure 1-5 Areas for palpating peripheral pulses. (Adapted from Tilkian AG, Conover MB. *Understanding Heart Sounds: With an Introduction to Lung Sounds.* 4th ed. Philadelphia: Saunders; 2001 [p. 51, Figure 6-2].)

Landmarks for Palpable Pulses (Figure 1-5)

- **Dorsalis pedis pulse:** Between the tendons of extensor hallucis longus and extensor digitorum longus.
- **Posterior tibial pulse:** 2 to 3 cm posterior to the medial malleolus.
- **Popliteal pulse:** Deep within the popliteal fossa (hold the knee in 15 degrees of flexion).
- **Femoral pulse:** Inferior to the inguinal ligament, midway between the pubic symphysis and anterior superior iliac spine—the lateral corners of the pubic hair triangle.
- **Radial pulse:** Anterolateral aspect of wrist (remember that the forearm is supinated in the anatomic position).
- **Ulnar pulse:** Anteromedial aspect of the wrist.
- **Brachial pulse:** Medial to the biceps tendon in the cubital fossa.
- **Carotid pulse:** Between the trachea and the sternocleidomastoid muscle at the level of the thyroid cartilage (ensure that there are no carotid bruits before you palpate the carotid pulse, and never palpate both carotid arteries simultaneously).

GLOSSARY OF SIGNS AND SYMPTOMS

Shortness of Breath

- **Orthopnea** is shortness of breath, which is brought on or exacerbated by lying flat.
- **Paroxysmal nocturnal dyspnea** is acute shortness of breath that appears suddenly at night, often waking the patient from sleep. It results from left-sided heart failure with mobilization of fluid from dependent areas after lying down, which leads to pulmonary congestion.

Swelling
- **Edema** is the accumulation of excessive fluid in cells or tissues. Edema may result from cardiac failure. Look for edema in dependent areas such as the lower extremities in mobile persons and the presacral region in persons who are bedridden.
- **Pitting edema** is edema that retains the indentation of your fingers when you apply pressure.

Loss of Consciousness
- **Syncope** is loss of consciousness and postural tone caused by decreased cerebral blood flow. Sudden syncope (i.e., syncope without warning) may be the presenting feature of dysrhythmia or severe aortic stenosis (AS).

Pulses
- **Pulsus tardus** is a pulse contour with slow upstroke and prolonged downstroke; the peak is blunted and forms a plateau (Figure 1-6).
- **Water-hammer pulse** is a pulse contour with rapid and forcible upstroke, followed by precipitous collapse, which is characteristic of aortic regurgitation (AR) (see Figure 1-6).
- **Pulsus bisferiens** is a double beat that may be perceived through light palpation of the carotid artery or auscultation of the compressed brachial artery (see Figure 1-6). It may occur in patients with significant AR or in mixed AS-AR in which AR is predominant.
- **Pulsus alternans** is a pulse that alternates in amplitude, varying from strong to weak. It often indicates serious myocardial dysfunction (see Figure 1-6).
- **Kussmaul's sign** is a jugular venous pressure (JVP) that paradoxically increases with inspiration.

Blood Pressure
- **Hypertension** is elevated blood pressure (BP) (Table 1-1). It is diagnosed clinically only when BP is measured accurately with a sphygmomanometer. Hypertension should be diagnosed only on the basis of the mean of two or more seated measurements during each of two or more examinations. The most common type of hypertension is primary idiopathic, or essential, hypertension. Secondary hypertension is rare but often correctable.

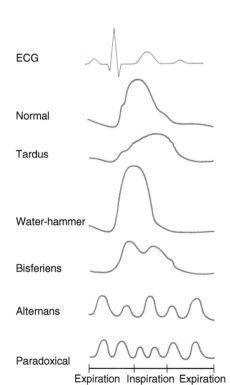

Figure 1-6 Pulse abnormalities. The electrocardiogram (ECG) demonstrates a P wave, a QRS interval, and a T wave so that the tracings for normal and pathologic pulses can be associated with the timing of the cardiac cycle. (Adapted from Swartz M. *Textbook of Physical Diagnosis: History and Examination.* 6th ed. Philadelphia: Elsevier; 2010 [p. 418, Figure 14-24].)

Table 1-1 2003 Classification of Hypertension

Blood Pressure Classification	Systolic Blood Pressure (mm Hg)		Diastolic Blood Pressure (mm Hg)
Normal	<120	and	<80
Prehypertension	120–139	or	80–89
Stage 1 hypertension	140–159	or	90–99
Stage 2 hypertension	≥160	or	≥100

Adapted from Chobanian AV, Bakris GL, Black HR, et al. The seventh report of the Joint National Committee on Prevention, Detection, Evaluation, and Treatment of High Blood Pressure: The JNC 7 report. *JAMA.* 2003;289:2561.

- **Secondary hypertension** is uncommon but often amenable to treatment. *Clues* that hypertension may be secondary to other disease are as follows:
  - Age <25 years or >55 years at onset
  - Hypertension that is severe, of sudden onset, and difficult to manage medically
- **Pulsus paradoxus** is an inspiratory decrease in systolic BP that is >20 mm Hg (see Figure 1-6). The exaggerated waxing and waning in pulse volume may be detected as a palpable decrease in pulse amplitude on quiet expiration, or by measurement with a sphygmomanometer. Pulsus paradoxus may be suggestive of severe asthma or chronic obstructive pulmonary disease (COPD), tension pneumothorax, pulmonary embolism, pericardial tamponade, or constrictive pericarditis.
- **Pulse pressure** is the difference between the systolic and diastolic values in millimeters of mercury. Pulse pressures <30 mm Hg are considered **narrow** and may occur in severe AS. Pulse pressures >30 to 40 mm Hg are considered **wide.**

Types of Pain
- **Claudication** is pain classically caused by ischemia of the muscles. It is most commonly characterized as calf pain brought on by walking; the condition may occur in other muscle groups.
- **Parietal chest pain** originates in the parietal pericardium and parietal pleura. It tends to be sharp and well localized over the involved structure. It is somatically innervated.
- **Referred pain** is pain that is felt at the level of somatic innervation (dermatome) that the sympathetic pain-carrying nerves innervate. Pain from thoracic viscera may be felt anywhere from the epigastrium to the mandible.
- **Visceral chest pain** originates in the thoracic organs and is carried by afferent fibers that enter the same thoracic dorsal ganglia. The pain from these organs (heart, lungs, and esophagus) is poorly localized and indistinct (gnawing, burning, stabbing, or achy).

ESSENTIAL SKILLS

APICAL IMPULSE: EXAMINATION

Patient Positioning
- Supine, with head of the bed elevated at 30 degrees

Inspection
- Inspect the precordium for the apical impulse. Tangential lighting may improve the visibility of impulses.

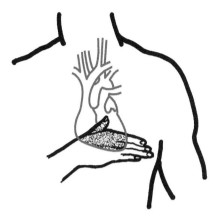

Figure 1-7 Palpation of the apical impulse. (From Tilkian AG, Conover MB. *Understanding Heart Sounds: With an Introduction to Lung Sounds.* 4th ed. Philadelphia: Saunders; 2001 [p. 50, Figure 6-1].)

Palpation

- Palpate the apical impulse with the pads of your fingers (Figure 1-7). Describe the location, amplitude, diameter, and duration of the apical impulse.
  - The apical impulse is usually found in the fifth ICS, at or just medial to the mid-clavicular line.
  - Normal **amplitude** is a gentle tap. Increases in amplitude may be caused by exercise, hyperthyroidism, severe anemia, and pressure or volume overload of the left ventricle.
  - The **diameter** is usually <2.5 cm, or the size of a nickel or quarter.
  - Estimate the proportion of systole occupied by the apical impulse. A normal apical impulse lasts through the first two thirds of systole.

Positional Maneuvers

- The following maneuvers may accentuate the apical impulse and are useful for identifying left ventricular hypertrophy (LVH). Ask the patient to perform *one* of the following maneuvers:
  - To exhale and hold his or her breath at the end of expiration
  - To turn onto his or her left side. When you locate the apex, ask the patient to return to a supine position.

CARDIAC AUSCULTATION: EXAMINATION

Patient Positioning

- Supine and upright, with the chest exposed

Auscultation

- The **diaphragm** of the stethoscope is best for auscultating relatively high-pitched sounds such as S_1, S_2, the murmurs of AR and mitral regurgitation (MR), AS, and pericardial friction rubs. The **bell** of the stethoscope is more sensitive to low-pitched sounds such as S_3, S_4, and the murmur of mitral stenosis (MS). Apply the bell lightly with just enough pressure to produce an air seal with its full rim. Applying too much pressure to the bell converts it to a diaphragm.
- Auscultate for high-pitched sounds by placing the diaphragm of the stethoscope firmly against the patient's chest at the right second ICS, close to the sternum. Listen for a few cycles to become accustomed to the rate and rhythm of the heart sounds. Make note of the following:
  - S_1 and S_2 (if you cannot tell which sound is S_1, continue to auscultate while you palpate the carotid pulse; S_1 just barely precedes the carotid pulsation)
  - Extra sounds in systole and diastole
  - Murmurs
  - Rubs

- Place the diaphragm of the stethoscope along the left sternal border at the left second ICS. Listen for each heart sound. Continue listening at the left third, fourth, and fifth ICSs and at the site of the apical impulse. Finally, listen in the axillae (where mitral murmurs may radiate) and over the carotid arteries (where aortic murmurs may radiate).
- Repeat this sequence for low-pitched sounds by using the bell of the stethoscope.

Positional Maneuvers

- Ask the patient to roll partly onto the left side into the left lateral decubitus position (Figure 1-8). Listen with the bell of the stethoscope over the apical impulse. This position accentuates left-sided S_3 and S_4 and the murmur of MS.
- Ask the patient to sit up, lean forward, exhale completely, and hold this position (Figure 1-9). Listen with the diaphragm of the stethoscope along the left sternal border and at the left second ICS. This position accentuates the murmur of AR.

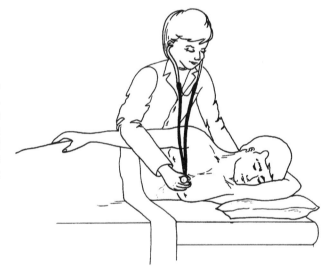

Figure 1-8 Auscultation with the patient in the left lateral decubitus position, to accentuate left-sided S_3 and S_4 and the murmur of mitral stenosis. (From Tilkian AG, Conover MB. *Understanding Heart Sounds: With an Introduction to Lung Sounds.* 4th ed. Philadelphia: Saunders; 2001 [p. 211, Figure 16-12].)

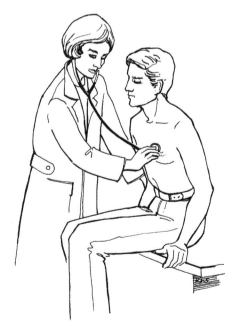

Figure 1-9 Auscultation with the patient seated and leaning forward to accentuate the murmur of aortic regurgitation. (From Tilkian AG, Conover MB. *Understanding Heart Sounds: With an Introduction to Lung Sounds.* 4th ed. Philadelphia: Saunders; 2001 [p. 202, Figure 16-6].)

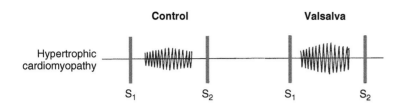

Control   Valsalva

Hypertrophic
cardiomyopathy

S_1 S_2 S_1 S_2

Figure 1-10 Effect of the performance of the Valsalva maneuver on the murmur of hypertrophic cardiomyopathy. (Adapted from Tilkian AG, Conover MB. *Understanding Heart Sounds: With an Introduction to Lung Sounds.* 4th ed. Philadelphia: Saunders; 2001 [p. 258, Figure 20-3].)

- To help identify murmurs associated with MR and hypertrophic cardiomyopathy, ask the patient to perform one of the following while you auscultate:
  - **Valsalva maneuver** (Figure 1-10): When a person takes a deep breath and bears down on a closed glottis (holding no longer than 8 to 10 seconds), venous return to the heart decreases, resulting in dynamic narrowing of the left ventricular (LV) outflow tract. A murmur that gets louder with performance of the Valsalva maneuver is almost diagnostic of hypertrophic cardiomyopathy.
  - **Squatting from a standing position:** Squatting improves venous return, causing increased stroke volume and widening of the LV outflow tract. This may accentuate the murmurs of MR and AR but diminish the murmur associated with hypertrophic cardiomyopathy.

Evidence
- Many clinical environments are noisy and distracting, which makes auscultation challenging. For example, emergency department studies have revealed noise levels in the range of 40 to 80 decibels.[1,2] In a simulated noisy environment, about half of health care practitioners who responded reported difficulty hearing heart and lung sounds.[1]

APPROACH TO A HEART MURMUR: EXAMINATION

Inspection
- Inspect for the apical impulse and the ventricular movements of a left-sided S_3 or S_4. Tangential lighting may improve the visibility of impulses.

Palpation
- Palpate the impulses with the pads of your fingers, exerting light pressure for an S_3 or S_4 and firmer pressure for S_1 or S_2. Thrills often accompany loud, harsh, or rumbling murmurs such as those of AS and MS. Thrills are best felt with the ball of your hand pressed firmly on the patient's chest.

Auscultation
- See pp. 7-8 for auscultatory techniques.
- Describe the following features of an identified murmur:
  - **Timing** (Figure 1-11): Relationship to systole and diastole (e.g., holosystolic versus mid- or late systolic). If you cannot tell which sound is S_1, continue to auscultate while palpating the carotid pulse. S_1 just barely precedes the carotid pulsation.
  - **Shape** (Figure 1-12): Crescendo, decrescendo, crescendo-decrescendo, decrescendo-crescendo, or plateau.
  - **Location** (Figure 1-13) of maximal intensity in relation to sternum, ICSs, and mid-clavicular line.
  - **Radiation** to carotids or axillae; this represents direction of blood flow and intensity.
  - **Pitch:** High, medium, or low.
  - **Quality:** Blowing, harsh, rumbling, or musical.
  - **Intensity:** Grades I through VI, ranging from faint to audible with the stethoscope entirely off the chest. The intensity of the murmur is not related to the severity of disease (e.g., AR).
  - **Effect of patient positioning** (upright, supine, left lateral decubitus) and respiratory maneuvers.

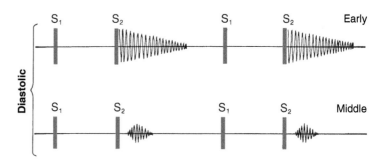

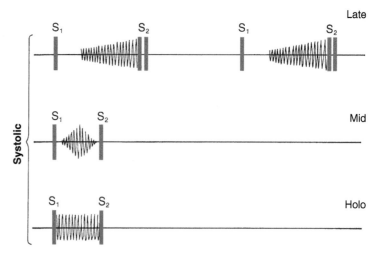

Figure 1-11 Description of the timing of murmurs in the cardiac cycle. (Adapted from Tilkian AG, Conover MB. *Understanding Heart Sounds: With an Introduction to Lung Sounds.* 4th ed. Philadelphia: Saunders; 2001 [p. 135, Figure 12-3].)

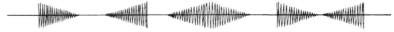

Figure 1-12 Description of the electrocardiographic "shape" of a murmur. (Adapted from Tilkian AG, Conover MB. *Understanding Heart Sounds: With an Introduction to Lung Sounds.* 4th ed. Philadelphia: Saunders; 2001 [p. 135, Figure 12-4].)

Figure 1-13 Auscultatory anatomy: "from **a**pe **t**o **m**an" is a mnemonic to help you remember where best to auscultate to detect **a**ortic, **p**ulmonic, **t**ricuspid, and **m**itral murmurs.

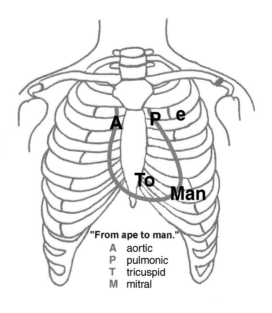

Table 1-2 Usefulness of Clinical Examination to Diagnose Valvular Murmurs

Clinical Feature	+LR (95% CI)	−LR (95% CI)
Fever >38.3°C	0.2 (0.09–0.6)	1.2 (1.1–1.4)
Systolic murmur grade >II/VI	4.5 (2.9–7.2)	0.4 (0.3–0.6)
Pathologic ECG*	2.1 (1.7–2.7)	0.2 (0.09–0.4)
Pathologic CXR†	2.0 (1.5–2.8)	0.4 (0.3–0.6)

From Reichlin S, Dieterle T, Camli C, et al. Initial clinical evaluation of cardiac systolic murmurs in the ED by noncardiologists. *Am J Emerg Med.* 2004 Mar;22(2):71-75.
*Pathologic electrocardiogram (ECG) (arrhythmia, conduction or repolarization disturbance).
†Pathologic chest x-ray (CXR) (cardiomegaly or signs of heart failure).
CI, Confidence interval; −LR, negative likelihood ratio; +LR, positive likelihood ratio.

Positional Maneuvers
- Listen at the apex with the patient in the left lateral decubitus position to accentuate the murmur of MS.
- Auscultate with the patient sitting up and leaning forward after exhaling completely, to accentuate AR.
- Maneuvers such as squatting and bearing down on a closed glottis help identify the murmurs of MR, hypertrophic cardiomyopathy, and AR.

Respiratory Maneuvers
- Inspiration may augment right-sided murmurs. Expiration accentuates the opening snap of MS.

Evidence
- Attending physicians (certified in internal medicine) clinically evaluated patients with systolic murmurs in the emergency department and determined whether they thought the murmur was "innocent" or "valvular" in origin.[3] In comparison to subsequent echocardiographic findings, physician judgment had a positive likelihood ratio (+LR) of 2.6 and a negative likelihood ratio (−LR) of 0.3. Table 1-2 shows the clinical indicators they studied that were helpful in discriminating patients with valvular murmurs.

APPROACH TO EXTRA HEART SOUNDS: EXAMINATION

Definition (Figure 1-14)
- S_3 is the sound produced by the period of ventricular filling in diastole after S_2 (follows the rhythm of "**To-ron-to**"). Its presence may be normal in children and young adults but is usually pathologic in persons >40 years old. It is often found in patients with heart failure (e.g., poor myocardial contractility).
- S_4 is the sound that occurs after atrial contraction, immediately before S_1 (follows the rhythm of "**Ken-tuck-y**"). It is often known as the *atrial gallop*. It is a marker for

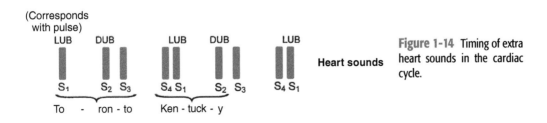

Figure 1-14 Timing of extra heart sounds in the cardiac cycle.

decreased ventricular compliance (i.e., "atrial kick" into a stiff ventricle). S_4 is *absent* in patients with atrial fibrillation because coordinated atrial contraction is absent.

Inspection
- Inspect for the apical impulse and the ventricular movements of a left-sided S_3 or S_4. Tangential lighting may improve the visibility of impulses.

Palpation
- Palpate by using light pressure to identify an S_3 or S_4.
  - **Left-sided S_3 and S_4:** These are best palpated at the apex with the patient in the left lateral decubitus position; they may be accentuated when the patient exhales and briefly stops breathing. A brief mid-diastolic impulse is indicative of an S_3. A presystolic movement that is maximal at the apex represents an S_4.
  - **Right-sided S_3 and S_4:** These are best palpated when the patient is supine. Place your index finger in the subxiphoid area and push gently toward the left shoulder.

Auscultation
- The bell of the stethoscope is more sensitive for detecting the low-pitched S_3 and S_4.
  - **Left-sided S_3 and S_4:** With the patient in the left lateral decubitus position, listen at the apex.
  - **Right-sided S_3 and S_4:** With the patient supine, listen over the lower left sternal border or subxiphoid.

Positional and Respiratory Maneuvers
- **Left-sided S_3 and S_4:** Accentuated by expiration
- **Right-sided S_3 and S_4:** Accentuated by inspiration.

Evidence
- Correlations between extra heart sounds and measures of LV function (LV end-diastolic pressure, LV ejection fraction, and levels of B-type natriuretic peptide) have shown that although neither S_3 nor S_4 is a sensitive marker of LV dysfunction, S_3 has higher specificity than S_4.[4]

JUGULAR VENOUS PRESSURE: EXAMINATION

Definition
- Pressure in the jugular veins reflects **right atrial pressure. JVP** is defined as the highest point of oscillation of the internal jugular vein measured as the vertical distance from the sternal angle **(angle of Louis).** The sternal angle is approximately 5 cm above the right atrium. A JVP of >3 to 4 cm is considered elevated and may be noted in right ventricular failure, pericardial tamponade, constrictive pericarditis, tension pneumothorax, or superior vena cava obstruction; it is decreased in hypovolemia. The JVP is not a reliable indicator of hydration status; however, in the setting of other physical findings and an appropriate history, it is a useful physical sign.
- **Waveform:** The JVP follows a biphasic waveform. The "a" wave corresponds to atrial contraction; the "v" wave is correlated with the filling of the atrium where the tricuspid valve remains closed (Figure 1-15).

Figure 1-15 Normal waveform of the jugular venous pulse. (Adapted from Hall T. *PACES for the MRCP with 250 Clinical Cases.* 2nd ed. Philadelphia: Churchill Livingstone; 2008 [p. 347, Figure 3.1].)

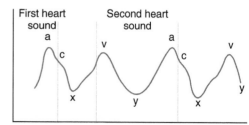

Patient Positioning
- Supine, with head on a pillow and sternocleidomastoid muscle relaxed (mouth open and head slightly away from inspecting side). The head of the bed is elevated initially to 30 degrees and then adjusted to maximize visibility of pulsations.

Inspection
- Use tangential lighting, and examine both sides of the neck. The right internal jugular vein is straighter than the left internal jugular vein. You should evaluate JVP by using the right internal jugular vein whenever possible.
- The internal jugular vein is located deep to the sternocleidomastoid muscle; look for pulsations between the heads of the sternocleidomastoid muscle as they are transmitted through surrounding soft tissues (Table 1-3). Identify the highest point of oscillation, and measure the vertical distance from the sternal angle (angle of Louis). Place the ruler vertically on the sternal angle, and place a long rectangular object perpendicularly and adjust so that it rests at the highest point of oscillation; read the vertical distance from the ruler. Round off to the nearest centimeter (Figure 1-16).

Table 1-3 Differentiating Internal Jugular Pulsations from Carotid Pulsations

Mnemonic: "POLICE"	Internal Jugular Pulsations	Carotid Pulsations
Palpability	Rarely palpable (e.g., severe tricuspid regurgitation)	Palpable
Occlusion	Pulsations eliminated by light pressure on the veins just above the sternal end of the clavicle	Cannot be occluded with light pressure
Location	Pulsations seen between heads of sternocleidomastoid muscle	Pulsations may be seen just medial to sternocleidomastoid muscle
Inspiration (effect of)	Level of pulsation descends with inspiration	Level of pulsation unaffected by inspiration
Contour	Rapid, undulating quality; two waveforms (two elevations: "a" wave and "v" wave)	Visible thrust with single elevation
Erect position (effect of)	Level of pulsation changes with position, decreasing as patient becomes more erect	Level of pulsation is unaffected by position

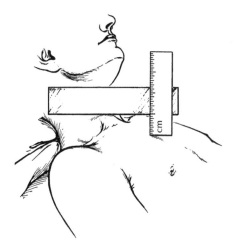

Figure 1-16 Measurement of the jugular venous pressure. (Adapted from Wilkins RL, Sheldon RL, Krider SJ. *Clinical Assessment in Respiratory Care.* 4th ed. St. Louis: Mosby; 2000 [p. 71, Figure 4-2].)

Palpation

- **Hepatojugular reflux:** Place your hand in the right upper quadrant of the patient's abdomen, and press firmly upward under the costal margin. A sustained increase in JVP (elevation >10 seconds or three respiratory cycles) is indicative of venous congestion. Carotid pulsation is unaffected by hepatojugular reflux.
- **Kussmaul's sign** is a JVP that paradoxically increases with inspiration.

Evidence

- The external jugular vein is often easier to identify than the internal jugular vein. In one study,[5] visual assessment of the external jugular vein ("high" or "low") was compared with catheter-measured central venous pressure ("low" ≤5 cm H_2O, "high" ≥10 cm H_2O) in a critical care setting. The investigators found that the external jugular vein was indeed easier to see and was useful for diagnosing aberrations in central venous pressure (+LR = 11.3 and −LR = 0.34 for low pressure; +LR = 4.9 and −LR = 0.4 for high pressure).

BLOOD PRESSURE: EXAMINATION

- The width of the bladder of the BP cuff should be approximately 40% of the circumference of the patient's arm; the length should be 80% of the circumference. Cuffs that are too short or too narrow give falsely high readings. A loose cuff may also yield falsely high readings.
- The patient should avoid smoking or ingesting caffeine for at least 30 minutes before BP measurement and should rest for at least 5 minutes.
- Position the patient comfortably sitting, with both feet on the floor. The brachial artery should be at heart level (approximately the fourth ICS). If the brachial artery is below heart level, BP measurements may be falsely high.
- The patient's own effort to support the arm may increase BP; therefore, the arm should be supported so as to relax in order to ensure accuracy in BP measurement.
- Anxiety is a frequent cause of high BP (otherwise known as "white coat syndrome"). Try to help the patient relax, and repeat measurements later in the encounter.
- Apply an appropriately selected BP cuff to the patient's arm, ensuring proper positioning with regard to the brachial artery.
- First estimate the systolic BP by palpation to avoid error caused by an auscultatory gap. Palpate the radial artery. Inflate the BP cuff beyond the point where the pulse is no longer palpable. Deflate the cuff at a rate of 2 to 3 mm Hg/sec. The estimated systolic BP is the point at which the pulse becomes palpable again.
- Wait 2 to 5 minutes before rechecking the BP (*this is not possible in an examination situation*). Position the stethoscope over the brachial artery. Inflate the cuff 20 to 30 mm Hg beyond the estimated systolic BP. Deflate the cuff at a rate of 2 to 3 mm Hg/sec. Note the point at which the first Korotkoff sound is heard (systolic BP). Continue to auscultate until the Korotkoff sounds disappear (diastolic BP).
- Measure BP in both arms. If the measurements are different, subsequent readings should be made on the arm with the higher pressure.
- BP may be measured with the patient sitting, standing, or supine. To detect orthostatic changes, first measure the BP with the patient supine. Then ask the patient to sit or stand up as you reassess the BP in this upright position.

CLAUDICATION: PHYSICAL EXAMINATION

INSTRUCTIONS TO CANDIDATE: A 60-year-old patient with diabetes has a 6-month history of calf pain when walking. The pain resolves with rest. Perform a focused physical examination.

Definition
- Intermittent **claudication** is characterized by attacks of pain, weakness, fatigue, or numbness in the calf brought on by exercise and relieved by rest. It may also occur in the foot, thigh, hip, or buttocks. In advanced disease, claudication may be present at rest.

DD$_X$: VITAMINS C
- **V**ascular: Peripheral vascular disease (occlusive arterial disease), deep venous thrombosis (DVT)
- **I**diopathic/**i**atrogenic: Thromboangiitis obliterans, spinal stenosis (lumbar)

6 Ps of Arterial Insufficiency
- **P**ain
- **P**ulselessness
- **P**allor
- **P**olar (cool temperature)
- **P**aresthesia
- **P**aralysis

Inspection (Table 1-4)
- Inspect both legs from the groin and buttocks to the feet, comparing both legs. Note the following:
  - Size and symmetry
  - Venous pattern and enlargement (varicose veins)
  - Integrity of skin and nails, including scars, ulcers, and atrophy (see Chapter 7, pp. 225-226)
  - Color of skin and nail beds
  - Distribution of hair growth

Table 1-4 Differentiating Arterial from Venous Insufficiency

Characteristic	Advanced Arterial Insufficiency	Advanced Venous Insufficiency
Pulses	Decreased or absent	Normal or difficult to palpate because of edema
Color	Marked pallor on elevation; dusky red on dependency	Brown pigmentation in chronic disease
Temperature	Cool	Normal
Edema	Absent to mild	May be marked
Skin	Thin and shiny with loss of hair; thick, rigid nails	Brown pigmentation; stasis dermatitis
Ulceration	At points of trauma (e.g., toes, plantar aspect of feet)	Medial aspect of ankles, anterior tibia
Capillary refill	Slow	Normal
Bruits	May be present	Absent
Buerger's test result	Positive	Negative
Trendelenburg's test result	Negative	Positive

Palpation (see Table 1-4)

- Pulses: Dorsalis pedis, posterior tibial, popliteal, and femoral (see Figure 1-5)
- Capillary refill (normal: <3 seconds)
- Temperature of feet and legs; evaluate by using back of your fingers, comparing one side with the other
- Pitting edema over dorsum of feet, behind medial malleoli, and over shins
- Tenderness of calves **(Homans' sign):** Flex the patient's knee. Forcefully and abruptly dorsiflex the ankle. This maneuver produces pain in 11% to 56% of patients with DVT, but such pain is also present in 11% to 61% of patients without DVT.[6] In theory, performing this examination exposes the patient to risk as such maneuvers could dislodge clot and precipitate pulmonary embolism.
- Ischemic peripheral neuropathy: Check **vibration sense** by using a tuning fork (128 Hz) placed over a bony prominence such as the medial malleolus. Check sensation of **light touch** by using a cotton swab.
- Test muscle power, tone, and reflexes in the lower extremities to assess for clinical signs of spinal stenosis.
- **Ankle-brachial index (ABI):** Measure the systolic BP in the arm and at the ankle. The systolic BP at the ankle is normally higher than the systolic BP in the arm. The ABI is calculated by dividing the ankle systolic BP by the arm systolic BP.
  - Normal ABI: 1.0 to 1.3
  - ABI > 1.3 indicates a calcified, noncompressible vessel in the lower extremity
  - ABI of 0.71 to 0.9 is indicative of mild peripheral arterial disease (PAD)
  - ABI of 0.41 to 0.7 is indicative of moderate PAD
  - ABI ≤ 0.4 is indicative of severe PAD
- **Buerger's test:** Ask the recumbent patient to elevate his or her legs to 60 degrees. Maintenance of color or slight pallor is normal, whereas marked pallor is a positive sign of arterial insufficiency. Ask the patient to sit up and dangle the legs over the side of the bed. Pink color normally returns in 10 seconds. Venous filling of the feet and ankle normally takes approximately 15 seconds. Persisting rubor and plethora on dependency are suggestive of arterial insufficiency. Normal findings with decreased arterial pulses are suggestive of good collateral circulation around an arterial occlusion.
- **Trendelenburg's test:** With the patient supine, elevate one of the patient's legs to 90 degrees, and stroke the veins toward the heart until they are empty. Manually occlude the great saphenous vein in the upper thigh with a tourniquet. Ask the patient to quickly stand, and watch for venous filling. Arterial blood flow from below normally fills the venous system over a period of 30 to 35 seconds. Rapid filling is indicative of incompetent valves in the communicating system (perforators). Release the tourniquet, and observe any further sudden venous filling, which is indicative of incompetent valves in the great saphenous vein.

Table 1-5	Usefulness of Clinical Examination in Diagnosing PAD in Symptomatic Patients	
Clinical Feature	**+LR (95% CI)**	**−LR (95% CI)**
Skin cooler to touch	**5.9 (4.1–8.6)**	0.92 (0.89–0.95)
Wounds or sores	**5.9 (2.6–13.4)**	0.98 (0.97–1.0)
Skin discoloration	2.8 (2.4–3.3)	0.74 (0.69–0.79)
At least one bruit (iliac, femoral, popliteal)	**5.6 (4.7–6.7)**	0.39 (0.34–0.45)
Palpable pulse abnormality	4.7 (2.2–9.9)	0.38 (0.23–0.64)

CI, Confidence interval; −LR, negative likelihood ratio; +LR, positive likelihood ratio; PAD, peripheral arterial disease.

Boldface represents findings associated with positive likelihood ratios ≥5 or with negative likelihood ratios ≤0.2. These are said to be moderate- to high-impact items.

Auscultation
- Listen for femoral and iliac bruits.

Evidence
- An ABI $\leq$ 0.9 is 95% sensitive and 100% specific for identifying angiogram-positive PAD. Table 1-5 lists other clinical features associated with PAD.[7]

HYPERTENSION: HISTORY AND PHYSICAL EXAMINATION

> **INSTRUCTIONS TO CANDIDATE: A 58-year-old man with a history of hypertension presents for a "check-up." Obtain a focused history and perform a physical examination.**

History
- Patients are usually **asymptomatic.** Ask the following questions:
  - "How are you feeling? Any changes in your health lately?"
  - "Do you have any headaches?" Suboccipital, pulsating headaches are common.
  - "Do you have any visual disturbance? Nausea or vomiting?"
  - "Do you have chest pain? Shortness of breath on exertion? How is your exercise tolerance?"
- **Risk factors** for cardiovascular disease:
  - Age (men >55 years; women >65 years)
  - Cigarette smoking
  - Hypertension
  - Diabetes mellitus (DM)
  - Hyperlipidemia
  - Obesity (especially around the waist)
  - Physical inactivity
  - Family history of premature cardiovascular disease (men <55 years; women <65 years)
- **Past medical history (PMH)/past surgical history (PSH):** Other medical or surgical problems
- **Medications (MEDS):** Nonsteroidal anti-inflammatory drugs (NSAIDs), cyclooxygenase-2 (COX-2) Inhibitors, steroids, or sympathomimetic agents
- Consider adherence with prescribed antihypertensive medications.
- **Social history (SH):** Diet (including sodium intake), exercise, smoking, use of alcohol (EtOH), use of street drugs, and psychosocial stressors
- **Family history (FH):** Lipid disorders, obesity, hypertension, endocrine disease, or polycystic kidney disease

Physical Examination
- To assess the effects of hypertension, you must evaluate end organs (e.g., eyes, heart, vasculature, brain, and kidneys).
- **Vital signs (Vitals):** measure heart rate (HR), BP, respiratory rate (RR), and temperature.
- **General:** Assess the patient's general appearance, noting body habitus.
  - Ascertain the **height** and **weight** of the patient. Body mass index (BMI) = weight (kg)/height^2 (m).
- **Head, eyes, ears, nose, and throat (HEENT):** Perform a careful funduscopic examination for signs of retinopathy (e.g., narrowed arterioles, copper/silver wire appearance, exudates, hemorrhages, and papilledema).
- **Respiratory (Resp):** Auscultate the lungs, noting breath sounds and adventitious sounds.
- **Cardiovascular system (CVS):** Measure the JVP (increased venous pressure in congestive heart failure [CHF]). Palpate peripheral pulses, and auscultate for bruits (e.g., carotid, aortic, renal, iliac, and femoral pulses). Inspect and palpate the apical impulse (note whether it is enlarged, sustained, and displaced as in LVH). Palpate

for thrills and heaves. Auscultate the heart, listening for an S_3 or a murmur. Examine for signs of arterial insufficiency in the lower limbs.
- **Abdomen:** Palpate the abdomen, and note any pulsatile masses.
- **Neurologic (Neuro):** Briefly assess the patient's mental status, which is altered when encephalopathy is present.

HYPERCHOLESTEROLEMIA: HISTORY AND PHYSICAL EXAMINATION

> **INSTRUCTIONS TO CANDIDATE: A 55-year-old man presents to his family physician for the results of routine blood work he had drawn last month. His total cholesterol level is 7.0 mmol/L, and his low-density lipoprotein (LDL) level is 4.5 mmol/L. Obtain a detailed history, and perform a focused physical examination.**

DD$_X$: VITAMINS C (Secondary Hypercholesterolemia)
- It is important to rule out treatable underlying causes of hypercholesterolemia.
- **Metabolic:** Hypothyroidism, DM, cholestasis
- **Idiopathic/iatrogenic:** Nephrotic syndrome, obesity (nonalcoholic steatohepatitis)

History
- Patients are usually **asymptomatic.** Ask the following questions:
  - "Have you ever been told you had high cholesterol?"
  - "How long have you had this problem?"
  - "Is it being treated (medications, lifestyle modifications)?"
  - "Is it improving, getting worse, or staying the same?"
  - "Any other problems (angina, stroke, abdominal pain, pancreatitis, liver disease, ischemic bowel, or claudication)?"
  - With regard to hypothyroidism: "Have you gained weight? Do you have cold intolerance? Constipation? Lethargy? Facial swelling?"
  - With regard to DM: "Do you pass a lot of urine (polyuria)? Are you often very thirsty (polydipsia)?"
  - With regard to nephrotic syndrome: "Do you have frothy urine? Swelling (edema)? Increased abdominal girth (ascites)?"
  - With regard to cholestasis: "Do you have jaundice? Excessive itching (pruritus)? Anorexia? Does your stool float and smell especially foul (steatorrhea)?"
- **Risk factors** for cardiovascular disease:
  - Age (men >55 years; women >65 years)
  - Cigarette smoking
  - Hypertension
  - DM
  - Hyperlipidemia
  - Obesity (especially around the waist)
  - Physical inactivity
  - Family history of premature cardiovascular disease (men <55 years; women <65 years)
- **PMH/PSH:** Pancreatitis
- **MEDS:** β-blockers, glucocorticoids, thiazides, oral contraceptive pill, estrogens, or progestin
- **SH:** Diet, exercise, smoking, use of EtOH, and use of street drugs
- **FH:** Lipid disorders, obesity, hypertension, DM, or liver disease

Physical Examination
- **Vitals:** Measure HR, BP, RR, and temperature.
- **General:** Assess the patient's general appearance, noting body habitus.
- Ascertain the **height** and **weight** of the patient. BMI = weight (kg)/height^2 (m).

- **Inspect** for signs associated with the following secondary causes of hypercholesterolemia:
  - Hypothyroidism: Narrowed pulse pressure, bradycardia; dry, coarse, sallow skin; nonpitting edema in face, hands, and feet; coarse, brittle hair; slow return phase of deep tendon reflexes, and carpal tunnel syndrome
  - Nephrotic syndrome: Anasarca, ascites, and muscle wasting
  - Cholestasis: Jaundice, excoriations
- **Skin:** Inspect for **tendon xanthoma** on ankles, extensor surface of elbows, and tendons of palms.
- **HEENT:** Inspect for **xanthelasma palpebrarum** (yellow deposits on the eyelids) and **corneal arcus** (granular fatty deposits on cornea). Examine the thyroid gland.
- **Resp:** Auscultate the lungs, noting breath sounds and adventitious sounds.
- **CVS:** Measure the JVP. Palpate peripheral pulses, and auscultate for bruits (carotid, aortic, renal, iliac, and femoral pulses). Note pulse volume, contour, and rhythm. Inspect and palpate the apical impulse (note whether it is enlarged, sustained, and displaced as in LVH). Palpate for thrills and heaves. Auscultate the heart, listening for extra heart sounds or murmurs.
- **Abdomen:** Examine the liver, spleen, and kidneys.

PALPITATIONS: HISTORY AND PHYSICAL EXAMINATION

INSTRUCTIONS TO CANDIDATE: A 35-year-old woman presents to the emergency department complaining that her "heart is beating out of her chest." This happened to her once before but resolved spontaneously. Obtain a detailed history, exploring possible causes, and perform a focused physical examination.

DD$_X$: VITAMINS C
- **Vascular:** Supraventricular tachycardia, rapid atrial fibrillation, ventricular tachycardia, and torsades de pointes
- **Metabolic:** Hypokalemia, hypomagnesemia, fever, anemia, hyper/hypothyroidism, and acromegaly
- **Neoplastic:** Pheochromocytoma
- **Substance abuse and psychiatric:** Drug ingestion (e.g., sympathomimetic agents), acquire long QT (e.g., antidysrhythmics, antidepressants, antiemetics, etc.) or drug withdrawal, anxiety, anorexia nervosa (electrolyte disturbance)
- **Congenital/genetic:** Wolff-Parkinson-White syndrome, Jervell and Lange-Nielsen syndrome, Romano-Ward syndrome

History
- Ask the patient the following questions:
  - **Character:** "Describe what happened. What do you mean when you say your heart was beating out of your chest? What were you doing when it started?"
  - **Onset:** "When did the palpitations begin? Did they start suddenly or gradually?"
  - **Intensity:** "How severe are the palpitations, on a scale of 1 to 10? How does it affect your activities of daily living?"
  - **Duration:** "How long do the palpitations last? How long has this been happening (acute versus chronic)?"
  - **Events associated:**
    - "How was your health before the palpitations began?"
    - "Do you have chest pain, shortness of breath, edema, diaphoresis, nausea or vomiting, or dizziness/syncope?"
    - Hyperthyroidism: "Have you had a goiter, weight loss, heat intolerance, diarrhea, or exophthalmos?"
    - Pheochromocytoma: "Have you had diaphoresis? Flushing?"

- ◆ Anxiety (diagnosis of exclusion): "Have you experienced lightheadedness, diaphoresis, trembling, choking sensation, palpitations, numbness or tingling in hands and feet, chest pain, nausea or abdominal pain, depersonalization/derealization, flushes or chills, fear of dying, fear of going crazy, or fear of doing something uncontrolled?"
  - ▪ Frequency: "How often do the palpitations occur? When was the last time this happened?"
  - ▪ Palliative factors: "Is there anything that makes these episodes better? If so, what?"
    - ◆ Carotid massage?
    - ◆ Valsalva maneuver?
  - ▪ Provocative factors: "Does anything make these episodes worse? If so, what?
    - ◆ Exercise? Other physical exertion?
- **PMH/PSH:** Arrhythmias, valvular disease, rheumatic fever, ischemic heart disease (IHD), multiple endocrine neoplasia (MEN; pheochromocytoma), hyperthyroidism, or psychiatric disorders
- **MEDS:** Thyroid replacement therapy, antiarrhythmics, salbutamol, or medication withdrawal (antidepressants, EtOH, opiates)
- **SH:** Caffeine, smoking, use of EtOH, and use of street drugs
- **FH:** Mitral valve prolapse (MVP), cardiomyopathy, multiple endocrine neoplasia (MEN), or psychiatric disorders

Physical Examination

- **Vitals:** Measure BP and HR while the patient is lying and either sitting or standing, RR, and temperature.
- **General:** Assess the patient's general appearance, noting signs of respiratory distress.
- **Skin:** Inspect the skin and nails, noting diaphoresis, flushing, cyanosis, or peripheral edema.
- **HEENT:** Examine the thyroid gland.
- **Resp:** Assess chest expansion for symmetry. Auscultate the chest, noting breath sounds and adventitious sounds.
- **CVS:** Measure the JVP. Palpate peripheral pulses. Note pulse volume, contour, and rhythm. Inspect and palpate the apical impulse (note whether it is enlarged, sustained, and displaced as in LVH). Palpate for thrills and heaves. Auscultate the heart, listening for extra heart sounds or murmurs.
- **Abdomen:** Examine for ascites and organomegaly.
- **Neuro:** Briefly assess the level of consciousness and mental status (adequate brain oxygenation).

HEART FAILURE: HISTORY AND PHYSICAL EXAMINATION

> **INSTRUCTIONS TO CANDIDATE: A 79-year-old man with a history of "heart failure" presents to the emergency department with worsening shortness of breath and swelling in his legs. Obtain a detailed history, exploring possible causes, and perform an appropriate physical examination.**

DD$_X$: VITAMINS C

- **V**ascular: CHF, acute coronary syndrome, and pulmonary embolism
- **I**nfectious: Pneumonia
- **T**raumatic: Pneumothorax
- **M**etabolic: Diabetic ketoacidosis (DKA)
- **I**diopathic/**i**atrogenic: COPD/asthma, massive atelectasis
- **N**eoplastic: Large pleural effusion
- **First evaluate a**irway, **b**reathing, and **c**irculation **(ABCs).** It may be necessary to perform an immediate intervention, such as administering supplemental O_2, establishing intravenous access, or initiating airway management.
  - ▪ Is the patient able to talk? Swallow? Cough?
  - ▪ Are both lungs ventilated? Is the patient oxygenating (check mentation, pulse oximetry)?

- Are vital signs abnormal? Is the peripheral circulation abnormal (check pulses, capillary refill)?
- If no immediate interventions are required, proceed to obtain the history, and perform the physical examination.

History (Table 1-6)
- Ask the patient the following questions:
  - **Character:** "Describe the nature of your breathing difficulty."
  - **Location:** "Where is the swelling in your legs? Both sides? Any other swelling?"
  - **Onset:** "How did the shortness of breath start (sudden versus gradual)? What were you doing when you became short of breath? Were you performing physical exertion? Lying down?"
  - **Intensity:** "How severe is your shortness of breath right now on a scale of 1 to 10, with 1 being mild and 10 being the worst? Has it gotten worse? Have your legs ever been this swollen?"
  - **Duration:** "How long have you been short of breath? How long have you had leg swelling?"
  - **Events associated:**
    - Decreased "Is your appetite decreased (liver and gastrointestinal [GI] congestion)? Do you have abdominal distension (ascites)?"
    - "Have you experienced weight gain (fluid retention), weakness, and fatigue (decreased cardiac output)?"
    - "Have you experienced orthopnea, paroxysmal nocturnal dyspnea, and pink frothy sputum (pulmonary edema)?"
    - "Have you had chest pain? Diaphoresis?"
    - Pulmonary embolism: "Have you experienced hemoptysis, pleuritic chest pain, DVT?"
    - Pneumonia, other infections: "Have you had fever or chills, rigors, increased sputum production, cough?"
  - **Frequency:** "Has this ever happened to you before? If so, how often does it happen? When was the last time you became short of breath?"
  - **Palliative factors:** "Does anything make your shortness of breath better? If so, what?"
  - **Provocative factors:** "Does anything make your shortness of breath worse? If so, what?"
    - Exertion
    - Position (sitting up versus lying down)
    - Exposure to cold air
    - Infection
    - Allergies

Table 1-6 Symptoms of Heart Failure

Symptoms of Right Ventricular Failure	Symptoms of Left Ventricular Failure
Exertional dyspnea	Dyspnea
Peripheral edema	Orthopnea
Abdominal distension (ascites)	Paroxysmal nocturnal dyspnea
Fullness in neck (jugular venous distension)	Coughing and wheezing (cardiac asthma)
Nocturia (increased venous return when supine increases venous return to kidneys)	Hemoptysis/pink froth (pulmonary congestion)
Wasting (cardiac cachexia), fatigue	Wasting (cardiac cachexia), fatigue
Right upper quadrant pain (hepatic congestion)	

- **Risk factors** for cardiovascular disease:
  - Age (men >55 years; women >65 years)
  - Cigarette smoking
  - Hypertension
  - DM
  - Hyperlipidemia
  - Obesity (especially around the waist)
  - Physical inactivity
  - Family history of premature cardiovascular disease (men <55 years; women <65 years)
- **PMH/PSH:** IHD, valvular disease, peripheral vascular disease, COPD, stroke, or malignancy
- **MEDS:** Calcium channel blockers, β-blockers, digitalis, diuretics, angiotensin-converting enzyme (ACE) inhibitors, or bronchodilators
  - Consider adherence with prescribed medications.
- **SH:** Smoking, use of EtOH, and use of street drugs
- **FH:** Cardiomyopathy, IHD, hypertension, increased cholesterol, obesity, or stroke
- **Immunizations:** Pneumococcal vaccine, influenza vaccine, childhood vaccinations, and bacille bilié de Calmette-Guérin (BCG) vaccine

Physical Examination (Table 1-7)
- **Vitals:** Evaluate HR, heart rhythm, RR (depth, effort, and pattern), BP, and temperature.
  - In end-stage heart failure, the patient may be hypothermic.
- **General:** Assess the patient's general appearance, noting signs of respiratory distress or apparent cachexia.
- **Skin:** Inspect the skin and nails, noting any diaphoresis, cyanosis, or pallor. Check capillary refill in distal extremities. Palpate for pitting edema over the tibia, behind medial malleolus, over dorsum of the foot, and in the presacral area.
- **HEENT:** Look in the mouth for central cyanosis. Assess tracheal position.
- **Resp:** Inspect for thoracic deformity and chest expansion (symmetry). Assess tactile fremitus, and perform percussion. Decreased tactile fremitus and flat percussion may be indicative of pleural effusion. Auscultate the lungs, and describe the breath sounds and adventitious sounds. You may note inspiratory crackles in pulmonary edema or expiratory wheezes (cardiac asthma).

Table 1-7 Physical Findings in Heart Failure

Signs of Right-Sided Heart Failure	Signs of Left-Sided Heart Failure

Increased venous pressure:
   Elevated jugular venous pressure (JVP), jugular venous distension (JVD)
   Positive hepatojugular reflux may be demonstrated even before elevated JVP
	Apical impulse:
	   Enlarged
	   Sustained
	   Displaced

Peripheral pitting edema:
   Feet and ankles, extending proximally
   Vulva/scrotum
   Presacral area
	Pulmonary edema:
	   Inspiratory crackles
	   Frothy, blood-tinged sputum

Hepatomegaly:
   Congested, tender liver
   Splenomegaly (may be a late finding)
	Pulsus alternans

Ascites	Pleural effusion (commonly right-sided)
Right-sided S_3	Left-sided S_3 or S_4

- **CVS:** Measure the JVP and hepatojugular reflux (increased venous pressure in CHF). Palpate peripheral pulses. Note pulse volume, contour, and rhythm. Pulses may be decreased, or pulsus alternans may be present. Inspect and palpate the apical impulse (note whether it is enlarged, sustained, and displaced as in LVH). Palpate for thrills and heaves. Auscultate the heart, listening for an S_3 or a murmur.
- **Abdomen:** Inspect for ascites (bulging flanks, protuberant abdomen, umbilical herniation). Percuss the abdomen, noting any shifting dullness. Assess liver span. Palpate the liver and spleen.
- **Neuro:** Briefly assess level of consciousness and mental status (adequate brain oxygenation).

Evidence
- Table 1-8 demonstrates the usefulness of clinical examination for diagnosing heart failure in the emergency department.

Pearl
- Manifestations of heart failure on chest radiography (Figure 1-17 demonstrates some of these features):
  - Alveolar infiltrates, usually symmetric bilaterally
  - Kerley B lines (engorged lymphatic vessels)
  - Pleural effusion (blunting of costophrenic angles)
  - Enlarged cardiac silhouette (chronic CHF)
  - Pulmonary vascular redistribution (enlarged vasculature in the apices)

Table 1-8	Usefulness of Clinical Examination for Diagnosing Heart Failure in the Emergency Department	
Clinical Feature	**+LR (95% CI)**	**−LR (95% CI)**
History of heart failure	**5.8 (4.1–8.0)**	0.45 (0.38–0.53)
History of myocardial infarction	3.1 (2.0–4.9)	0.69 (0.58–0.82)
Paroxysmal nocturnal dyspnea	2.6 (1.5–4.5)	0.70 (0.54–0.91)
Orthopnea	2.2 (1.2–3.9)	0.65 (0.45–0.92)
Edema	2.1 (0.92–5.0)	0.64 (0.39–1.1)
Dyspnea on exertion	1.3 (1.2–1.4)	0.48 (0.35–0.67)
Presence of an S_3*	**11 (4.9–25.0)**	0.88 (0.83–0.94)
Hepatojugular reflux	**6.4 (0.81–51.0)**	0.79 (0.62–1.0)
JVD	**5.1 (3.2–7.9)**	0.66 (0.57–0.77)
Crackles	2.8 (1.9–4.1)	0.51 (0.37–0.70)
Any murmur	2.6 (1.7–4.1)	0.81 (0.73–0.90)
Lower extremity edema	2.3 (1.5–3.7)	0.64 (0.47–0.87)

From Wang CS, FitzGerald JM, Schulzer M, et al. Does this dyspneic patient in the emergency department have congestive heart failure? *JAMA.* 2005;294:1944-1956.

*In patients with chronic obstructive pulmonary disease (COPD) or asthma, the presence of an S_3 is a reliable indicator of heart failure (+LR 57.0; 95% CI 7.6 to 425).

CI, Confidence interval; JVD, jugular venous distension; −LR, negative likelihood ratio; +LR, positive likelihood ratio.

Boldface represents findings associated with positive likelihood ratios ≥5 or with negative likelihood ratios ≤0.2. These are said to be moderate- to high-impact items.

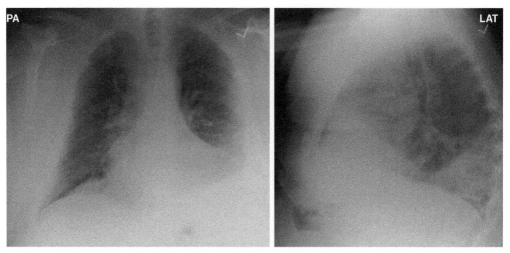

Figure 1-17 Posteroanterior **(left)** and lateral **(right)** views of the chest. The heart is moderately enlarged. A left-sided pleural effusion is present, and the lungs demonstrate vascular redistribution with increased interstitial and air space disease at the lung bases, all of which are consistent with congestive heart failure.

PERICARDITIS: HISTORY AND PHYSICAL EXAMINATION

INSTRUCTIONS TO CANDIDATE: A 39-year-old man presents to the emergency department with sharp chest pain that is most severe when he is lying down. He feels unwell and is having "trouble breathing." Obtain a detailed history, exploring possible causes, and perform a focused physical examination.

DD$_X$: VITAMINS C (Chest Pain)
- **V**ascular: Aortic dissection, myocardial infarction (MI), pulmonary embolism, and pulmonary infarction
- **I**nfectious: Pericarditis, pneumonia, bronchiectasis, tuberculosis, empyema, subphrenic abscess, and herpes zoster
- **T**raumatic: Pneumothorax, fractured rib, and chest wall injury
- **A**utoimmune/allergic: Systemic lupus erythematosus (serositis)
- **M**etabolic: Diabetic ketoacidosis
- **I**diopathic/iatrogenic: Dressler syndrome, esophageal spasm, peptic ulcer disease, and gastroesophageal reflux
- **N**eoplastic: Malignant pericarditis
- **S**ubstance abuse and psychiatric: Cocaine ingestion (coronary vasospasm), other sympathomimetic ingestion, and anxiety
- **C**ongenital/genetic: Hiatal hernia
- **First evaluate ABCs.** It may be necessary to perform an immediate intervention, such as administering supplemental O$_2$, establishing intravenous access, or initiating airway management.
  - Is the patient able to talk? Swallow? Cough?
  - Are both lungs ventilated? Is the patient oxygenating (check mentation, pulse oximetry)?
  - Are vital signs abnormal? Is the peripheral circulation abnormal (check pulses, capillary refill)?
  - If no immediate interventions are required, proceed to obtain the history, and perform the physical examination.

History
- Ask the patient the following questions:
  - **Character:** "How would you describe the pain?"
  - **Location:** "Where exactly is the pain?"
  - **Onset:** "When did the pain begin (sudden versus insidious)?"

- ■ Radiation: "Does the pain go anywhere else?"
- ■ Intensity: "How bad is the pain on a scale of 1 to 10, with 1 being mild pain and 10 being the worst pain?"
- ■ Duration: "How long has the pain lasted (acute versus chronic)?"
- ■ Events associated:
  - ◆ Tamponade/constrictive pericarditis: "Have you experienced dyspnea, orthopnea, palpitations, and distension of neck veins?"
  - ◆ MI: "Have you had nausea or vomiting? Have you experienced diaphoresis?"
  - ◆ Pneumonia: "Have you had fever or chills, rigors, increased sputum production, or cough?"
  - ◆ Trauma: "Have you suffered any significant injuries recently (specifically abdominothoracic)?"
- ■ Frequency: "How often does this pain occur? When was the last time this happened?"
- ■ Palliative factors: "Does anything make the pain better? If so, what?"
  - ◆ Sitting up
  - ◆ Leaning forward
  - ◆ NSAIDs
- ■ Provocative factors: "Does anything make the pain worse? If so, what?"
  - ◆ Lying down (especially on left side)
  - ◆ Coughing or deep inspiration
  - ◆ Swallowing (proximity of the esophagus to the pericardium)
- **PMH/PSH:** MI, malignancy, radiation, renal failure, or systemic lupus erythematosus
- **MEDS:** Procainamide, hydralazine, dantrolene, cromolyn sodium, or if patient is female, oral contraceptive pill
- **SH:** Smoking, use of EtOH, and use of street drugs

Physical Examination
- **Vitals:** Measure HR, BP, RR, and temperature.
- **General:** Assess the patient's general appearance, noting position and posture and any signs of respiratory distress.
- **Resp:** Assess chest expansion for symmetry. Auscultate the lungs, noting breath sounds and adventitious sounds.
- **CVS:** Measure the JVP. Palpate peripheral pulses. Note pulse volume, contour, and rhythm. Inspect and palpate the apical impulse. Palpate for thrills, heaves, and pericardial friction rub. Auscultate the heart, listening for extra heart sounds or murmurs. Use the diaphragm of the stethoscope to listen for the high-pitched, inconstant pericardial friction rub. The rub is best heard in the sitting position and is described as "Velcro-like."
  - ■ Using a sphygmomanometer, assess for **pulsus paradoxus.** As the patient breathes quietly, lower the cuff pressure to the level of the first Korotkoff sound, which identifies the *highest systolic BP* during the respiratory cycle. Then lower the pressure slowly until sounds can be heard throughout the respiratory cycle; note the pressure level as that of the *lowest systolic BP.* The difference between the highest and lowest systolic pressures is *normally* no greater than 8 to 12 mm Hg.
- **Abdomen:** Examine for ascites and organomegaly.
- **Neuro:** Briefly assess level of consciousness and mental status (adequate brain oxygenation).

Evidence
- Table 1-9 demonstrates the usefulness of clinical examination for diagnosing pericardial tamponade.

Pearl
- **Cardiac tamponade** is a life-threatening complication of pericarditis. It is characterized by the following:
  - **Beck's triad:** Hypotension, jugular venous distension (JVD), and muffled heart sounds
  - **Electrocardiographic signs:** Electrical alternans (variation in the QRS axis seen on ECG as the heart moves within the fluid-filled pericardium), low voltages

Table 1-9	Usefulness of Clinical Examination for Diagnosing Pericardial Tamponade	
Clinical Feature	**Sensitivity (95% CI)**
Dyspnea	87–88%
Pulsus paradoxus >10 mm Hg	82% (72%–92%)
Tachycardia	77% (69%–85%)
Hypotension	26% (16%–36%)
Diminished heart sounds	28% (21%–35%)
Elevated JVP	76% (62%–90%)

From Roy CL, Minor MA, Brookhart MA, et al. Does this patient with a pericardial effusion have cardiac tamponade? *JAMA.* 2007;297:1810-1818.
CI, Confidence interval; JVP, jugular venous pressure.

MYOCARDIAL INFARCTION: HISTORY, PHYSICAL EXAMINATION, AND INTERPRETATION OF THE ELECTROCARDIOGRAM

INSTRUCTIONS TO CANDIDATE: A 56-year-old woman presents to the emergency department complaining of 3 hours of severe left-sided chest pain. The nurse hands you an ECG. Obtain a detailed history, exploring possible causes, and perform an appropriate physical examination. Interpret the ECG (Figure 1-18).

Interpretation of the Electrocardiogram
- Normal sinus rhythm, 55 beats/minute
- Four to 5 mm of ST elevation in leads I, aV_L, and V_2 to V_4
- Two to 3 mm of ST elevation in V_5 and reciprocal ST depression in leads II, III, and aV_F
- These electrocardiographic changes are consistent with an anterolateral MI.

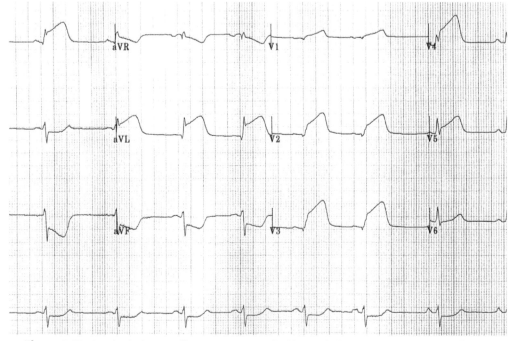

Figure 1-18 A 12-lead electrocardiogram (ECG). (Used with permission of Dr. Arik Drucker, Dalhousie University, Halifax, Nova Scotia.)

DD$_X$: VITAMINS C (Chest Pain)

- **V**ascular: MI, acute coronary syndrome, aortic dissection, pulmonary embolism, and pulmonary infarction
- **I**nfectious: Pericarditis, pneumonia, bronchiectasis, tuberculosis, empyema, subphrenic abscess, and herpes zoster
- **T**raumatic: Pneumothorax, fractured rib, and chest wall injury
- **A**utoimmune/**a**llergic: Systemic lupus erythematosus (serositis)
- **M**etabolic: Diabetic ketoacidosis
- **I**diopathic/**i**atrogenic: Dressler syndrome, esophageal spasm, peptic ulcer disease, and gastroesophageal reflux
- **N**eoplastic: Malignant pericarditis
- **S**ubstance abuse and psychiatric: Cocaine ingestion (coronary vasospasm), other sympathomimetic ingestion, and anxiety
- **C**ongenital/genetic: Hiatal hernia
- **First evaluate ABCs.** It may be necessary to perform an immediate intervention, such as administering supplemental O_2, establishing intravenous access, or initiating airway management.
  - Is the patient able to talk? Swallow? Cough?
  - Are both lungs ventilated? Is the patient oxygenating (check mentation, pulse oximetry)?
  - Are vital signs abnormal? Is the peripheral circulation abnormal (check pulses, capillary refill)?
  - If no immediate interventions are required, proceed to obtain the history, and perform the physical examination.

History

- Ask the patient the following questions:
  - Character: "Describe the pain. Is it crushing, squeezing, tight, heavy, or burning? Tearing? Sharp?"
  - Location: "Where exactly is the pain?"
  - Onset: "When did it start? Was it gradual or sudden? What events led up to this episode of pain?"
  - Radiation: "Does the pain go anywhere else? Shoulder, neck, jaw, or arms? Back?"
  - Intensity: "How bad is it on a scale of 1 to 10, with 1 being mild pain and 10 being the worst pain? Does it hinder you from performing daily tasks?"
  - Duration: "How long has the pain been there?"
  - Events associated:
    - "Do you have nausea or vomiting, diaphoresis, weakness, or anxiety?"
    - "Do you have shortness of breath, orthopnea, or paroxysmal nocturnal dyspnea?"
    - Pulmonary embolism: "Do you have hemoptysis, pleuritic chest pain, or leg swelling/pain (DVT)?"
    - Pneumonia, other infections: "Have you experienced fever or chills, rigors, increased sputum production, and cough?"
  - Frequency: "How often does this pain occur?"
  - Palliative factors: "Does anything make the pain better? If so, what?"
    - Nitroglycerin
    - Rest
    - Antacids
    - Sitting forward
- Provocative factors: "Does anything make the pain worse? If so, what?"
  - Exercise/exertion
  - Movement
  - Deep inspiration
  - Eating

- **Risk factors** for cardiovascular disease:
  - Age (men >55 years; women >65 years)
  - Cigarette smoking
  - Hypertension
  - DM
  - Hyperlipidemia
  - Obesity (especially around the waist)
  - Physical inactivity
  - Family history of premature cardiovascular disease (men <55 years; women <65 years)
- **PMH/PSH:** IHD, COPD, or stroke
- **MEDS:** Antihypertensive agents, acetylsalicylic acid (ASA), nitroglycerin, or anticoagulants
- **FH:** IHD, stroke

Physical Examination

- **Vitals:** Evaluate HR, heart rhythm, RR (depth, effort, and pattern), BP, and temperature.
- **General:** Assess the patient's general appearance, noting any signs of respiratory distress, including restlessness or apprehension.
- **Skin:** Inspect the skin and nails, noting any diaphoresis, cyanosis, or pallor. Check capillary refill in distal extremities. Palpate for pitting edema over the tibia, behind the medial malleolus, over the dorsum of the foot, and in the presacral area.
- **HEENT:** Look in the mouth for central cyanosis.
- **Resp:** Inspect for thoracic deformity and chest expansion (symmetry). Auscultate the lungs, and describe the breath sounds and adventitious sounds. You may note inspiratory crackles in pulmonary edema or expiratory wheezes (cardiac asthma).
- **CVS:** Measure the JVP and hepatojugular reflux (increased venous pressure in CHF). Palpate peripheral pulses. Note pulse volume, contour, and rhythm. Inspect and palpate the apical impulse (note whether it is enlarged, sustained, and displaced as in LVH). Palpate for thrills and heaves. Auscultate the heart, listening for an S_3, an S_4, or a murmur. A pericardial friction rub over the infarcted area occurs in some cases of MI. Listen for the murmur of AR and for asymmetric pulses to distinguish aortic dissection.
- **Abdomen:** Inspect for ascites (bulging flanks, protuberant abdomen, umbilical herniation). Percuss the abdomen, noting any shifting dullness. Assess liver span. Palpate the liver and spleen.
- **Neuro:** Briefly assess level of consciousness and mental status (adequate brain oxygenation).

Evidence (Tables 1-10, 1-11, and 1-12)

- Prediction rules and scores using features of the clinical assessment have not been well validated.[8]
- In one study of patients in the emergency department with chest pain, the presence of pain that radiated to the right arm or both arms, vomiting, and observed diaphoresis increased the likelihood that acute coronary syndrome was present. Central chest pain was also a predictive factor (+LR 3.3; 95% CI 1.9 to 5.6). In contrast, pain that radiated to the left arm was not predictive of acute coronary syndrome (+LR 1.4; 95% CI 0.9 to 2.1).[9]
- Chest pain that is described as pleuritic, sharp, or stabbing is less likely to be associated with acute MI, as is positional pain and pain that is reproduced by palpation.[10]
- The modified Thrombolysis In Myocardial Infarction (TIMI) risk score (see Table 1-11) is useful for risk stratifying patients with chest pain.[11]

Table 1-10 Usefulness of the Clinical Examination for Diagnosing Acute Coronary Syndrome

Clinical Feature	+LR (95% CI)
Chest pain radiating to right arm or shoulder*	4.7 (1.9–12)
Chest pain radiating to left arm†	2.3 (1.7–3.1)
Chest pain radiating to both left and right arm*	4.1 (2.5–6.5)
Nausea/vomiting†	1.9 (1.7–2.3)
Diaphoresis†	2.0 (1.9–2.2)
Presence of S_3†	3.2 (1.6–6.5)
Systolic BP ≤ 80 mm Hg†	3.1 (1.8–5.2)

*Data from Swap CJ, Nagurney JT. Value and limitations of chest pain history in the evaluation of patients with suspected acute coronary syndromes. *JAMA.* 2005;294:2623-2629.

†Data from Panju AA, Hemmelgarn BR, Guyatt GH, et al. The rational clinical examination: Is this patient having a myocardial infarction? *JAMA.* 1998;280:1256-1263.

BP, Blood pressure; CI, confidence ratio; +LR, positive likelihood ratio.

Table 1-11 The Modified TIMI Risk Score

Predictor	Score	Definition
Age ≥65	1	
≥3 cardiac risk factors	1	Risk factors: Family history of CAD Hypertension Hypercholesterolemia Diabetes Current smoker
ASA use in last 7 days	1	
Recent severe symptoms of angina	1	≥2 Anginal episodes in last 24 hours
Elevated serum cardiac markers OR	5	Elevations in CK-MB or cardiac-specific troponin level
Ischemic ECG changes		ST deviation ≥0.5 mm
Prior coronary artery stenosis ≥50%	1	

From Body R, Carley S, McDowell G, et al. Can a modified Thrombolysis in Myocardial Infarction risk score outperform the original for risk stratifying emergency department patients with chest pain? *Emerg Med J.* 2009;26:95-99.

ASA, Acetylsalicylic acid; CAD, coronary artery disease; CK-MB, creatine kinase–muscle-brain isoenzyme; ECG, electrocardiographic; TIMI, Thrombolysis In Myocardial Infarction.

Table 1-12 Frequency of Cardiac Events Within the Modified TIMI Risk Strata

Modified TIMI Score	Frequency of Death, AMI, or Revascularization
0 or 1	2%
2	7%
3	15%
4	23%
5	24%
>5	44%

From Hess EP, Perry JJ, Calder LA, et al. Prospective validation of a modified Thrombolysis In Myocardial Infarction risk score in emergency department patients with chest pain and possible acute coronary syndrome. *Acad Emerg Med.* 2010;17:368-375.

AMI, Acute myocardial infarction; TIMI, Thrombolysis In Myocardial Infarction.

SAMPLE CHECKLISTS

Hypertension: Measure Blood Pressure

INSTRUCTIONS TO CANDIDATE: Demonstrate how you would measure BP in a patient referred to you for evaluation of hypertension. Explain what you are doing, and document the patient's BP measurement.

Key Points	Satisfactorily Completed
Introduces self to the patient	❏
Determines how the patient wishes to be addressed	❏
Washes hands	❏
Explains nature of the examination to the patient	❏
Selects correctly sized cuff	❏
Places cuff in correct position	❏
Estimates systolic BP by palpating radial or brachial pulse	❏
Positions arm at heart level	❏
Supports the patient's arm	❏
BP auscultation: arms	
• Positions stethoscope	❏
• Inflates to 20 to 30 mm Hg above estimated systolic BP	❏
• Deflates cuff at a rate of 2 to 3 mm Hg/sec	❏
• Positions patient supine	❏
• Positions patient standing/sitting	❏
• States that BP would be measured in both arms	❏
BP reading	
• States systolic pressure	❏
• States diastolic pressure	❏
Makes appropriate closing remarks	❏

Peripheral Vascular Disease: Physical Examination

INSTRUCTIONS TO CANDIDATE: Examine this patient's lower extremities for evidence of peripheral arterial insufficiency. Describe your findings.

Key Points	Satisfactorily Completed
Introduces self to the patient	❏
Determines how the patient wishes to be addressed	❏
Washes hands	❏
Explains nature of the examination to the patient	❏
Inspects lower extremities comparatively, noting:	
• Color/pigmentation of skin	❏
• Texture of skin	❏
• Hair distribution	❏
• Skin breakdown or ulcers	❏
• Infarction of distal extremity (e.g., toes)	❏
• Nails	❏

Key Points	Satisfactorily Completed
Palpates lower extremities, noting:	
• Temperature	❑
• Edema (absent or mild)	❑
• Capillary refill	❑
Auscultates for bruit in the lower extremities:	
• Femoral	❑
• Popliteal	❑
Palpates pulses in the lower extremities:	
• Femoral	❑
• Popliteal	❑
• Dorsalis pedis	❑
• Posterior tibial	❑
Evaluates color of extremity	
• With elevation of leg	❑
• With leg dangling down	❑
Measures BP in upper and lower extremities to calculate the ABI	❑
Performs Buerger's test	❑
Performs Trendelenburg's test	❑
Drapes the patient appropriately	❑
Makes appropriate closing remarks	❑

Abdominal Aortic Aneurysm: Physical Examination

INSTRUCTIONS TO CANDIDATE: A 62-year-old man presents to his family doctor for refill of his BP medications. He is disturbed by his brother's recent sudden death from a ruptured abdominal aortic aneurysm and wonders whether he too might be a "ticking time bomb." Perform a focused physical examination, and describe your findings.

Key Points	Satisfactorily Completed
Introduces self to the patient	❑
Determines how the patient wishes to be addressed	❑
Washes hands	❑
Explains nature of the examination to the patient	❑
Examines the patient in a logical manner	❑
Vitals:	
• Requests a complete set of vital signs	❑
• Notes any abnormalities such as tachycardia or hypotension	❑
• Palpates peripheral pulses in lower extremities, noting volume, contour, and rhythm	❑
Inspection:	
• Abdominal contour	❑
• Scars indicating previous surgery	❑
• Visible pulsations	❑
Auscultates the abdomen, noting any bruits	❑
Palpation:	
• Positions the patient supine	❑
• Lightly palpates abdomen, noting areas of tenderness	❑
• Palpates deeper, noting tenderness and masses	❑
• Attempts to identify central pulsatile mass	❑
Drapes the patient appropriately	❑
Makes appropriate closing remarks	❑

Evidence

- Palpation is a fairly well-studied physical examination technique for identifying abdominal aortic aneurysm[12] (Table 1-13).

Pearl

- To palpate the aorta, first identify the aortic pulsation (central and superior to the umbilicus). Position both hands on the abdomen at either side of the aortic pulsation and estimate its width (>2.5 cm is abnormal). Abdominal obesity may limit the usefulness of the examination.

Table 1-13	Usefulness of Palpation for Identifying Abdominal Aortic Aneurysm in Asymptomatic Patients*

Size of AAA	Sensitivity
3.0–3.9 cm	29%
4.0–4.9 cm	50%
≥5.0 cm	76%

From Lederle FA, Simel DL. The rational clinical examination. Does this patient have abdominal aortic aneurysm? *JAMA*. 1999;281:77-82.

*Note that palpation in these studies was performed for the purpose of identifying abdominal aortic aneurysm (AAA); therefore, these sensitivities cannot be extrapolated to routine physical examination.

Chest Pain: History

> **INSTRUCTIONS TO CANDIDATE: A 59-year-old man presents to the emergency department with chest pain that started about 1 hour ago. Obtain a focused history.**

Key Points	Satisfactorily Completed
Introduces self to the patient	❑
Determines how the patient wishes to be addressed	❑
Washes hands	❑
Establishes the purpose of the encounter	❑
Establishes the presenting concern in the patient's own words	❑
History of chest pain:	
• Characterizes the pain	❑
• Establishes the location of pain	❑
• Ascertains whether and to where pain radiates	❑
• Establishes the onset and pattern of the pain (e.g., pleuritic)	❑
• Asks about the patient's activities at time of pain onset	❑
• Establishes the duration of this particular episode of pain	❑
• Asks about the severity of the pain on a scale	❑
• Asks about previous episodes of similar pain	❑
• Asks about the frequency with which the pain occurs	❑
• Asks about palliative factors (e.g., nitroglycerin, rest, position)	❑
• Asks about provocative factors (e.g., exertion, movement)	❑
Assesses associated symptoms:	
• Fever	❑
• Dyspnea: At rest? Exertional? Supine (orthopnea)? Nighttime (paroxysmal nocturnal dyspnea)?	❑
• Diaphoresis	❑
• Nausea, vomiting, or both	❑
Ascertains relevant social history:	
• Smoking	❑
• EtOH use	❑
• Physical activity	❑
Ascertains past medical and surgical history:	
• Diabetes	❑
• Hypertension	❑
• Hyperlipidemia	❑
• Coronary artery disease (past MI, angina, angioplasty)	❑
• Vascular disease (e.g., aortic, cerebrovascular, peripheral vascular)	❑
Asks about medications:	
• Prescription drugs (including anticoagulants)	❑
• Over-the-counter drugs (including ASA)	❑
Asks about allergies	❑
Makes appropriate closing remarks	❑

ADVANCED SKILLS

AORTIC STENOSIS: EXAMINATION

DD_X: VITAMINS C
- **A**utoimmune/**a**llergic: Rheumatic valvular disease
- **I**diopathic/**i**atrogenic: Degenerative valve calcification, hypertrophic cardiomyopathy
- **C**ongenital/genetic: Congenital bicuspid valve

Patient Positioning
- To accentuate the murmur of AS, examine the patient while he or she is seated and leaning forward.

Inspection
- Inspect for the apical impulse and the ventricular movements of a left-sided S_3 or S_4. Tangential lighting may improve the visibility of impulses.

Palpation
- Palpate the carotid pulse, noting its contour and volume (**pulses tardus et parvus:** slow upstroke and a small amplitude). Simultaneously palpate the apical impulse and right carotid pulsation, noting any apical-carotid delay.
- Palpate for systolic thrills over the base of the heart and at the carotid arteries. Thrills are best felt with the ball of your hand pressed firmly on the patient's chest.
- Palpate the impulses with the pads of your fingers, exerting light pressure for S_3 or S_4 and firmer pressure for S_1 and S_2. The apical impulse may be enlarged, sustained, and displaced because of LVH.

Auscultation
- Listen for high-pitched murmurs with the diaphragm of the stethoscope held firmly against the chest wall. Also, with the patient in the left lateral decubitus position, listen at the apex with the bell of the stethoscope.
  - Expect a loud systolic crescendo-decrescendo murmur of medium pitch (higher pitch at the apex). It is often described as harsh and is best heard in the second right ICS. It is also often heard along the left sternal border and radiates to the neck.
  - During expiration, S_2 may be split; this phenomenon is known as **paradoxical splitting.** In severe fixed AS, A_2 is diminished or absent. If a normal split S_2 is present, severe AS is very unlikely. An S_4 may be audible.

Other Signs of Aortic Stenosis
- Narrowed pulse pressure

Evidence
- Useful findings for the clinical diagnosis of AS include slow upstroke of the carotid pulse (+LR 2.8 to 130); middle to late peak intensity of the systolic murmur (+LR 8.0 to 101); and decreased intensity of S_2 (+LR 3.1 to 50). Poorer quality studies indicate that apical-carotid delay and brachioradial delay *may* be useful. The absence of a systolic murmur that radiates to the right carotid artery is a strong indicator against a diagnosis of AS (−LR 0.05 to 0.10).[13]

AORTIC REGURGITATION: EXAMINATION

DD_X: VITAMINS C
- **V**ascular: Acute aortic dissection, dilatation of the aortic root (Marfan syndrome)
- **I**nfectious: Bacterial endocarditis, syphilis of the aorta
- **T**raumatic: Chest trauma (acute AR)

- **Autoimmune/allergic:** Rheumatic valvular disease, ankylosing spondylitis, collagen vascular disease
- **Idiopathic/iatrogenic:** Idiopathic valvular degeneration
- **Congenital/genetic:** Congenital bicuspid valve

Patient Positioning
- To accentuate the murmur of AR, examine the patient while seated and leaning forward.

Inspection
- Inspect for the apical impulse and the ventricular movements of a left-sided S_3 or S_4. Tangential lighting may improve the visibility of impulses.

Palpation
- Palpate the carotid pulse, noting its contour and volume **(water-hammer pulse, pulsus bisferiens).**
- Palpate for systolic thrills over the base of the heart and at the carotid arteries. Thrills are best felt with the ball of your hand pressed firmly on the patient's chest.
- Palpate the impulses with the pads of your fingers, exerting light pressure for an S_3 or S_4 and firmer pressure for S_1 and S_2. The apical impulse may be enlarged, sustained, and displaced because of LVH.

Auscultation
- Listen for the high-pitched murmur with the diaphragm of the stethoscope held firmly against the chest wall. Also, with the patient in the left lateral decubitus position, listen at the apex with the bell of the stethoscope.
  - Expect an early, blowing, decrescendo diastolic murmur that is high pitched. It is heard with maximal intensity in the second to fourth left ICSs. If the murmur is loud, it may radiate to the apex or right sternal border. The intensity of the murmur is not correlated with severity of AR.
  - A_2 is often absent, and the presence of an S_3 or S_4 may be suggestive of severe disease accompanied by LV dysfunction.

Positional and Respiratory Maneuvers
- The murmur of AR is accentuated by squatting and is decreased during the Valsalva maneuver.

Other Signs of Aortic Regurgitation
- Widened pulse pressure
- **Corrigan's sign:** A prominent carotid pulsation characterized by *bounding* and *increased volume*; similar to the *water-hammer pulse*
- **de Musset's sign:** Head nodding that accompanies carotid pulsations
- **Hills' sign:** BP that is higher in the legs than in the arms (difference > 60 mm Hg).
- **Duroziez's sign:** A femoral diastolic murmur with slight compression; it reflects flow backward up the aorta, is indicative of severe disease, and is related to *pulsus bisferiens*
- **Pistol shot sound** (Traube's sign) over the femoral arteries: Produced by the high-pressure arterial pulse wave striking the femoral arterial wall
- Systolic pulsations may also be noted in the liver **(Rosenbach's sign)**, spleen **(Gerhard's sign)**, uvula **(Mueller's sign)**, retinal vessels **(Becker's sign)**, or nail beds **(Quincke's sign)**

Evidence
- The early diastolic murmur of AR has been well studied and appears to be the best physical sign for diagnosing AR (+LR 8.8 to 32.0; −LR 0.2 to 0.3).[14] Transient arterial occlusion is also useful. To perform this test, inflate the sphygmomanometer on

both arms simultaneously to a pressure that is about 20 mm Hg higher than the patient's systolic BP. Auscultate the heart, noting any changes in the intensity of the murmur about 20 seconds after cuff inflation. In a small study of transient arterial occlusion, investigators found a +LR of 8.4 (95% CI 1.3 to 81) and a −LR of 0.3 (95% CI 0.1 to 0.8).[15] Most of the peripheral signs of AR are not well studied.

MITRAL STENOSIS: EXAMINATION

DD$_X$: VITAMINS C
- **A**utoimmune/**a**llergic: Rheumatic valvular disease
- **I**diopathic/**i**atrogenic: Idiopathic valvular degeneration
- **N**eoplastic: Left atrial myxoma
- **C**ongenital/genetic: Congenital valvular lesion

Patient Positioning
- To accentuate the murmur of MS, position the patient in the left lateral decubitus position.

Inspection
- Inspect for the apical impulse. Tangential lighting may improve the visibility of impulses.

Palpation
- Palpate the carotid pulse, noting its contour and volume. Pulses in MS are generally diminished in amplitude as a result of reduced stroke volume.
- Palpate the apical impulse with the pads of your fingers. If right ventricular hypertrophy develops because of pulmonary hypertension, a right ventricular heave may be palpable.

Auscultation
- This murmur is low pitched and heard best with the bell of the stethoscope at the apex.
  - An opening snap often follows S_2 and initiates the murmur of MS. The opening snap is best heard along the left sternal border, second to fourth ICSs, with the diaphragm of the stethoscope.
  - Expect a low-pitched **rumbling** murmur, resembling the roll of a drum and best heard with the bell of the stethoscope. The murmur may have two components: mid-diastolic decrescendo (during rapid ventricular filling) and a presystolic crescendo that disappears in the presence of atrial fibrillation. S_1 is usually accentuated, and P_2 is also accentuated if pulmonary hypertension is present.
  - An associated murmur termed **Graham Steell's murmur** is indicative of pulmonic regurgitation. It is virtually indistinguishable from the murmur of AR, but it is usually not as loud, is transmitted less widely, and is not associated with peripheral signs of AR. It is caused by dilation of the pulmonic valve in pulmonary hypertension.

Positional and Respiratory Maneuvers
- The murmur of MS is accentuated by maneuvers that increase venous return, such as mild exercise. The murmur of MS is best heard in full expiration in the left lateral decubitus position.

Other Signs of Mitral Stenosis
- Irregularly irregular pulse (in the presence of atrial fibrillation)
- Increased JVP (in presence of right ventricular failure)
  - In sinus rhythm: Prominent "a" wave
  - In atrial fibrillation: Absence of "a" wave and prominent "v" wave

- Mitral facies: Malar flush in the setting of severe MS with low cardiac output
- Ortner syndrome: Hoarseness caused by left vocal cord paralysis that results from compression of left recurrent laryngeal nerve by a dilated left atrium

MITRAL REGURGITATION: EXAMINATION

DD$_X$: VITAMINS C
- **V**ascular: Ruptured chordae tendineae or papillary muscles (secondary to ischemia)
- **I**nfectious: Bacterial endocarditis
- **A**utoimmune/allergic: Rheumatic valvular disease, rheumatoid arthritis
- **I**diopathic/iatrogenic: MVP
- **C**ongenital/genetic: Dilation of the mitral ring

Patient Positioning
- To accentuate the murmur of MR, position the patient in the left lateral decubitus position.

Inspection
- Inspect for the apical impulse and the ventricular movements of a left-sided S$_3$ or S$_4$. Tangential lighting may improve the visibility of impulses.

Palpation
- Palpate the carotid pulse, noting its contour and volume. In chronic MR, the pulses are typically **bounding** in nature with a brisk upstroke, a rapid downstroke, and overall decreased volume (similar to those in AR but with lower pulse volume and a normal pulse pressure).
- Palpate for systolic thrills over the base of the heart. Thrills are best felt with the ball of your hand pressed firmly on the patient's chest, and they may occur in severe or acutely exacerbated MR.
- Palpate the impulses with the pads of your fingers, exerting light pressure for an S$_3$ or S$_4$ and firmer pressure for S$_1$ and S$_2$. The apical impulse may be enlarged, sustained, and displaced because of LVH.

Auscultation
- Auscultate the precordium, and listen for the medium- to high-pitched murmur of MR with the diaphragm of the stethoscope held firmly against the apex. Unlike the murmur of tricuspid regurgitation, the murmur of MR does not change in intensity with respiration.
  - A loud, blowing, pansystolic (holosystolic) murmur with maximal intensity at the apex and radiating to the axilla is typical. S$_1$ is often decreased; the presence of an apical S$_3$ is indicative of LVH.
  - In extreme cases, there may be wide splitting of S$_2$, caused by premature emptying of the left ventricle and resulting in an early A$_2$. In rare cases, an apical diastolic rumble is present.

Positional and Respiratory Maneuvers
- Maneuvers that decrease venous return (e.g., Valsalva) diminish the intensity of the murmur of MR, whereas maneuvers that increase ventricular volume (e.g., squatting) intensify the murmur. The murmur of MR does not vary with respiration.

Other Signs of Mitral Regurgitation
- Irregularly irregular pulse (in the presence of atrial fibrillation)
- Normal pulse pressure

Evidence
- In one study, transient arterial occlusion performed by cardiologists appeared to be useful in diagnosis of MR (+LR 7.5; 95% CI 2.5 to 23; −LR 0.28; 95% CI 0.13 to 0.6).[13]

MITRAL VALVE PROLAPSE: EXAMINATION

Patient Positioning

* To accentuate the murmur of MVP, examine the patient while standing erect.
* Auscultation after exercise may elicit a murmur not audible at rest.

Inspection

* Inspect for the apical impulse and the ventricular movements of a left-sided S_3 or S_4. Tangential lighting may improve the visibility of impulses. Unless MVP is associated with MR, LVH should not occur.

Palpation

* Palpate the carotid pulse, noting its contour and volume.
* Palpate the impulses with the pads of your fingers, exerting light pressure for an S_3 or S_4 and firmer pressure for S_1 and S_2. Thrills are best felt with the ball of your hand pressed firmly on the patient's chest.

Auscultation

* Auscultate the precordium. Listen for the high-pitched murmur with the diaphragm of the stethoscope held firmly against the chest wall.
  * This murmur is heard best at the apex and is a short, high-pitched murmur that occurs late in systole, giving an impression of a crescendo sound and described as a "cooing" or a "whooping." Heard best at the apex, it may radiate to the back to the left of the spine. The intensity is variable.
  * Wide splitting of S_2 may occur with an audible S_3. A snapping or clicking sound is sometimes heard in midsystole, corresponding to an observable retraction in the apical region.

Positional and Respiratory Maneuvers

* The murmur is softer and shorter when the patient is squatting and becomes more pronounced after the patient stands again (Figure 1-19).

Other Signs of Mitral Valve Prolapse

* The patient may have signs and symptoms associated with dysrhythmia. Associated dysrhythmias include premature ventricular contractions (PVCs), paroxysmal atrial tachycardia, atrial fibrillation/flutter, sinus bradycardia, and sick sinus syndrome.
* MVP is sometimes associated with connective tissue diseases such as *Marfan syndrome*. Stigmata of Marfan syndrome include arachnodactylism, hyperextensible joints, ectomorph build, and dislocated lenses.

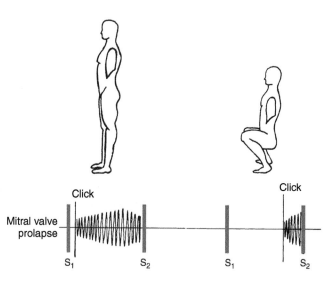

Figure 1-19 Effect of standing and squatting on the murmur of mitral valve prolapse. (Adapted from Tilkian AG, Conover MB. *Understanding Heart Sounds: With an Introduction to Lung Sounds.* 4th ed. Philadelphia: Saunders; 2001 [p. 255, Figure 20-2].)

SECONDARY HYPERTENSION: HISTORY AND PHYSICAL EXAMINATION

> **INSTRUCTIONS TO CANDIDATE: A 22-year-old woman presents to her family doctor after checking her BP at a local pharmacy. She is worried that she has "high blood pressure." Obtain a detailed history, exploring possible causes, and perform a focused physical examination.**

DD$_X$: VITAMINS C

- **V**ascular: Renal vascular disease (e.g., fibromuscular dysplasia), coarctation of the aorta
- **M**etabolic: Drugs, endocrine disease (Conn syndrome, Cushing syndrome, hyperthyroidism, acromegaly, or congenital adrenal hyperplasia)
- **I**diopathic/**i**atrogenic: Sleep apnea, renal parenchymal disease
- **N**eoplastic: Pheochromocytoma

History

- Patients are usually **asymptomatic.** Ask the following questions:
  - "How are you feeling? Any changes in your health lately?"
  - "Do you have headaches?" Suboccipital, pulsating headaches are common.
  - "Do you have visual disturbance? Nausea or vomiting? Weakness?"
  - "Do you have chest pain? Shortness of breath on exertion? How is your exercise tolerance?"
  - For women: "When was your last menstrual period? Are you pregnant?"
  - Cushing syndrome: "Have you experienced weight gain? Do you have stretch marks? Do you bruise easily?"
  - Pheochromocytoma: "Do you experience palpitations? Sweating? Flushing?"
  - Hyperthyroidism: "Have you lost weight? Do you have heat intolerance? Diarrhea?"
  - Acromegaly: "Are your hands or feet enlarged? Do you have hyperpigmentation? Carpal tunnel syndrome?"
- **Risk factors** for cardiovascular disease:
  - Age (men >55 years; women >65 years)
  - Cigarette smoking
  - Hypertension
  - DM
  - Hyperlipidemia
  - Obesity (especially around the waist)
  - Physical inactivity
  - Family history of premature cardiovascular disease (men <55 years; women <65 years)
- **PMH/PSH:** Systemic lupus erythematosus, hyperthyroidism, acromegaly, congenital heart disease, post-streptococcal glomerulonephritis, or coarctation of the aorta
- **MEDS:** NSAIDs, COX-2 inhibitors, sympathomimetic agents, oral contraceptive pill, or steroids
- **SH:** Diet (including sodium intake), exercise, smoking, use of EtOH, and use of street drugs
- **FH:** MEN, obesity, hypertension, DM, polycystic kidney disease, or collagen vascular diseases

Physical Examination

- **Vitals:** Measure HR, BP (use accurate technique via sphygmomanometer in at least one arm and leg), RR, and temperature.
- **General:** Assess the patient's general appearance, noting body habitus.
- Ascertain the **height** and **weight** of the patient. BMI = weight (kg)/height^2 (m).

- **Examine** for signs associated with the following secondary causes of hypertension:
  - Cushing syndrome: Moon facies, buffalo hump, supraclavicular fat pad, central obesity, purplish striae on abdomen and in axillae, acne, and proximal muscle wasting
  - Pheochromocytoma: Paroxysmal tachycardia, diaphoresis, and flushing
  - Coarctation of the aorta: Decreased femoral pulses, radial-femoral delay, aortic bruits, and arm BP > leg BP
  - Acromegaly: Enlarged hands, feet, mandible, nose, lips, and tongue; increased space between the teeth; coarse facial features; oily skin; bitemporal hemianopsia; hyperpigmentation; and carpal tunnel syndrome
  - Hyperthyroidism: Goiter, hyperreflexia, atrial fibrillation, widened pulse pressure, exophthalmos, lid lag, and periorbital edema
- **HEENT:** Perform a careful funduscopic examination for signs of retinopathy (narrowed arterioles, copper/silver wire appearance, exudates, hemorrhages, and papilledema). Inspect the neck for any masses, and palpate the thyroid gland.
- **Resp:** Auscultate the chest, noting breath sounds and adventitious sounds.
- **CVS:** Measure the JVP. Palpate peripheral pulses, and auscultate for bruits (carotid, aortic, renal, iliac, and femoral pulses). Note any radial-radial delay or radial-femoral delay. Note pulse volume, contour, and rhythm. Inspect and palpate the apical impulse (note whether it is enlarged, sustained, and displaced as in LVH). Palpate for thrills and heaves. Auscultate the heart, listening for extra heart sounds or murmurs. Coarctation is associated with a soft bruit heard in the second left or right ICS and radiating to the thoracic spine.
- **Abdomen:** Palpate the abdomen for masses. Palpate the kidneys (polycystic kidney, aldosterone/renin-secreting neoplasms).

SAMPLE CHECKLISTS

Aortic Regurgitation: Physical Examination

INSTRUCTIONS TO CANDIDATE: A 40-year-old man with ankylosing spondylitis has been referred to the cardiology clinic for evaluation of possible AR. Perform a focused physical examination, and describe your findings.

Key Points	Satisfactorily Completed
Introduces self to the patient	❏
Determines how the patient wishes to be addressed	❏
Washes hands	❏
Explains nature of the examination to the patient	❏
Examines the patient in a logical manner	❏
Pulses:	
• Palpates for systolic thrills at the carotid artery	❏
• Palpates carotid pulse (notes contour and volume: water-hammer pulse, pulsus bisferiens)	❏
• Notes de Musset's sign	❏
BP:	
• Comments on pulse pressure (widened)	❏
• If measuring lower limb BP, notes any discrepancy in comparison with upper limbs (Hill's sign)	❏
Precordium:	
• Inspects precordium for apical impulse and left-sided S_3 or S_4	❏
• Palpates for systolic thrills at base of heart	❏
• Palpates the apical impulse (notes location, amplitude, and diameter)	❏
Auscultation:	
• Auscultates with diaphragm and bell of stethoscope	❏
• Positions patient seated and leaning forward, to accentuate the murmur	❏
• Describes early, blowing, decrescendo diastolic murmur	❏
• Listens for murmur, which is best heard in second to fourth ICSs	❏
Other	
• Listens for Duroziez's sign (femoral diastolic murmur with slight compression)	❏
• Listens for Traube's sign (pistol shot sound over the femoral arteries)	❏
• Notes systolic pulsations in other areas: liver, spleen, uvula, retinal vessels, or nail beds	❏
Drapes the patient appropriately	❏
Makes appropriate closing remarks	❏

Aortic Dissection: History and Physical Examination

> **INSTRUCTIONS TO CANDIDATE: A 21-year-old man with Marfan syndrome presents to the emergency department with acute onset of severe, tearing chest pain during a hockey game. Obtain a focused history and physical examination, and describe your findings.**

Key Points	Satisfactorily Completed
Introduces self to the patient	❑
Determines how the patient wishes to be addressed	❑
Washes hands	❑
Establishes the purpose of the encounter	❑
Establishes the presenting concern in the patient's own words	❑
History of chest pain:	
• Characterizes the pain	❑
• Establishes the location of pain	❑
• Ascertains whether and to where pain radiates	❑
• Establishes the onset and pattern of the pain (e.g., pleuritic)	❑
• Asks about the patient's activities at time of pain onset	❑
• Establishes the duration of this particular episode of pain	❑
• Asks the patient to rate the severity of the pain on a scale	❑
• Asks whether he was able to continue playing hockey	❑
• Asks about previous episodes of similar pain	❑
• Asks about the frequency with which the pain occurs	❑
• Asks about palliative factors (e.g., rest, position)	❑
• Asks about provocative factors (e.g., exertion, movement)	❑
Checks for associated symptoms:	
• Fever	❑
• Dyspnea: At rest? Exertional?	❑
• Diaphoresis	❑
• Nausea, vomiting, or both	❑
• Back pain	❑
• Abdominal pain	❑
• Syncope	❑
Documents relevant social history:	
• Smoking	❑
Documents past medical and surgical history:	
• Hypertension	❑
• Known aortic disease (e.g., aneurysm, prior dissection, or surgery)	❑
Documents medications:	
• Prescription drugs (including anticoagulants)	❑
• Over-the-counter drugs (including ASA)	❑
Documents allergies	❑
Explains nature of the examination to the patient	❑
Documents vital signs:	
• Requests a complete set of vital signs	❑
• Notes any abnormalities such as tachycardia and hypertension	❑

Key Points	Satisfactorily Completed
• Palpates peripheral pulses, noting volume, contour, and rhythm	❏
• Compares pulses in the upper extremities and lower extremities	❏
Performs inspection:	
• Assesses the patient's general appearance, noting diaphoresis, posture, and any apparent distress	❏
• Inspects precordium for apical impulse	❏
Performs palpation:	
• Palpates for systolic thrills at base of heart	❏
• Palpates the apical impulse (notes location, amplitude, and diameter)	❏
Performs auscultation:	
• Auscultates with diaphragm and bell of stethoscope	❏
• Positions patient seated and leaning forward, to assess for the murmur of AR (best heard in second to fourth ICSs)	❏
Performs cursory neurologic evaluation:	
• Tests power in upper and lower extremities	❏
• Performs a cranial nerve examination	❏
Drapes the patient appropriately	❏
Makes appropriate closing remarks	❏

Evidence

- The sudden onset of pain (sensitivity 84%; 95% CI 80% to 89%) and the presence of severe pain (sensitivity 90%; 95% CI 88% to 92%) are the most sensitive historical features of aortic dissection. Descriptors such as "tearing" or "ripping" sensations or the migratory nature of the pain may also be informative, but study results have been variable.[16]
- The problem with the "classic" physical findings of aortic dissection, such as the murmur of AR, is that they occur in a third or fewer cases.[17] However, when present, these signs can be of prognostic significance. For example, in one study, pulse deficits were found in 30% of patients, and these patients were more likely to suffer serious in-hospital complications such as coma, renal failure, and limb ischemia[18] (Table 1-14).

Table 1-14	Usefulness of Clinical Examination for Diagnosing Acute Thoracic Aortic Dissection When Clinical Suspicion Is High	
Clinical Feature	**+LR (95% CI)**	**−LR (95% CI)**
Sudden chest pain	1.6 (1.0–2.4)	0.3 (0.2–0.5)
Pulse deficit	**5.7 (1.4–23.0)**	0.7 (0.6–0.9)
Diastolic murmur	1.4 (1.0–2.0)	0.9 (0.8–1.0)

CI, confidence interval; +LR, positive likelihood ratio; −LR, negative likelihood ratio.
Boldface represents findings associated with positive likelihood ratios ≥5 or with negative likelihood ratios ≤0.2. These are said to be moderate- to high-impact items.

REFERENCES

1. Zun LS, Downey L. The effect of noise in the emergency department. *Acad Emerg Med.* 2005;12:663-666.
2. Tijunelis MA, Fitzsullivan E, Henderson SO. Noise in the ED. *Am J Emerg Med.* 2005;23: 332-335.
3. Reichlin S, Dieterle T, Camli C, et al. Initial clinical evaluation of cardiac systolic murmurs in the ED by noncardiologists. *Am J Emerg Med.* 2004;22(2):71-75.
4. Marcus GM, Gerber IL, McKeown BH, et al. Association between phonocardiographic third and fourth heart sounds and objective measures of left ventricular function. *JAMA.* 2005;293:2238-2244.
5. Vinayak AG, Levitt J, Gehlbach B, et al. Usefulness of the external jugular vein examination in detecting abnormal central venous pressure in critically ill patients. *Arch Intern Med.* 2006;166:2132-2137.
6. Anand SS, Wells PS, Hunt D, et al. Does this patient have deep vein thrombosis? *JAMA.* 1998;279:1094-1099.
7. Khan NA, Rahim SA, Anand SS, et al. Does the clinical examination predict lower extremity peripheral arterial disease? *JAMA.* 2006;295:536-546.
8. Hess EP, Thiruganasambandamoorthy V, Wells GA, et al. Diagnostic accuracy of clinical prediction rules to exclude acute coronary syndrome in the emergency department setting: A systematic review. *CJEM.* 2008;10:373-382.
9. Body R, Carley S, Wibberley C, et al. The value of symptoms and signs in the emergent diagnosis of acute coronary syndromes. *Resuscitation.* 2010;81:281-286.
10. Swap CJ, Nagurney JT. Value and limitations of chest pain history in the evaluation of patients with suspected acute coronary syndromes. *JAMA.* 2005;294:2623-2629.
11. Body R, Carley S, McDowell G, et al. Can a modified Thrombolysis In Myocardial Infarction risk score outperform the original for risk stratifying emergency department patients with chest pain? *Emerg Med J.* 2009;26(2):95-99.
12. Lederle FA, Simel DL. The rational clinical examination. Does this patient have abdominal aortic aneurysm? *JAMA.* 1999;281:77-82.

13. Etchells E, Bell C, Robb K. Does this patient have an abnormal systolic murmur? *JAMA*. 1997;277:564-571.

14. Choudhry NK, Etchells EE. The rational clinical examination. Does this patient have aortic regurgitation? *JAMA*. 1999;281:2231-2238.

15. Lembo NJ, Dell'Italia LJ, Crawford MH, et al. Diagnosis of left-sided regurgitant murmurs by transient arterial occlusion: A new maneuver using blood pressure cuffs. *Ann Intern Med*. 1986;105:368-370.

16. Klompas M. Does this patient have an acute thoracic aortic dissection? *JAMA*. 2002;287: 2262-2272.

17. Hagan PG, Nienaber CA, Isselbacher EM, et al. The International Registry of Acute Aortic Dissection (IRAD): new insights into an old disease. *JAMA*. 2000;283:897-903.

18. Bossone E, Rampoldi V, Nienaber CA, et al. Usefulness of pulse deficit to predict in-hospital complications and mortality in patients with acute type A aortic dissection. *Am J Cardiol*. 2002;89:851-855.

CHAPTER 2

Respiratory System

ANATOMY

- The human body has 12 ribs. The costal cartilages of the first seven ribs articulate with the sternum. The second rib articulates at the manubriosternal joint **(angle of Louis)**. Ribs 8, 9, and 10 articulate with the costal cartilages above them. Ribs 11 and 12 are "floating." Each of the intercostal spaces (ICSs) is named for the rib above it.
- The trachea bifurcates into its mainstem bronchi at the angle of Louis.
- The pleurae are serous membranes that cover the outer surface of the lungs **(visceral pleura)** and line the inner rib cage and dome of the diaphragm **(parietal pleura)**. A thin layer of pleural fluid lubricates the pleural space between the visceral and parietal pleurae.

Surface Anatomy

- Angle of Louis: articulation of the second costal cartilage.
- Nipple: fifth ICS.
- Inferior tip of the scapula: seventh ICS.
- Spinous prominence: spinous process of C7.
- The right lung is divided into three lobes (upper, middle, and lower), whereas the left lung has just two lobes (the upper and lower lobes; Figure 2-1).
  - **Apex:** 2 to 4 cm above inner third of the clavicle.
  - **Lower border:** crosses the sixth rib at the midclavicular line (MCL) and the eighth rib at the midaxillary line (MAL). Posteriorly, the lower border is at T10, and on inspiration it descends further (T12).
  - **Oblique fissure:** runs like a string connecting T3 posteriorly to the fifth rib at the MAL and to the sixth rib at the MCL.
  - **Horizontal fissure:** runs anteriorly close to the fourth rib and meets the oblique fissure in the MAL near the fifth rib.
- The parietal pleura and costophrenic recesses generally extend about two ribs inferior to the lung.

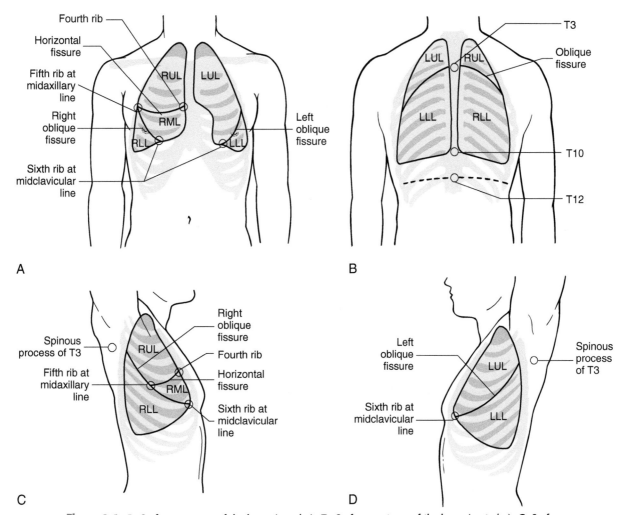

Figure 2-1 A, Surface anatomy of the lungs (anterior). **B,** Surface anatomy of the lungs (posterior). **C,** Surface anatomy of the lungs (right lateral). **D,** Surface anatomy of the lungs (left lateral). LLL, left lower lobe; LUL, left upper lobe; RLL, right lower lobe; RML, right middle lobe; RUL, right upper lobe. (From Seidel HM, Ball JW, Dains JE, et al. *Mosby's Guide to Physical Examination.* 5th ed. St. Louis: Mosby; 2003 [p. 361].)

Breathing

- The diaphragm is the primary muscle of inspiration. When it contracts, it descends and enlarges the thoracic cavity, causing a decrease in intrathoracic pressure and allowing air to enter the tracheobronchial tree and expand the lungs. O_2 diffuses into blood from the alveoli to the capillary bed, and CO_2 diffuses from the blood into the alveoli. At the end of inspiration, the chest wall and lungs recoil, forcing air outward. The most important accessory muscle of inspiration is the sternocleidomastoid; abdominal muscles *may* assist in forced expiration.

GLOSSARY OF SIGNS AND SYMPTOMS

Respiratory Distress

- **Respiratory distress** is a subjective term that is poorly defined. Signs consistent with distress include the following:
  - Apprehension
  - Inability to speak in full sentences without stopping for breath
  - Tachypnea
  - Pursed lips
  - Nasal flare
  - Tripod positioning: patient holds on to an object to fix pectoral girdle
  - Tracheal tug
  - Accessory muscle use
  - Intercostal/subcostal retractions
  - Thoracoabdominal dissociation
- **Dyspnea** is the subjective sensation of shortness of breath that is inappropriate for the circumstances.

Cyanosis

- **Cyanosis** is bluish discoloration of the skin or mucosa.
- **Central cyanosis** occurs when the amount of reduced hemoglobin in the blood is excessive. Thus, central cyanosis occurs more readily in patients with polycythemia than in those with anemia. It is best detected by inspection of the tongue. Causes of central cyanosis are as follows:
  - Inadequate O_2 transfer caused by lung disease (e.g., chronic obstructive pulmonary disease [COPD]) or hypoventilation. This is usually at least partially reversed by optimizing inspired O_2.
  - Shunting from pulmonary to systemic circulation (e.g., transposition of the great arteries). Optimizing inspired O_2 does not correct cyanosis caused by shunting.
  - Hemoglobinopathies such as methemoglobinemia.
- **Peripheral cyanosis** is detected by inspection of the lips or extremities. Because of the array of causes, peripheral cyanosis is a nonspecific sign. In patients with normal hemoglobin saturation, peripheral cyanosis occurs when impairment of peripheral or cutaneous circulation leads to increased uptake of O_2 by the tissues, which causes a localized increase in desaturated hemoglobin. Cold, anxiety, and vascular disease may contribute to peripheral cyanosis. Underlying causes of central cyanosis can also result in peripheral cyanosis.

Clubbing

- **Clubbing** is an exaggerated longitudinal curvature of the fingernail (>180 degrees) and loss of the angle between the nail and the nail bed (Figure 2-2). The distal phalanx is rounded and bulbous; the nail fold may feel "boggy." Clubbing is also known as *hypertrophic peripheral arthropathy.*
- Observe the angle between the nail bed and base of the finger. This is known as the *ungual-phalangeal angle,* or *Lovibond's angle.* Place the dorsal surfaces of the right and

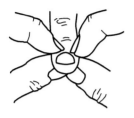

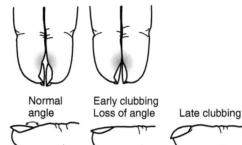

Testing for fluctuation at the base of the nail

Testing for loss of normal angle

Normal angle

Early clubbing Loss of angle

Late clubbing

Figure 2-2 Tests for clubbing. (From Lehrer S. *Understanding Lung Sounds.* 3rd ed. Philadelphia: Saunders; 2002 [p. 39, Figure 3-4].)

left fingers against each other, knuckle to knuckle and tip to tip. A definite rhombus should be seen in normal individuals; no rhombus is seen if clubbing is present.

* The reliability of the clinical examination for clubbing is only fair to moderate.[1] Clubbing is a nonspecific sign with numerous possible causes (Table 2-1). Some of these associations have been studied. For example, the presence of clubbing increases the risk of lung cancer (positive likelihood ratio [+LR], 3.9; 95% confidence interval [CI] 1.6 to 9.4), Crohn disease (+LR 2.8; 95% CI 1.8 to 4.1), and ulcerative colitis (+LR 3.7; 95% CI 1.4 to 9.4).

Table 2-1 Causes of Clubbing

Malignancy	Chronic Suppurative Disease	Cyanotic Disease	Other
Bronchogenic carcinoma	Cystic fibrosis	Congenital heart disease	Inflammatory bowel disease, celiac disease
Mesothelioma	Bronchiectasis	Sequelae of infective endocarditis	Familial clubbing (often before puberty)
Gastrointestinal lymphoma	Empyema	Unilateral clubbing	Chronic renal failure
Myelogenous leukemia	Abscess	Brachial arteriovenous malformation	Cirrhotic liver disease
		Axillary artery aneurysm	Thyrotoxicosis, Graves disease
		Thoracic outlet syndrome	

Thoracic Deformities (Figure 2-3)
* **Barrel chest:** Increased anteroposterior (AP) diameter
* **Kyphosis:** Excessive flexion of the spine (humpback)
* **Scoliosis:** Abnormal lateral curvature of the spine
* **Kyphoscoliosis:** Coexistence of both kyphosis and scoliosis
* **Pectus excavatum:** Backward displacement of the sternum (funnel chest)
* **Pectus carinatum:** Forward projection of the sternum (pigeon chest)

Patterns of Abnormal Breathing (Figure 2-4)
* **Apnea** is the absence of breathing.
* **Bradypnea** is abnormal slowness of respirations (<12 breaths/minute).
* **Tachypnea** is abnormal increase in frequency of respirations (>20 breaths/minute).
* **Cheyne-Stokes respiration** is a cyclic breathing pattern with periods of increased depth of respiration, followed by decreased depth, down to a period of apnea. Causes include brainstem lesions, bilateral cerebral lesions, increased intracranial pressure, metabolic encephalopathy, poor cardiac output, and respiratory depression induced by drugs (e.g., narcotics).

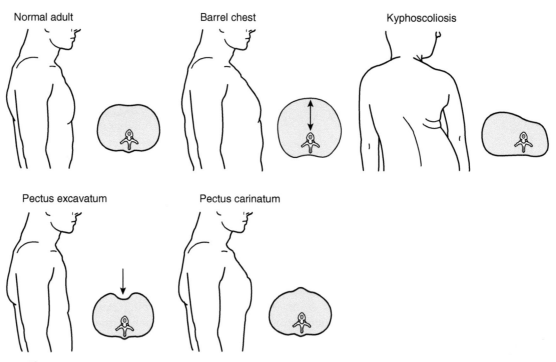

Figure 2-3 Thoracic deformities. (Adapted from Lehrer S. *Understanding Lung Sounds*. 3rd ed. Philadelphia: Saunders; 2002 [p. 42, Figure 3-7].)

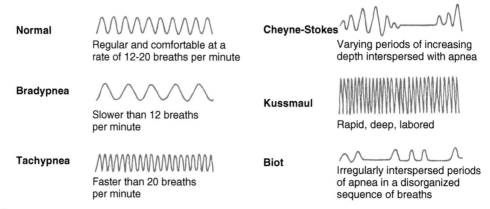

Figure 2-4 Patterns of abnormal breathing. (Adapted from Seidel HM, Ball JW, Dains JE, et al. *Mosby's Guide to Physical Examination*. 5th ed. St. Louis: Mosby; 2003 [p. 372, Figure 12-13].)

- **Kussmaul respiration** is deep, rapid breathing characteristic of metabolic acidosis (e.g., diabetic ketoacidosis).
- **Biot respiration** is an irregular breathing pattern with variable rate and depth and with periods of apnea. It may result from medullary brain lesions, increased intracranial pressure, or drug-induced respiratory depression.
- **Stridor** is a high-pitched sound reflecting some degree of upper airway obstruction. Obstruction above the cords results in inspiratory stridor, whereas obstruction below the cords may produce expiratory or mixed stridor. Causes include foreign body, tumor, edema, croup, and external compression by goiter or enlarged lymph nodes.

Pathologic Transmission of Voice Sounds
- **Bronchophony** is the increased transmission of the spoken voice. On auscultation, words are noted to have increased intensity and clarity.
- If the "EE" sound is heard as an "AY" on auscultation, **egophony** is said to be present.
- **Whispering pectoriloquy** is the increased transmission of the whispered voice so that it is clearly heard on auscultation.

Pulsus Paradoxus (see Figure 1-6)
- **Pulsus paradoxus** refers to an inspiratory decrease in systolic blood pressure that is >20 mm Hg (see Figure 1-6). The exaggerated waxing and waning in pulse volume may be detected as a palpable decrease in pulse amplitude on quiet expiration, or it may be measured by a sphygmomanometer. Pulses paradoxus may be suggestive of severe asthma or COPD, tension pneumothorax, pulmonary embolism, pericardial tamponade, or constrictive pericarditis.

ESSENTIAL SKILLS

APPROACH TO THE RESPIRATORY HISTORY

- Use the mnemonic **ChLORIDE FPP** to delineate the presenting complaint:
  - **C**haracter
  - **L**ocation
  - **O**nset
  - **R**adiation
  - **I**ntensity
  - **D**uration
  - **E**vents
  - **F**requency
  - **P**alliative factors
  - **P**rovocative factors

Functional Respiratory Inquiry
- Use the mnemonic **SPACED** to obtain further information:
  - **S**moking (quantify pack-years), **s**hortness of breath on expiration (SOBOE), **s**putum production (mucus, pus, or blood)
  - **P**ain (pleuritic, bony/musculoskeletal, tracheobronchial), **p**igeons (associated with psittacosis, cryptococcosis, and extrinsic allergic alveolitis)
  - **A**sthma (wheeze, nocturnal/morning cough), **a**topy, α_1-antitrypsin deficiency
  - **C**ough (nocturnal/morning), **c**hest radiograph (CXR) (known abnormalities)
  - **E**xercise tolerance (quantify: ability to dress oneself, distance walked, and climbing stairs), **e**nvironmental/occupational **e**xposures (allergies, tuberculosis [TB], asbestos, vapors, dust, or farms)
  - **D**yspnea (provocative/palliative factors)
- Upper respiratory tract: Nasal polyps, rhinitis, and sneezing
- Sleeping patterns: Snoring, apnea
- Constitutional symptoms: Fever, chills, night sweats, weight loss, anorexia, and asthenia
- Differentiate from cardiac causes (see pp. 4-5): Paroxysmal nocturnal dyspnea (PND), orthopnea, and peripheral edema
- Immunization status: Pneumococcal vaccine, influenza vaccine, childhood vaccinations, and bacille bilié de Calmette-Guérin (BCG) vaccine
- Previous history of respiratory problems: TB, COPD, deep venous thrombosis (DVT)/pulmonary embolism, bronchiectasis, recurrent infections such as bronchitis or pneumonia, lung cancer, and cystic fibrosis

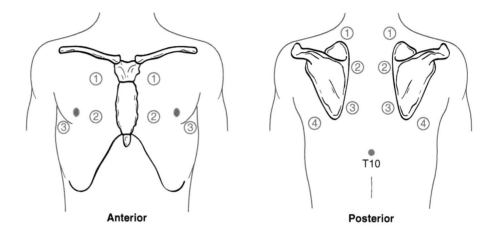

Figure 2-5 Sites for tactile fremitus.

Anterior   Posterior

TACTILE FREMITUS: EXAMINATION

- **Fremitus** refers to the vibrations transmitted through the bronchopulmonary tree to the chest wall when the patient speaks.

Palpation
- Ask the patient to repeat the words "ninety-nine" or "one-to-one." Palpate the patient's chest wall with the hypothenar aspect of your hand (the vibratory sensitivity of the bones in your hand detects the fremitus) (Figure 2-5). The simultaneous use of both hands, to compare sides, may be beneficial in terms of speed and detection of asymmetry.

Decreased Fremitus
- Voice is too soft.
- Transmission of vibrations is impeded: obstructed bronchus, COPD, pleural effusion, pleural thickening, pneumothorax, infiltrating tumor, or thickened chest wall.

Increased Fremitus
- Consolidation (pneumonia)
- Atelectasis

Evidence
- Although the technique of assessing vocal fremitus still finds its way into textbooks and classrooms, it is uncommonly used in clinical practice.[2]

Pearl
- Fremitus is often more prominent on the right side, and it disappears below the diaphragm.

PERCUSSION: EXAMINATION

- **Percussion** is the act of striking a surface to determine whether underlying tissues are filled with air, filled with fluid, or solid. The vibrations penetrate only 5 to 7 cm, so the technique is unreliable for detecting deep lesions. You should interpret the percussion note by using both sound and tactile sense (Table 2-2, Figure 2-6).

Percussion
- Percuss posteriorly with both arms of the patient crossed in front to displace the scapulae. Place the palmar surface of your left hand on the patient's chest wall, hyperextending the distal interphalangeal joint of your middle finger. Remember that the action of percussion is at the wrist. Using the middle finger of your right hand,

strike the distal interphalangeal joint of your left middle finger (this requires short fingernails for your own comfort) (Figure 2-7, *A*). Percussion of the chest should be performed over the ICSs (to avoid the "dullness" of percussing the ribs). This technique can be difficult to master. An alternative technique is to use your reflex hammer to strike the hyperextended distal interphalangeal joint of your left middle finger. (see Figure 2-7, *B*)
* Compare the percussion notes for symmetry (Figure 2-8).
* **Diaphragmatic excursion** is the difference between the level of dullness on inspiration and the level of dullness on expiration, estimated by percussion (Figure 2-9). Normal excursion is 5 to 6 cm.

Table 2-2 Percussion Notes

Percussion Note	Example	Pathologic Process
Flat	Extremity (e.g., thigh, forearm)	Large pleural effusion
Dull	Liver or spleen	Consolidation (e.g., pneumonia)
Resonant	Normal lung	
Hyperresonant	—*	Emphysema, pneumothorax
Tympanitic	Gastric air bubble	

*There is no location where hyperresonance (very loud, hollow sound) is normally found.

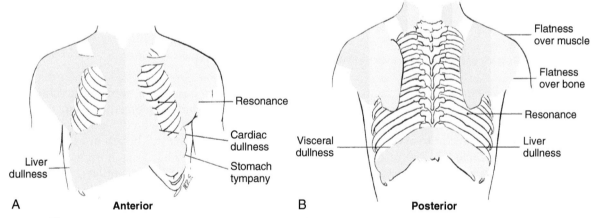

Figure 2-6 Expected percussion notes. **A,** Anterior locations. **B,** Posterior locations. (From Barkauskas VH, Baumann LC, Darling-Fisher CS. *Health & Physical Assessment.* 3rd ed. St Louis: Mosby; 2002 [p. 326, Figure 15-15].)

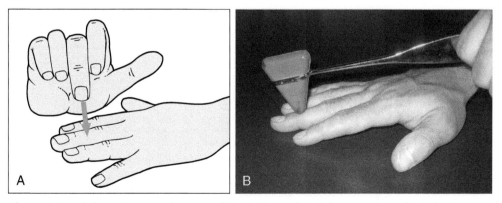

Figure 2-7 Techniques for percussion. **A,** Traditional (bimanual) technique. **B,** Alternative (reflex hammer) technique. (**A,** From Munro JF, Campbell IW, eds. *Macleod's Clinical Examination.* 10th ed. Edinburgh: Churchill Livingstone; 2000 [p. 134, Figure 4-16].)

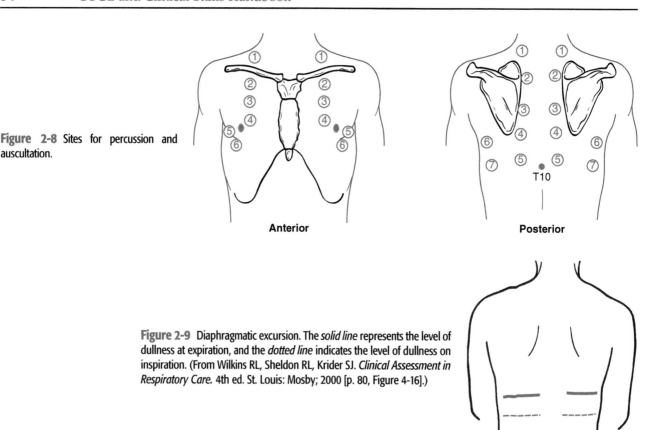

Figure 2-8 Sites for percussion and auscultation.

Anterior   Posterior

Figure 2-9 Diaphragmatic excursion. The *solid line* represents the level of dullness at expiration, and the *dotted line* indicates the level of dullness on inspiration. (From Wilkins RL, Sheldon RL, Krider SJ. *Clinical Assessment in Respiratory Care.* 4th ed. St. Louis: Mosby; 2000 [p. 80, Figure 4-16].)

RESPIRATORY AUSCULTATION: EXAMINATION

- Using the diaphragm of the stethoscope, listen for breath sounds, adventitious sounds, and transmitted voice sounds. Instruct the patient to breathe deeply through an open mouth. Use the same pattern suggested for percussion in Figure 2-8, moving from side to side for comparison. Listen to at least one full breath at each location (Table 2-3, Figure 2-10). Ask the patient to cross his or her arms in front when you auscultate posteriorly. Ensure that the patient does not hyperventilate, which may cause lightheadedness.
- Breath sounds may be louder at the base posteriorly. Breath sounds are decreased when airflow is decreased (as with COPD) or when sound transmission is poor (as with pleural effusion).

Adventitia
- **Adventitious sounds** are extra sounds (e.g., crackles, wheezes, and pleural rub) that are superimposed on normal breath sounds (Figure 2-11). Describe the location at which these sounds were identified and their timing within the respiratory cycle. Note the persistence of these sounds from breath to breath and any changes after cough or change in position.

Transmitted Voice Sounds
- Assess transmitted voice sounds if abnormally located bronchial or bronchovesicular sounds are identified. Increased transmission of voice sounds is indicative of an "airless lung," as in consolidation. Auscultate in symmetric areas over the chest wall as for percussion in Figure 2-8.
  - Ask the patient to say "ninety-nine"; sound should be transmitted as muffled and indistinct.
  - Ask the patient to say "EE"; normally you will hear a muffled long "E" sound.

Table 2-3 Normal Breath Sounds

Normal Breath Sounds	Duration	Relative Intensity	Example
Vesicular	Inspiration > expiration	Soft	Over most of both lungs
Bronchovesicular	Inspiration = expiration	Intermediate	First and second ICSs anteriorly and between the scapulae
Bronchial	Inspiration < expiration	Loud	Over the manubrium, if heard at all

ICS, Intercostal space.

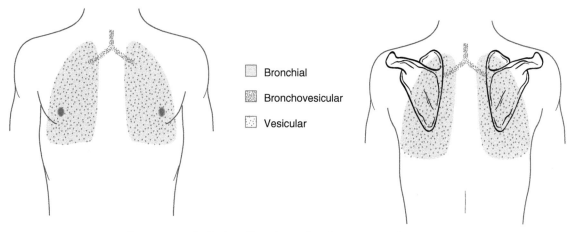

Figure 2-10 Distribution of breath sounds. **Left,** Anterior. **Right,** Posterior.

Bronchial
Bronchovesicular
Vesicular

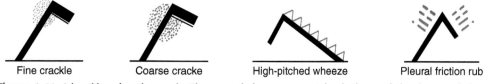

Fine crackle   Coarse cracke   High-pitched wheeze   Pleural friction rub

Figure 2-11 Adventitious breath sounds. The upward slopes represent inspiration, and the downward slopes represent expiration. (Adapted from Lehrer S. *Understanding Lung Sounds.* 3rd ed. Philadelphia: Saunders; 2000 [p. 121, Figure 5-29].)

- ▪ Ask the patient to whisper "ninety-nine" or "one-two-three"; normally this is heard faintly if at all.

Evidence

- Although the stethoscope is widely regarded as a symbol of medicine and the clinical examination, it appears to add little to the diagnostic value of the examination. Normal sounds heard on lung auscultation do imply reduced odds of heart or lung disease (odds ratio 0.12; 95% confidence ratio [CI] 0.05 to 0.29), and wheezing implies increased odds of lung disease (odds ratio 7.4; 95% CI 3.3 to 16.8).[3]
- Many clinical environments, however, are noisy and distracting, which makes auscultation challenging. For example, emergency department studies have revealed that noise levels are in the range of 40 to 80 decibels.[4,5] In a simulated noisy environment, about half of health care practitioners who responded reported difficulty hearing heart and lung sounds.[4]

ASTHMA: HISTORY

> **INSTRUCTIONS TO CANDIDATE: A 20-year-old woman with a long history of asthma presents to her family doctor complaining of frequent exacerbations since moving out of her parents' home. Obtain a detailed history, exploring possible causes.**

History

- Ask the patient the following:
  - ▪ **Character:** "How has your asthma changed since moving to your new apartment? Cough? Dyspnea? Wheezing? Chest pain? Sleep disturbance? Night cough? When are symptoms most severe (time of day, time of week)? Do the symptoms show diurnal variation (worse in early morning)?"
  - ▪ **Onset:** "How long have you been known to have asthma? When did you notice that your asthma had gotten worse?"
  - ▪ **Intensity:** "Please rate the severity of your asthma on a scale of 1 to 10, with 1 being mild and 10 being the worst."
  - ▪ **Duration:** "How long do your asthma attacks typically last?"
  - ▪ **Events associated:**
    - ◆ "How has your adjustment to living away from home been going?"
    - ◆ "How much time have you lost from school or work?"
    - ◆ "Have you had any asthma attacks for which you required treatment in a hospital? How were you treated?"
    - ◆ "Have you ever been intubated?"
    - ◆ "Do you keep records of your peak flow? How has it changed in the past year?"
  - ▪ **Frequency:** "How frequently are you having asthma attacks?"
  - ▪ **Palliative factors:** "What improves your asthma?"
  - ▪ **Provocative factors:** "What brings on the attacks?"
    - ◆ Exposure to known allergens: "Are you exposed to animal dander, dust mites, pollen, or feathers?"
    - ◆ "Do you live in a basement apartment? Do you have a roommate with pets or stuffed animals? Do you have carpets? What kind of pillows do you use?"
    - ◆ Environment: "Are you exposed to cold air, an industrialized area, air pollution or smog, or scented products?"
    - ◆ "Do you smoke? Does your roommate smoke?"
    - ◆ Occupational: "Are you exposed to industrial chemicals, plastics, detergents, or plush materials?"
    - ◆ Infections: "Have you recently had an upper respiratory tract infection, pneumonia, or influenza?"
    - ◆ Exercise: "Are your symptoms induced by exercise? What about outdoor activities (e.g., running)?"

> ◆ Emotional stress: "Are your symptoms triggered by excessive crying, scream-ing, or hard laughing?"
- **Functional respiratory inquiry:** Use the SPACED mnemonic.
- **Past medical history (PMH)/past surgical history (PSH):** Asthma, atopy, eczema, or gastroesophageal reflux
- **Medications (MEDS):** Nonsteroidal anti-inflammatory drugs (NSAIDs), acetylsali-cylic acid (ASA), β-blockers, or sulfa drugs
  - Check for any increase/decrease in medication dosage and for more frequent use of inhalers. Verify the type of inhalers the patient uses. If a metered dose inhaler is used, check that the patient is using a holding chamber.
  - Check whether any new medications have been prescribed.
  - Consider the patient's adherence to the prescribed medication regimen.
- **Social history (SH):** Smoking, use of alcohol (EtOH), and use of street drugs
- **Family history (FH):** Asthma, allergic rhinitis, atopy, or eczema

Pearls
- Symptoms of asthma are variable. Episodes may be mild and brief. Some cases are characterized by mild coughing and wheezing much of the time, punctuated by severe exacerbations. An attack may begin suddenly with wheezing, coughing, shortness of breath, and chest tightness, or it may begin insidiously with slowly in-creasing manifestations of respiratory distress. The cough during an acute attack sounds "tight" and generally does not produce sputum. Dry cough, particularly at night and during exercise, may be the sole presenting symptom.
- The **asthma triad** consists of atopy, ASA sensitivity, and nasal polyps.

ACUTE ASTHMA EXACERBATION: PHYSICAL EXAMINATION

> **INSTRUCTIONS TO CANDIDATE: A 26-year-old woman presents to the emergency department with an "asthma attack." She has used her albuterol puffer several times today but is having difficulty speaking in full sentences without pausing to take a breath. Treatment was initiated in triage. Perform a focused physical examination.**

- **First evaluate a**irway, breathing, and circulation **(ABCs).** It may be necessary to per-form an immediate intervention, such as administering supplemental O_2, establishing intravenous access, or initiating airway management.
  - Is the patient able to talk? Swallow? Cough?
  - Are both lungs ventilated? Is the patient oxygenating (check mentation, pulse oximetry)?
  - Are vital signs abnormal? Is the peripheral circulation abnormal (check pulses, capillary refill)?
  - If no immediate interventions are required, proceed to perform an appropriate physical examination.

Physical Examination
- **Vital signs (Vitals):** Evaluate heart rate (HR), heart rhythm, respiratory rate (RR) (depth, effort, and pattern), blood pressure (BP), and temperature, and evaluate for pulsus paradoxus.
- **General:** Assess the patient's general appearance, noting any signs of respiratory distress.
- **Respiratory system (Resp)** (Table 2-4): Inspect for thoracic deformity. Assess chest expansion for symmetry. Evaluate tracheal position (tracheal tug may be noted). Assess tactile fremitus and perform percussion, noting diaphragmatic excursion. Auscultate the lungs, noting breath sounds and adventitious sounds.
- **Cardiovascular system (CVS):** Measure the jugular venous pressure (JVP), and assess for hepatojugular reflux (signs of venous congestion may herald a pneumothorax).

Palpate peripheral pulses, noting contour, volume, and rhythm. Inspect and palpate the apical impulse. Auscultate the heart, listening for a P_2, S_3, or murmurs.

- **Neurologic system (Neuro):** Briefly assess level of consciousness and mental status (adequate brain oxygenation).
- If no signs of distress are apparent, then proceed with the remainder of the examination:
  - **Skin:** Inspect the skin and nails, noting cyanosis, clubbing, or eczema.

Evidence

- Physicians' ability to predict degree of airway obstruction by using auscultation—in comparison with forced expiratory volume in 1 second (FEV_1)/ forced vital capacity (FVC)—is modest at best (+LR 1.4; negative likelihood ratio [−LR] 0.59).[6]

Pearls

- A quiet-sounding chest in a patient having an acute asthma exacerbation may be a *warning* of patient fatigue or obstruction of small airways. It can quickly become *life-threatening.*
- The most reliable signs of a severe attack are dyspnea at rest, inability to speak, accessory muscle use, cyanosis, and pulsus paradoxus. An asthma attack may begin with cough and wheezing and rapidly progress to dyspnea and respiratory distress. Confusion and lethargy may indicate respiratory failure and CO_2 narcosis. A normal or increased partial pressure of arterial CO_2 ($Paco_2$) on a blood gas may indicate respiratory failure, since hyperventilation should result in a decrease in $Paco_2$.

Table 2-4 Expected Findings in an Acute Exacerbation of Asthma

Examination	Expected Findings
Thoracic deformity	Barrel chest: hyperinflation
Chest movement	May be asymmetric in case of associated pneumothorax
Trachea	Midline; tracheal tug may be noted
Tactile fremitus	Decreased
Percussion	Hyperresonant, flattened diaphragms
Breath sounds	Prolonged expiratory phase; localized disappearance of breath sounds can occur temporarily as a result of bronchial plugging
Adventitious sounds	High-pitched wheezes

SHORTNESS OF BREATH: HISTORY AND PHYSICAL EXAMINATION

> **INSTRUCTIONS TO CANDIDATE: A 62-year-old man presents to the emergency department with new onset of shortness of breath. Obtain a detailed history, exploring possible causes, and perform a focused physical examination.**

DD$_X$: VITAMINS C

- **Vascular:** Pulmonary embolism, congestive heart failure (CHF) (pulmonary edema, large pleural effusion, significant ascites), and acute coronary syndrome
- **Infectious:** Pneumonia
- **Traumatic:** Pneumothorax, aspiration of foreign body
- **Metabolic:** Diabetic ketoacidosis
- **Idiopathic/iatrogenic:** Exacerbation of COPD/asthma, massive atelectasis
- **Neoplastic:** Large pleural effusion, significant ascites

- Substance abuse and psychiatric: Sympathomimetic ingestion, drug withdrawal syndrome, anxiety (diagnosis of exclusion)
- **First evaluate ABCs.** It may be necessary to perform an immediate intervention, such as administering supplemental O_2, establishing intravenous access, or initiating airway management.
  - Is the patient able to talk? Swallow? Cough?
  - Are both lungs ventilated? Is the patient oxygenating (check mentation, pulse oximetry)?
  - Are vital signs abnormal? Is the peripheral circulation abnormal (check pulses, capillary refill)?
  - If no immediate interventions are required, proceed to obtain the history, and perform the physical examination.

History

- Ask the patient the following:
  - **Character:** "Describe the nature of your breathing difficulty."
  - **Onset:** "How did the shortness of breath start (sudden versus gradual)? What were you doing when you became short of breath?"
  - **Intensity:** "How severe is your shortness of breath right now, on a scale of 1 to 10 with 1 being mild and 10 being the worst? Has it gotten worse?"
  - **Duration:** "How long have you been short of breath?"
  - **Events associated:**
    - Pulmonary embolism: "Have you experienced hemoptysis, pleuritic chest pain, or leg swelling/tenderness (DVT)?"
    - Pulmonary edema/acute coronary syndrome: "Have you experienced exertional chest pain, PND, orthopnea, and peripheral edema?"
    - COPD: "Have you had cough, wheeze, and progressively worsening shortness of breath on exertion?"
    - Pneumonia, other infections: "Have you had fever or chills, rigors, increased sputum production, or cough?"
    - Ascites: "Have you experienced abdominal distension?"
    - Anxiety (diagnosis of exclusion): "Have you experienced lightheadedness, diaphoresis, trembling, choking sensation, palpitations, numbness or tingling in hands or feet, chest pain, nausea, abdominal pain, depersonalization or derealization, flushes or chills, fear of dying, or fear of going crazy or doing something uncontrolled?"
    - Constitutional symptoms: "Have you experienced fever, chills, night sweats, weight loss, anorexia, or asthenia?"
  - **Frequency:** "Has this ever happened to you before? If so, how often does it happen? When was the last time you became short of breath?"
  - **Palliative factors:** "Does anything make your shortness of breath better? If so, what?"
  - **Provocative factors:** "Does anything make your shortness of breath worse? If so, what?"
    - Exertion
    - Position (sitting up versus lying down)
    - Exposure to cold air
    - Infection
    - Allergies
- **Functional respiratory inquiry:** Use the SPACED mnemonic.
- **PMH/PSH:** Thromboembolic disease, ischemic heart disease (IHD), valvular disease, COPD, diabetes mellitus, or systemic disease that causes immunosuppression
- **Previous investigations:** Ask about prior pulmonary function tests, peak flow measurements, electrocardiogram (ECG), or CXR. What were the results?
- **MEDS:** Bronchodilators, inhaled steroids, cardiac medications, or antihypertensive agents
  - Consider the patient's adherence to the prescribed medication regimen.

- **SH:** Smoking, use of EtOH, and use of street drugs
- **Immunizations:** Pneumococcal vaccine, influenza vaccine, childhood vaccinations, and BCG vaccine
- **FH:** Thromboembolic disease, premature IHD

Physical Examination

- **Vitals:** Evaluate HR, heart rhythm, RR (depth, effort, and pattern), BP, and temperature, and evaluate for pulsus paradoxus.
- **General:** Assess the patient's general appearance, noting signs of respiratory distress.
- **Skin:** Inspect the skin and nails, noting any diaphoresis, peripheral edema, cyanosis, or clubbing.
- **Head, eyes, ears, nose, and throat (HEENT):** Inspect for central cyanosis. Examine the lymph nodes in the head and neck.
- **Resp:** Inspect for thoracic deformity (barrel chest with COPD). Assess chest expansion for symmetry (Figure 2-12). Evaluate tracheal position. Assess tactile fremitus and perform percussion. Auscultate the lungs, noting breath sounds, transmitted voice sounds, and adventitious sounds. You may note a prolonged expiratory phase in obstructive disease.
- **CVS:** Measure the JVP, and assess for hepatojugular reflux (indicative of increased venous pressure in CHF). Palpate peripheral pulses, noting contour, volume, and rhythm. Inspect and palpate the apical impulse. Auscultate the heart, listening for an S_3 or murmurs.
- **Abdomen:** Examine for ascites and organomegaly.
- **Neuro:** Briefly assess level of consciousness and mental status (adequate brain oxygenation).

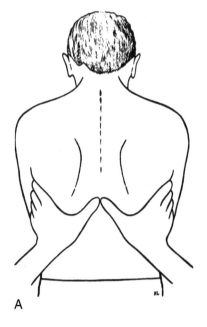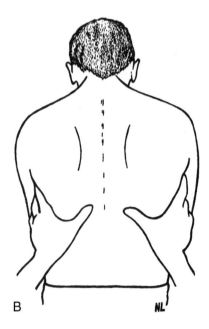

Figure 2-12 Technique for palpating chest expansion. **A,** Exhalation. **B,** Maximal inhalation. (From Wilkins RL, Sheldon RL, Krider SJ. *Clinical Assessment in Respiratory Care.* 4th ed. St. Louis: Mosby; 2002 [p. 79, Figure 4-14].)

SHORTNESS OF BREATH ON EXERTION: HISTORY AND PHYSICAL EXAMINATION

> **INSTRUCTIONS TO CANDIDATE: A 58-year-old male smoker presents to his family physician with increasing shortness of breath on exertion. Obtain a detailed history, exploring possible causes, and perform a focused physical examination.**

DD$_X$: VITAMINS C
- **V**ascular: CHF (pulmonary edema, pleural effusion)
- **I**nfectious: TB
- **A**utoimmune/**a**llergic: Sarcoidosis
- **M**etabolic: Anemia, asbestosis
- **I**diopathic/**i**atrogenic: COPD, massive atelectasis, pulmonary fibrosis, and abdominal distension (ascites, organomegaly)
- **N**eoplastic: Large pleural effusion

History
- Ask the patient the following:
  - **Character:** "Describe the nature of your breathing difficulty."
  - **Onset:** "How does the shortness of breath start (sudden versus gradual)? In what type of activity are you engaged when you become short of breath?"
  - **Intensity:** "How severe is your shortness of breath? Do you need to stop and rest during activity? How far can you walk before you must rest? How many stairs can you climb? Has it gotten worse? Over what period of time has it changed?"
  - **Duration:** "When did these episodes start? How long do these episodes last?"
  - **Events associated:**
    - COPD: "Have you experienced cough, wheeze, and progressively worsening shortness of breath on exertion?"
    - CHF: "Have you experienced PND, orthopnea, peripheral edema, or exertional chest pain?"
    - Anemia: "Have you noticed pallor, weakness, fatigue, or palpitations?"
    - "Have you experienced hemoptysis?" This may be a sign of pulmonary malignancy or TB. It is highly unusual in COPD.
    - Ascites: "Have you experienced abdominal distension?"
    - Constitutional symptoms: "Have you experienced fever, chills, night sweats, weight loss, anorexia, or asthenia?"
  - **Frequency:** "How often do you become short of breath? When was the last time it happened?"
  - **Palliative factors:** "Does anything make your shortness of breath better? If so, what?"
  - **Provocative factors:** "Does anything make your shortness of breath worse? If so, what?"
    - Exertion
    - Lying down
    - Exposure to cold air
    - Infection
    - Allergies
- **Functional respiratory inquiry:** Use the SPACED mnemonic.
- **PMH/PSH:** COPD/asthma, IHD, valvular disease, or malignancy
- **Previous investigations:** Ask about prior pulmonary function tests, peak flow measurements, ECG, or CXR. What were the results?
- **MEDS:** Bronchodilators, inhaled steroids, or cardiac medications
  - Consider the patient's adherence to the prescribed medication regimen.
  - Pulmonary fibrosis: Ask about use of amiodarone, sulfonamides (long-term), intravenous street drugs, and use of antineoplastic agents such as bleomycin and chlorambucil.

- **SH:** Smoking, use of EtOH, use of street drugs, occupational history, and TB contacts
- **Immunizations:** Pneumococcal vaccine, influenza vaccine, childhood vaccinations, and BCG vaccine
- **FH:** α_1-antitrypsin deficiency, atopy (eczema, allergic rhinitis, asthma), cystic fibrosis, or premature IHD

Physical Examination
- **Vitals:** Evaluate HR, heart rhythm, RR (depth, effort, and pattern), BP, and temperature.
- **General:** Assess the patient's general appearance, noting any signs of respiratory distress.
- **Skin:** Inspect the skin and nails, noting any diaphoresis, peripheral edema, plethora (may arise secondary to erythrocytosis), cyanosis, or clubbing.
- **HEENT:** Inspect for central cyanosis. Examine the lymph nodes in the head and neck.
- **Resp:** Inspect for thoracic deformity (barrel chest with COPD). Assess chest expansion for symmetry. Evaluate tracheal position. Assess tactile fremitus and perform percussion, noting diaphragmatic excursion (low diaphragm in COPD). Auscultate the lungs, noting breath sounds, transmitted voice sounds, and adventitious sounds. You may note a prolonged expiratory phase in obstructive disease.
- **CVS:** Measure the JVP, and assess for hepatojugular reflux (indicative of increased venous pressure in CHF). Palpate peripheral pulses, noting contour, volume, and rhythm. Inspect and palpate the apical impulse. Auscultate the heart, listening for an S_3 or murmurs.
- **Abdomen:** Examine for ascites and organomegaly.

Pearls
- **COPD** includes several disease entities: chronic bronchitis, emphysema, asthma, and bronchiectasis. It is characterized by progressive airway obstruction, punctuated by acute exacerbations of increasing dyspnea and sputum production or acute respiratory failure. FEV_1 and FEV_1/FVC decrease as severity of disease increases. Severe disease may result in cor pulmonale. Cigarette smoking is the major risk factor. Most patients have a combination of chronic bronchitis and emphysema rather than exclusively one or the other.
- Table 2-5 contains information about how the clinical examination can help differentiate emphysema from atelectasis, pulmonary fibrosis, and pneumonia.

COUGH: HISTORY AND PHYSICAL EXAMINATION

> **INSTRUCTIONS TO CANDIDATE: A 67-year-old woman complains of a bothersome cough. Obtain a detailed history, exploring possible causes, and perform a focused physical examination.**

DD$_X$: VITAMINS C
- **Vascular:** CHF, pulmonary embolism
- **Infectious:** Pneumonia, upper respiratory tract infection (pharyngitis, laryngitis, tracheitis, tracheobronchitis), pertussis, and TB
- **Traumatic:** Inhalational injury, aspiration of foreign body
- **Autoimmune/allergic:** Sarcoidosis
- **Idiopathic/iatrogenic:** Postnasal drip, gastroesophageal reflux, aspiration pneumonitis, COPD/asthma, and angiotensin-converting enzyme (ACE) inhibitor
- **Neoplasm**
- **Congenital/genetic:** Anatomic abnormalities in the tracheobronchial tree or compressing the tracheobronchial tree; cystic fibrosis, α_1-antitrypsin deficiency

Table 2-5 Signs and Symptoms: Emphysema, Atelectasis, Pulmonary Fibrosis, and Pneumonia

	Normal	Emphysema	Atelectasis	Pulmonary Fibrosis	Pneumonia
Definition		Characterized by loss of interstitial elasticity and permanent abnormal enlargement of air spaces distal to terminal bronchioles with destructive changes in alveolar walls	A shrunken, airless state affecting all or part of a lung; may be acute or chronic The chief cause is intraluminal bronchial obstruction	Chronic inflammation of the alveolar walls with progressive fibrosis of unknown cause	An acute infection of lung parenchyma, including alveolar spaces and interstitial tissue; may affect an entire lobe or a segment (lobar pneumonia), alveoli contiguous to bronchi (bronchopneumonia), or interstitial tissue
		Dilated alveoli with septal destruction	Bronchial obstruction with distal collapse of alveoli	Thickened and irregularly dilated alveoli	Alveoli consolidated with fluid, bacteria, and cells (e.g., white blood cells [pus])
Symptoms	—	Exertional dyspnea is the most common symptom Chronic hypercapnia, polycythemia, and right-sided heart failure may develop	Symptoms depend on the rate of bronchial occlusion and percentage of affected lung Rapid occlusion with massive collapse may cause sudden pain, dyspnea, cyanosis, and shock Slowly developing collapse may be asymptomatic	Exertional dyspnea and nonproductive cough In advanced disease, cor pulmonale, digital clubbing, and cyanosis may occur	Typical symptoms include cough, fever, and sputum production, usually developing over days and sometimes accompanied by pleuritic chest pain; signs of respiratory distress may develop
Percussion	Resonant	Hyperresonant	Absent in affected area	Resonant to hyperresonant	Dullness over consolidated area
Tactile fremitus	Normal	Decreased	Usually absent	Normal	Increased over consolidated area
Breath sounds	Vesicular	Diminished or not audible	Diminished or not audible	Bronchovesicular	Bronchial over consolidated area

Continued

Table 2-5 Signs and Symptoms: Emphysema, Atelectasis, Pulmonary Fibrosis, and Pneumonia—cont'd

	Normal	Emphysema	Atelectasis	Pulmonary Fibrosis	Pneumonia
Adventitious sounds	None	When audible, breath sounds are faint and harsh	None	Velcro-type inspiratory crackles	Late inspiratory crackles over consolidated area
Other	—	Barrel chest, accessory muscle use, pursed lips, and tripod positioning may be present	Decreased or delayed chest expansion on affected side	—	Bronchophony, egophony, whispered pectoriloquy, and decreased chest expansion on affected side

Adapted from Jarvis C. *Physical Examination and Health Assessment*. Philadelphia: Saunders; 1992. Illustrations from Tilkian AG, Conover MB. *Understanding Heart Sounds: With an Introduction to Lung Sounds*. 4th ed. Philadelphia: Saunders; 2001 (pp. 285-287).

History
- Ask the patient the following:
  - **Character:** "What is the cough like?"
    - Clearing of the throat: Gastroesophageal reflux and postnasal drip
    - Brassy cough (hard and metallic): Conditions that narrow the trachea or larynx
    - Barking cough (like a seal): Croup
    - Hacking cough: Pharyngitis, tracheobronchitis, and early pneumonia
    - Whooping cough: Pertussis
    - Sputum production: If present, check color, amount, and content (mucus, blood, pus, pink froth).
  - **Onset:** "How did it start (sudden versus gradual)?"
  - **Intensity:** "At what time of day is your cough at its worst? Does it keep you awake at night?" (Asthma and chronic bronchitis may be associated with nocturnal or morning cough.)
  - **Duration:** "How long has it been going on (acute versus chronic versus paroxysmal versus seasonal versus perennial)? If cough is chronic, how has it changed recently? Is it getting better, getting worse, or staying the same?"
  - **Events associated:**
    - Pneumonia: "Do you have fever, chills, rigors, or increased sputum production?"
    - Upper respiratory tract infection: "Do you have malaise, sore throat, rhinorrhea, myalgias, headache, or ear pain?"
    - Tracheitis: "Do you have retrosternal pain like a hot poker?"
    - TB/malignancy: "Are you experiencing hemoptysis or constitutional symptoms (fever, chills, night sweats, weight loss, anorexia, or asthenia)?"
    - CHF: "Do you have exertional dyspnea, orthopnea, or PND?"
    - Gastroesophageal reflux: "Do you have heartburn or epigastric pain?"
  - **Frequency:** "Have you ever had a cough before? When? How often?"
  - **Palliative factors:** "Does anything make the cough better? If so, what?"
  - **Provocative factors:** "What brings on the cough? What makes the cough worse?"
- **Functional respiratory inquiry:** Use the SPACED mnemonic.
- **PMH/PSH:** Previous pneumonia, CHF, COPD/asthma, TB exposure, immunosuppression, or previous aspiration
- **MEDS:** Use of ACE inhibitors, for which cough is known to be a side effect
- **SH:** Travel history, smoking, use of EtOH (which increases risk for aspiration) and use of street drugs

- **Immunizations:** Pneumococcal vaccine, influenza vaccine, childhood vaccinations, and BCG vaccine
- **FH:** COPD, IHD, α_1-antitrypsin deficiency, cystic fibrosis, or TB

Physical Examination
- **Vitals:** Evaluate HR, heart rhythm, RR (depth, effort, and pattern), BP, and temperature.
- **General:** Assess the patient's general appearance, noting any signs of respiratory distress. Characterize any cough observed during the assessment.
- **Skin:** Inspect the skin and nails, noting peripheral edema, cyanosis, or clubbing.
- **HEENT:** Inspect for central cyanosis. Inspect the tympanic membranes and oropharynx. Examine the lymph nodes in the head and neck.
- **Resp:** Inspect for thoracic deformity. Assess chest expansion for symmetry. Evaluate tracheal position. Assess tactile fremitus and perform percussion, noting diaphragmatic excursion. Auscultate the lungs, noting breath sounds, transmitted voice sounds, and adventitious sounds. You may note a prolonged expiratory phase in obstructive disease.
- **CVS:** Measure the JVP, and assess for hepatojugular reflux (indicative of increased venous pressure in CHF). Palpate peripheral pulses, noting contour, volume, and rhythm. Inspect and palpate the apical impulse. Auscultate the heart, listening for an S_3 or murmurs.
- **Abdomen:** Examine for ascites and organomegaly.

HEMOPTYSIS: HISTORY AND PHYSICAL EXAMINATION

> **INSTRUCTIONS TO CANDIDATE: A 70-year-old man presents to the emergency department after coughing up some blood. Obtain a detailed history, exploring possible causes, and perform a focused physical examination.**

Definition
- **Hemoptysis** is the coughing or "spitting" up of blood originating from lungs or airways.

DD$_X$: VITAMINS C
- **V**ascular: Pulmonary embolism, pulmonary hypertension (e.g., mitral stenosis), arteriovenous malformation, and vasculitis
- **I**nfectious: TB, lung abscess, pneumonia, and bronchitis
- **T**raumatic: Aspiration of foreign body
- **A**utoimmune/**a**llergic: Goodpasture syndrome, Wegener granulomatosis
- **M**etabolic: Coagulopathy
- **I**diopathic/**i**atrogenic: Bronchiectasis
- **N**eoplastic: Bronchogenic carcinoma
- **First evaluate ABCs.** It may be necessary to perform an immediate intervention, such as administering supplemental O_2, establishing intravenous access, or initiating airway management.
  - Is the patient able to talk? Swallow? Cough?
  - Are both lungs ventilated? Is the patient oxygenating (check mentation, pulse oximetry)?
  - Are vital signs abnormal? Is the peripheral circulation abnormal (check pulses, capillary refill)?
  - If no immediate interventions are required, proceed to obtain the history, and perform the physical examination

History
- Ask the patient the following:
  - **Character:** "Did you vomit blood or cough up blood? Was it pure blood or blood-tinged mucus? What color was it: bright red, rust, brown, pink and frothy, coffee ground appearance?"

- Onset: "What were you doing when this coughing first happened?"
- Intensity: "How much blood did you cough up?"
- Duration: "How long has this been happening? Is it getting better, getting worse, or staying the same?"
- Events associated:
  - "Have you had any recent infections? Have you been exposed to TB?"
  - Lung cancer: "Do you have pain, shortness of breath, or constitutional symptoms (fever, chills, night sweats, weight loss, anorexia, or asthenia)?"
  - CHF: "Do you have PND, orthopnea, peripheral edema, exertional chest pain or dyspnea?"
  - Pulmonary embolism: "Have you experienced sudden shortness of breath, pleuritic chest pain, or calf swelling/tenderness (DVT)?"
  - Goodpasture syndrome: "Have you experienced shortness of breath, hematuria, or renal failure?"
  - Wegener granulomatosis: "Have you experienced epistaxis, sinusitis, hematuria, constitutional symptoms, or skin lesions?"
  - Differentiate from gastrointestinal bleeding, aspirated blood from epistaxis, bleeding gums, and so on.
- Frequency: "Have you ever coughed or spit up blood before? When? How often?"
- Palliative factors: "Has anything helped make this better? If so, what?"
- Provocative factors: "What brought on previous episodes, if anything?"
- **Functional respiratory inquiry:** Use the SPACED mnemonic
- **PMH/PSH:** Lung cancer, bleeding diathesis, CHF, human immunodeficiency virus (HIV) infection, TB, poor dental hygiene, or peptic ulcer disease
- **MEDS:** Anticoagulants (warfarin, heparin), ASA, or NSAIDs
- **SH:** Smoking, use of EtOH (Mallory-Weiss tears are caused by severe retching or esophageal varices), use of street drugs, and exposure to occupational hazards (e.g., asbestos, coal, hay)
- **FH:** Bleeding disorders, lung cancer, other lung disease, or TB

Physical Examination
- **Vitals:** Evaluate HR, heart rhythm, RR (depth, effort, pattern), BP (hypotension occurs in massive hemoptysis), and temperature.
- **General:** Assess the patient's general appearance, noting any signs of respiratory distress.
- **Skin:** Inspect the skin and nails, noting clubbing, cyanosis, peripheral edema, purple plaques (Kaposi sarcoma), eruptions (paraneoplastic syndromes), petechiae, or ecchymosis.
- **HEENT:** Inspect the nose and oropharynx, noting any evidence of trauma, ulceration, or gingivitis. Examine the lymph nodes in the head and neck.
- **Resp:** Assess chest expansion for symmetry. Evaluate tracheal position. Assess tactile fremitus and perform percussion, noting diaphragmatic excursion. Auscultate the lungs, noting breath sounds, transmitted voice sounds, and adventitious sounds such as apical crackles in TB or a friction rub from pulmonary infarct in pulmonary embolism. You may note a prolonged expiratory phase in obstructive disease.
- **CVS:** Measure the JVP, and assess for hepatojugular reflux (indicative of increased venous pressure in CHF). Palpate peripheral pulses, noting contour, volume, and rhythm. Inspect and palpate the apical impulse. Auscultate the heart, listening for P_2 (pulmonary hypertension), S_3, or murmurs.
- **Abdomen:** Palpate the abdomen, assessing organomegaly and any tenderness.
- **Musculoskeletal system (MSK):** Inspect the lower extremities, noting any asymmetry. Measure the calf circumference.

Pearl
- Blood originating from the stomach is usually darker than that from the respiratory tract. Blood originating from the gastrointestinal tract can be aspirated and coughed up.

SAMPLE CHECKLISTS

Right Middle Lobe Consolidation: Auscultatory Findings

INSTRUCTIONS TO CANDIDATE: Demonstrate the boundaries of the right middle lobe (RML) of the lung. Auscultate the lung, and verbalize over which lobe you are listening. Describe auscultatory findings consistent with RML consolidation.

Key Points	Satisfactorily Completed
Introduces self to the patient	❏
Determines how the patient wishes to be addressed	❏
Washes hands	❏
Explains nature of the examination to the patient	❏
Examines the patient in a logical manner	❏
Demonstrates boundaries of the RML of the lung:	
• Oblique fissure: Like a string connecting T3 posteriorly to the fifth rib at the MAL and the sixth rib at the MCL	❏
• Horizontal fissure: Anteriorly, runs close to the fourth rib and meets the oblique fissure in the MAL near the fifth rib	❏
Performs auscultation:	
• Uses diaphragm of stethoscope	❏
• Instructs patient to breathe deeply through an open mouth	❏
• Listens first on one side and then on the other side for comparison	❏
• Listens for at least one full breath in each location	❏
• Auscultates posteriorly with both arms of the patient crossed in front to displace scapulae	❏
• States that at least five locations should be auscultated anteriorly and posteriorly	❏
Describes expected findings:	
• Breath sounds: bronchial or bronchovesicular sounds over consolidated area; breath sounds may be decreased	❏
• Adventitious sounds: late inspiratory crackles over consolidated area	❏
Transmitted voice sounds:	
• Spoken "EE": heard as "AY" (*egophony*)	❏
• Whispered words: louder and clearer (*whispered pectoriloquy*)	❏
• Spoken words: louder and clearer (*bronchophony*)	❏
Drapes the patient appropriately	❏
Makes appropriate closing remarks	❏

Asthma: History and Physical Examination

> **INSTRUCTIONS TO CANDIDATE:** A 24-year-old man with a long history of well-controlled asthma presents to a walk-in clinic for a prescription refill. The physician notes that he is tachypneic. The patient admits that he has been using his albuterol quite frequently in the past 2 weeks since beginning a summer job at a construction site. Perform a focused history and physical examination.

Key Points	Satisfactorily Completed
Introduces self to the patient	❏
Determines how the patient wishes to be addressed	❏
Washes hands	❏
Establishes the purpose of the encounter	❏
Establishes the presenting concern in the patient's own words	❏
Symptom history:	
• Asks about current symptoms (shortness of breath)	❏
• Asks about onset of difficulty breathing	❏
• Asks whether it is getting better, getting worse, or staying the same	❏
• Asks patient to rate symptom severity on a scale	❏
• Asks patient to compare today's symptom rating to his "norm"	❏
• Asks about most recent use of albuterol (time and dose)	❏
• Asks about frequency of albuterol use	❏
• Asks about evolution of symptoms since starting new job: Cough Shortness of breath Wheezing	❏
• Asks when symptoms tend to be most severe	❏
• Asks whether he tracks his peak flow (if so, how has it changed in the past month?)	❏
• Asks about the type of work he is doing and the kinds of materials he works with	❏
• Asks about lost time from work	❏
• Asks about changes to his living arrangements (e.g., new apartment, new pet)	❏
Asthma history:	
• Asks about known asthma triggers	❏
• Asks about his asthma management plan	❏
• Asks whether he has ever been treated for asthma in hospital	❏
• Asks whether he has ever been intubated	❏
Associated symptoms:	
• Fever	❏
• Chest pain	❏
• Nausea and/or vomiting	❏
• Allergy: rhinitis, eczema, itchy watery eyes	❏
Relevant social history:	
• Smoking	❏

Key Points	Satisfactorily Completed
Past medical and surgical history	❏
Medications:	
• Prescription and over-the-counter drugs	❏
• Asks about patient's adherence to prescribed medicine regimen to control asthma	❏
• Asks about formulation of respiratory medications (e.g., puffer, disc, holding chamber)	❏
Allergies	❏
Explains nature of the examination to the patient	❏
Vital signs:	
• Requests a complete set of vital signs	❏
• Notes any abnormalities such as tachypnea and tachycardia	❏
• Palpates peripheral pulses, noting volume, contour, and rhythm	❏
Inspection:	
• Assesses the patient's general appearance, noting diaphoresis, posture, and any apparent distress	❏
• Inspects chest wall for asymmetry during respiration	❏
Palpation:	
• Assesses position of the trachea	❏
• Places hands on the patient's chest to assess for asymmetry during respiration	❏
• Assesses tactile fremitus	❏
Percussion:	
• Percusses the chest	❏
• Percusses first one side and then the other side for comparison	❏
• Percusses posteriorly with both arms of the patient crossed in front to displace scapulae	❏
• States that at least five locations should be percussed anteriorly and posteriorly	❏
• Notes whether the expected hyperresonance is present	❏
Auscultation:	
• Uses diaphragm of stethoscope	❏
• Instructs patient to breathe deeply through an open mouth	❏
• Auscultates first one side and then the other side for comparison	❏
• Listens for at least one full breath in each location	❏
• Auscultates posteriorly with both arms of the patient crossed in front to displace scapulae	❏
• States that at least five locations should be auscultated anteriorly and posteriorly	❏
• Notes prolonged expiratory phase and whether the expected high-pitched wheezes are present	❏
Drapes the patient appropriately	❏
Makes appropriate closing remarks	❏

ADVANCED SKILLS

INTERPRETATION OF CHEST RADIOGRAPH

- Start by checking the name and date on the film.
- Note the orientation of the film and adequacy of penetration.
  - Two views are needed to localize lesions.
  - Heart size and mediastinal size should be assessed on a posteroanterior (PA) view of the chest rather than an AP view, on which they appear larger. On a PA film, the cardiothoracic ratio should not be >50% (Figure 2-13, *A* and *B*).
  - Assess extent of inspiration by counting the ribs. Poor inspiratory effort leads to vascular crowding and widened central shadow.
  - Assess rotation by looking at the relationship of the sternoclavicular joints to the midline.
  - Note patient position: upright versus supine.
  - The lateral film is particularly useful for assessing the size of the right ventricle, which extends retrosternally when enlarged.

Interpretation (ABCS)

- **A**irway
  - Trachea and mainstem bronchi
- **B**reathing
  - Lung fields (apex, upper and lower lobes, RML, and lingula)
  - Fissures
  - Costophrenic angles
  - Peribronchial changes
  - Pleura: thickening, effusion
- **C**irculation (Figure 2-14)
  - Vasculature in the lungs
  - Pulmonary artery and aortic knuckle
  - Left ventricle and heart size
  - Hila
- **S**oft tissues and skeleton
  - Bilateral breast shadows in women
  - Subcutaneous emphysema
  - Mediastinal enlargement
  - Ribs, clavicle, and humerus

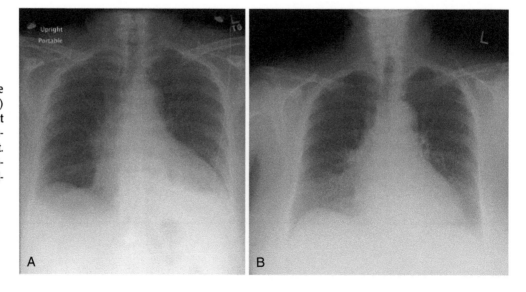

Figure 2-13 A, Portable upright anteroposterior (AP) chest radiograph. **B,** Upright posteroanterior (PA) chest radiograph of the same patient. Note the difference in the appearance of the cardiac silhouette.

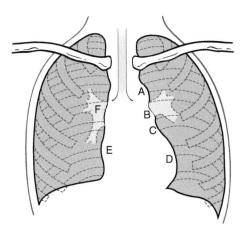

Figure 2-14 Diagram of normal findings on chest radiograph. *A,* Aortic knuckle; *B,* pulmonary artery; *C,* depression over left auricle; *D,* left ventricle; *E,* right atrium; *F,* position of the horizontal fissure. (Used with the permission of Dr. Tom Scott, Memorial University of Newfoundland, St. John's, Canada.)

SOLITARY LUNG NODULE: HISTORY AND DIFFERENTIAL DIAGNOSIS

INSTRUCTIONS TO CANDIDATE: One of your patients recently had a "screening chest x-ray" (Figure 2-15). Your assistant hands you a report saying there is a solitary nodule in the left lung. This 56-year-old man is now in your office. Perform an appropriate functional inquiry. List the differential diagnosis of a solitary pulmonary nodule.

DD$_X$: VITAMINS C
- **V**ascular: Infarct, vascular lesion
- **I**nfectious: TB (granuloma), histoplasmosis, aspergilloma, abscess, and consolidation
- **T**raumatic: Hematoma
- **I**diopathic/**i**atrogenic: Fluid-filled cyst, artifact
- **N**eoplastic: Bronchial carcinoma (squamous cell carcinoma, adenocarcinoma, small cell carcinoma, large cell carcinoma), metastatic disease, and benign neoplasm (bronchial adenoma, hamartoma)

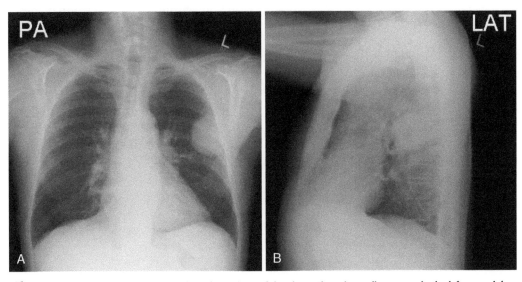

Figure 2-15 Posteroanterior **(A)** and lateral **(B)** views of the chest. There is a solitary mass in the left upper lobe of the lung.

History

- Screen for the following symptoms. Use the mnemonic **ChLORIDE FPP** to delineate any further symptoms.
  - Hemoptysis
  - Wheeze: Obstructing lesion
  - Chest infections: Post-obstructive process, pneumonia, TB, and abscess
  - Alcoholism: Increased risk of aspiration
  - Constitutional symptoms: Fever, chills, night sweats, weight loss, anorexia, and asthenia
- **Functional respiratory inquiry:** Use the SPACED mnemonic

Symptoms Associated with Malignant Spread

- Hoarseness (recurrent laryngeal nerve)
- Superior vena cava syndrome (increased JVP, dyspnea, congestion of face and neck)
- Dysphagia (esophageal compression)
- Horner syndrome and brachial plexus invasion (Pancoast tumor)
- Hepatomegaly and lymphadenopathy (metastasis)
- Bone pain (bone metastases)
- Seizures or neurologic deficits (brain metastases)

Paraneoplastic Syndromes

- **Endocrine:** Hypercalcemia (bone metastases or parathyroid hormone–related protein [PTHrp] secretion by squamous cell carcinoma), Cushing syndrome (secretion of adrenocorticotropic hormone [ACTH] by small cell carcinoma), and hyponatremia (syndrome of inappropriate antidiuretic hormone [SIADH])
- **Neuromuscular:** Sensory neuropathy, cerebellar ataxia, and Eaton-Lambert myasthenic syndrome (small cell carcinoma; characterized by progressive proximal myopathy with absence of reflexes that develops after brief periods of isometric contractions; bulbar muscles are unaffected)
- **Cutaneous:** Acanthosis nigricans in body folds such as in the axillae (adenocarcinoma)
- **MSK:** Hypertrophic osteoarthropathy—clubbing, arthralgias of the wrists and ankles (squamous cell carcinoma)

Risk Factors for Malignancy

- Cigarette smoking is the major risk factor for developing lung malignancy. Adenocarcinoma, however, is *not* related to cigarette smoking. Other risk factors include increasing age and exposure to asbestos, radiation, chromium, iron, or iron oxides.

Pearl

- **Tuberculosis (TB)** is an infection caused by *Mycobacterium tuberculosis* or *Mycobacterium bovis.* TB is usually transmitted through inhalation of droplet nuclei from a person who has active pulmonary TB. Initial infection leaves **nodular scars** in the apex of the lung; immunity rapidly develops, and infection is walled off **(Ghon complex).**

PLEURAL EFFUSION: PHYSICAL EXAMINATION AND INTERPRETATION OF CHEST RADIOGRAPH

INSTRUCTIONS TO CANDIDATE: A 48-year-old man with unresectable bronchogenic carcinoma presents with worsening shortness of breath. Perform a focused physical examination. Interpret this patient's chest radiograph (Figure 2-16), and describe expected physical findings.

- **First evaluate ABCs.** It may be necessary to perform an immediate intervention, such as administering supplemental O_2, establishing intravenous access, or initiating airway management.
  - Is the patient able to talk? Swallow? Cough?
  - Are both lungs ventilated? Is the patient oxygenating (check mentation, pulse oximetry)?
  - Are vital signs abnormal? Is the peripheral circulation abnormal (check pulses, capillary refill)?
  - If no immediate interventions are required, proceed to obtain the history, and perform the physical examination.

Interpretation of Chest Radiograph
- Start by checking the name and date on the film. Figure 2-16 is an AP view of the chest that is adequately penetrated. The right hemidiaphragm is not visible, and the right heart border is obliterated. There is some tracking at the pleural margin, suggestive of a right-sided pleural effusion.
- **Transudates** may be caused by increased venous pressure or hypoproteinemic states that result in reduced capillary oncotic pressure. Transudates are often bilateral. Causes include the following:
  - Hypoproteinemia: Nephrotic syndrome, protein-losing enteropathy
  - Increased venous pressure: CHF, constrictive pericarditis, fluid overload, cirrhosis, pulmonary embolism, and myxedema
- **Exudates** may be caused by increased leakiness of pleural capillaries or inflammation. Effusions are unilateral in focal diseases and bilateral in systemic and diffuse lung diseases. Causes include the following:
  - Infectious: Pneumonia, TB, fungal infection, viral infection, and abscess
  - Inflammatory: Pulmonary infarction, collagen vascular disease, pancreatitis, and Dressler syndrome

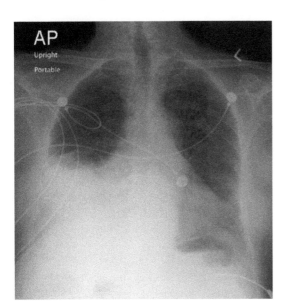

Figure 2-16 Anteroposterior radiographic view of the chest (portable).

- Neoplastic: Lung cancer, mesothelioma, lymphoma, and metastatic disease
- Miscellaneous: Asbestos exposure, drugs, and Meige syndrome

Physical Examination
- **Vitals:** Evaluate HR, heart rhythm, RR (depth, effort, and pattern), BP, and temperature.
- **General:** Assess the patient's general appearance, noting any signs of respiratory distress.
- **Skin:** Inspect the skin and nails, noting any diaphoresis, peripheral edema, cyanosis, or clubbing.
- **HEENT:** Inspect for central cyanosis. Examine the lymph nodes in the head and neck.
- **Resp** (Table 2-6): Assess chest expansion for symmetry. Evaluate tracheal position. Assess tactile fremitus and perform percussion, noting diaphragmatic excursion. Auscultate the lungs, noting breath sounds and adventitious sounds.
- **CVS:** Measure the JVP and assess for hepatojugular reflux (indicative of increased venous pressure in CHF). Palpate peripheral pulses, noting contour, volume, and rhythm. Inspect and palpate the apical impulse. Auscultate the heart, listening for an S_3 or murmurs.
- **Neuro:** Briefly assess level of consciousness and mental status (adequate brain oxygenation).

Evidence
- Table 2-7 lists clinical features that are useful in diagnosing pleural effusion.

Table 2-6 Expected Findings in Pleural Effusion

Examination	Expected Findings
Chest expansion	May be decreased ipsilaterally
Trachea	Deviation toward opposite side with large effusions
Tactile fremitus	Decreased to absent; may be increased near top of a large effusion
Percussion	Dull to flat over fluid
Breath sounds	Decreased to absent; bronchial sounds may be heard near the top of a large effusion
Adventitious sounds	None except for possible pleural rub

Table 2-7 Usefulness of Clinical Examination for Diagnosing Pleural Effusion

Clinical Feature	+LR (95% CI)	−LR (95% CI)
Asymmetric chest expansion*	**8.1 (5.2–12.7)**	0.29 (0.19–0.45)
Decreased tactile fremitus*	**5.7 (4.0–8.0)**	0.21 (0.12–0.37)
Percussion dullness*	**8.7 (2.2–33.8)**	0.31 (0.03–3.3)
Diminished breath sounds†	**5.2 (3.8–7.1)**	**0.15 (0.07–0.30)**
Pleural rub†	3.9 (0.80–18.7)	0.96 (0.90–1.0)

*Data from Wong CL, Holroyd-Leduc J, Straus SE. Does this patient have a pleural effusion? *JAMA.* 2009;301:309-317.

†Data from Kalantri S, Joshi R, Lokhande T, et al. Accuracy and reliability of physical signs in the diagnosis of pleural effusion. *Respir Med.* 2007;101:431-438.

CI, Confidence interval; +LR, positive likelihood ratio; −LR, negative likelihood ratio.

Boldface represents findings associated with positive likelihood ratios ≥5 or with negative likelihood ratios ≤0.2. These are said to be moderate- to high-impact items.

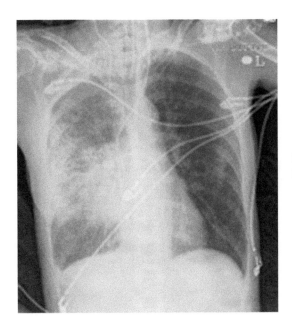

Figure 2-17 Anteroposterior radiographic view of the chest (portable).

PNEUMONIA: PHYSICAL EXAMINATION AND INTERPRETATION OF CHEST RADIOGRAPH

INSTRUCTIONS TO CANDIDATE: A 32-year-old woman presents with fever, rigors, and green sputum. Perform a focused physical examination. Interpret this patient's chest radiograph (Figure 2-17), and describe expected physical findings.

- **First evaluate ABCs.** It may be necessary to perform an immediate intervention, such as administering supplemental O_2, establishing intravenous access, or initiating airway management.
  - Is the patient able to talk? Swallow? Cough?
  - Are both lungs ventilated? Is the patient oxygenating (check mentation, pulse oximetry)?
  - Are vital signs abnormal? Is the peripheral circulation abnormal (check pulses, capillary refill)?
  - If no immediate interventions are required, proceed to obtain the history, and perform the physical examination.

Interpretation of Chest Radiograph
- Start by checking the name and date on the film. Figure 2-17 is an AP view of the chest that is adequately penetrated. There is an infiltrate throughout the right lung with lobar consolidation of the RML. The right costophrenic angle is blunted.
- At the time of this CXR, the patient had already been admitted to the intensive care unit because of respiratory failure and septic shock. The CXR shows that the patient is intubated with a right internal jugular central line and a left internal jugular line through which a pulmonary artery catheter has been inserted. Cardiac monitor leads also are visible.

Physical Examination
- **Vitals:** Evaluate HR, heart rhythm, RR (depth, effort, and pattern), BP, and temperature.
  - The patient was febrile, tachypneic, tachycardic, and hypotensive.
- **General:** Assess the patient's general appearance, noting any signs of respiratory distress.

- **Skin:** Inspect the skin and nails, noting any diaphoresis, cyanosis, or clubbing.
- **Resp** (Table 2-8): Assess chest expansion for symmetry. Evaluate tracheal position. Assess tactile fremitus, and perform percussion. Auscultate the lungs, noting breath sounds, transmitted voice sounds, and adventitious sounds. Expect positive findings in the area of the RML (some findings may be evident throughout the right lung).
- **CVS:** Measure the JVP (may be decreased because of distributive shock). Palpate peripheral pulses, noting contour, volume, and rhythm. Inspect and palpate the apical impulse. Auscultate the heart, listening for an S_3 or murmurs.
- **Neuro:** Briefly assess level of consciousness and mental status (adequate brain oxygenation).

Evidence

- The reliability of the clinical examination for pneumonia is moderate at best.[7,8] No individual clinical features can be used to definitively diagnose pneumonia (Table 2-9).

Table 2-8 Expected Findings in Consolidation

Examination	Expected Findings
Chest movement	May be asymmetric because of pleuritic chest pain
Trachea	Midline
Tactile fremitus	Increased
Percussion	Dull over airless area
Breath sounds	Bronchial or bronchovesicular over consolidated area; breath sounds may be decreased
Adventitious sounds	Late inspiratory crackles over consolidated area
Transmitted voice sounds (ask patient to speak while you listen with stethoscope)	Spoken words: louder and clearer (*bronchophony*) Spoken "EE": heard as "AY" (*egophony*) Whispered words: louder and clearer (*whispered pectoriloquy*)

Table 2-9 Usefulness of Clinical Examination for Diagnosing Pneumonia

Clinical Feature	+LR Range	−LR Range
Temperature >37.8° C	1.4–4.4	0.58–0.78
Asymmetric chest expansion	No data	0.96
Increased tactile fremitus	No data	No data
Percussion dullness	2.2–4.3	0.79–0.93
Bronchial breath sounds	3.5	0.9
Decreased breath sounds	2.3–2.5	0.64–0.78
Crackles	1.6–2.7	0.62–0.87
Egophony	2.0–8.6	0.76–0.96

From Metlay JP, Kapoor WN, Fine MJ. Does this patient have community-acquired pneumonia? Diagnosing pneumonia by history and physical examination. *JAMA.* 1997;278:1440-1445.
−LR, Negative likelihood ratio; +LR, positive likelihood ratio.

PNEUMOTHORAX: PHYSICAL EXAMINATION AND INTERPRETATION OF CHEST RADIOGRAPH

INSTRUCTIONS TO CANDIDATE: A 24-year-old woman presents to the emergency department with sudden onset of left-sided chest pain and mild shortness of breath. She has had two previous pneumothoraces. Perform a focused physical examination. Interpret this patient's chest radiograph (Figure 2-18), and describe expected physical findings.

- **First evaluate ABCs.** It may be necessary to perform an immediate intervention, such as administering supplemental O_2, establishing intravenous access, or initiating airway management.
  - Is the patient able to talk? Swallow? Cough?
  - Are both lungs ventilated? Is the patient oxygenating (check mentation, pulse oximetry)?
  - Are vital signs abnormal? Is the peripheral circulation abnormal (check pulses, capillary refill)?
  - If no immediate interventions are required, proceed to obtain the history, and perform the physical examination.

Interpretation of Chest Radiograph
- Start by checking the name and date on the film. The PA expiratory and inspiratory films shown in Figure 2-18 are adequately penetrated. The pulmonary vascular markings do not extend to the left chest wall in either film, and the left hemithorax is particularly lucent. This appearance is enhanced on the expiratory film, in which shift of the trachea and mediastinum is notable. The pneumothorax appears larger in the expiratory view in relation to the lung; the size of the pneumothorax remains stable, but the lung is reduced in volume during expiration, which makes the pneumothorax *appear* larger.

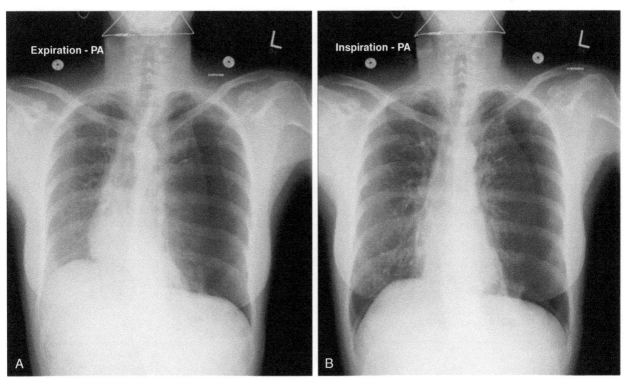

Figure 2-18 (A) Expiratory and **(B)** inspiratory posteroanterior (PA) radiographic views of the chest.

DD$_X$: VITAMINS C
- Infectious: Abscess, pneumonia, and TB
- Traumatic: Puncture by a fractured rib, penetrating injury (stab wound, gunshot wound), mechanical ventilation, barotrauma
- Idiopathic/iatrogenic: Spontaneous pneumothorax, COPD/asthma (bleb rupture), central line insertion, thoracentesis, ascent in airplane
- Neoplasm
- Congenital/genetic: Rupture of subpleural bleb, cystic fibrosis

Physical Examination
- **Vitals:** Evaluate HR, heart rhythm, RR (depth, effort, and pattern), BP, and temperature, and assess for pulsus paradoxus.
- **General:** Assess the patient's general appearance, noting any signs of respiratory distress.
- **Skin:** Inspect the skin and nails, noting any diaphoresis, peripheral edema, cyanosis, or clubbing.
- **Resp** (Table 2-10): Inspect for thoracic deformity (e.g., pectus excavatum associated with Marfan syndrome). Assess chest expansion for symmetry. Evaluate tracheal position. Assess tactile fremitus, and perform percussion. Auscultate the lungs, noting breath sounds and adventitious sounds.
- **CVS:** Measure the JVP, and assess for hepatojugular reflux (signs of venous congestion are consistent with tension pneumothorax). Palpate peripheral pulses, noting contour, volume, and rhythm. Inspect and palpate the apical impulse. Auscultate the heart.
- **Neuro:** Briefly assess level of consciousness and mental status (adequate brain oxygenation).

Pearls
- A **tension pneumothorax** is an *emergency* and occurs when a pleural defect forms a one-way valve, allowing air to enter during inspiration but preventing escape of air during expiration. Positive pressure in the pleural space escalates, which results in extreme shift of the trachea and mediastinum. Both lungs and heart are compressed, which causes severe dyspnea and decreases in venous return, cardiac output, and BP. This is a *clinical diagnosis* rather than a radiologic one.
  - **Signs and symptoms:** Severe dyspnea, deep cyanosis, ipsilateral hyperresonance to percussion and absence of breath sounds, contralateral tracheal and mediastinal deviation, distension of neck veins, hypotension, and tachycardia
  - **Treatment:** Insertion of large-bore needle into the second ICS at the MCL to release pressure; definitive management includes subsequent insertion of a chest tube

Table 2-10 Expected Findings in Pneumothorax

Examination	Expected Findings
Chest movement	May be decreased ipsilaterally
Trachea	Deviation toward the opposite side
Tactile fremitus	Decreased to absent ipsilaterally
Percussion	Hyperresonant or tympanitic over pleural air
Breath sounds	Decreased to absent ipsilaterally
Adventitious sounds	None except for possible pleural rub

SAMPLE CHECKLIST

Hemothorax: Physical Examination and Interpretation of Chest Radiograph

> **INSTRUCTIONS TO CANDIDATE:** An 18-year-old male inpatient is noted to be tachypneic (RR, 24/minute) by his nurse. Yesterday he had surgery to repair curvature in his spine. He has good pain control and complains only of breathlessness. You are called to assess him after he has a chest radiograph. Interpret the radiograph (Figure 2-19, *A* and *B*), and perform a focused physical examination.

Key Points	Satisfactorily Completed
CXR interpretation:	
• Verifies the CXR belongs to the correct patient	❏
• Identifies the films as portable AP supine and right lateral decubitus chest views	❏
• Notes complete opacification ("white-out") of the left hemithorax	❏
• Looks for left mainstem bronchus (barely visible)	❏
• Notes absence of fluid level on decubitus view (no apparent fluid shift)	❏
• Notes surgical hardware	❏
• Articulates most likely diagnosis in this patient is large hemothorax	❏
• Also considers mucous plugging with significant atelectasis	❏
Introduces self to the patient	❏
Determines how the patient wishes to be addressed	❏
Washes hands	❏
Establishes the purpose of the encounter	❏
Explains nature of the examination to the patient	❏

Continued

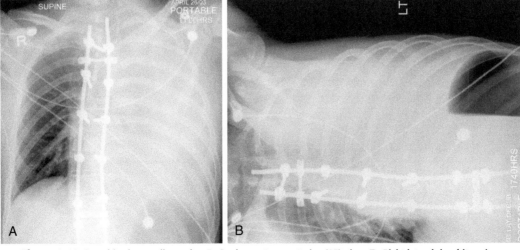

Figure 2-19 Portable chest radiographs. **A,** Supine, anteroposterior (AP) view. **B,** Right lateral decubitus view.

Key Points	Satisfactorily Completed
Vital signs:	
• Requests a complete set of vital signs	❑
• Notes any abnormalities such as tachypnea and tachycardia	❑
• Palpates peripheral pulses, noting volume, contour, and rhythm	❑
Inspection:	
• Assesses the patient's general appearance, noting diaphoresis, posture, and any apparent distress	❑
• Inspects chest wall for asymmetry during respiration	❑
Palpation:	
• Assesses position of the trachea	❑
• Places hands on the patient's chest to assess for asymmetry during respiration	❑
• Assesses tactile fremitus	❑
Percussion:	
• Percusses the chest	❑
• Percusses first one side and then the other side for comparison	❑
• Percusses posteriorly with both arms of the patient crossed in front to displace scapulae	❑
• States that at least five locations should be percussed anteriorly and posteriorly	❑
Auscultation:	
• Uses diaphragm of stethoscope	❑
• Instructs patient to breathe deeply through an open mouth	❑
• Auscultates first one side and then the other side for comparison	❑
• Listens for at least one full breath in each location	❑
• Auscultates posteriorly with both arms of the patient crossed in front to displace scapulae	❑
• States that at least five locations should be auscultated anteriorly and posteriorly	❑
Notes expected findings for hemothorax and atelectasis, which are similar:	
• Decreased chest expansion on left	❑
• Decreased or absent tactile fremitus on left	❑
• Dullness to percussion on left	❑
• Decreased or absent breath sounds on left	❑
• Large left-sided effusion, which may cause trachea to deviate to the right	❑
Drapes the patient appropriately	❑
Makes appropriate closing remarks	❑

- Hemothorax was confirmed later by a computed tomographic (CT) scan (Figure 2-20).

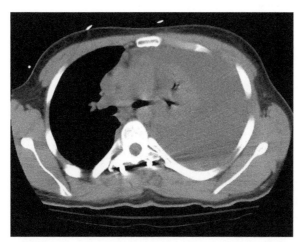

Figure 2-20 Subsequent computed tomographic (CT) scan confirmed a large hemothorax.

REFERENCES

1. Myers KA, Farquhar DR. The rational clinical examination: does this patient have clubbing? *JAMA.* 2001;286:341-347.
2. Hla KS. Clinical usefulness of "vocal fremitus" and "vocal resonance"—GP perceptions and practice. *Aust Fam Physician.* 2007;36:573, 576.
3. Leuppi JD, Dieterle T, Koch G, et al. Diagnostic value of lung auscultation in an emergency room setting. *Swiss Med Wkly.* 2005;135:520-524.
4. Zun LS, Downey L. The effect of noise in the emergency department. *Acad Emerg Med.* 2005;12:663-666.
5. Tijunelis MA, Fitzsullivan E, Henderson SO. Noise in the ED. *Am J Emerg Med.* 2005;23:332-335.
6. Leuppi JD, Dieterle T, Wildeisen I, et al. Can airway obstruction be estimated by lung auscultation in an emergency room setting? *Respir Med.* 2006;100:279-285.
7. Wipf JE, Lipsky BA, Hirschmann JV, et al. Diagnosing pneumonia by physical examination: relevant or relic? *Arch Intern Med.* 1999;159:1082-1087.
8. Metlay JP, Kapoor WN, Fine MJ. Does this patient have community-acquired pneumonia? Diagnosing pneumonia by history and physical examination. *JAMA.* 1997;278:1440-1445.

Gastrointestinal System

ANATOMY

- The **liver** is in the right upper quadrant (RUQ) and is almost entirely covered by the rib cage (Figure 3-1). It moves inferiorly with inspiration, making it easier to palpate. Because of its soft consistency, the liver may be difficult to palpate through the abdominal wall.
- The **spleen** (see Figure 3-1) is in the left upper quadrant (LUQ), posterior to the stomach and anterior to the upper pole of the left kidney. It lies in the curve of the

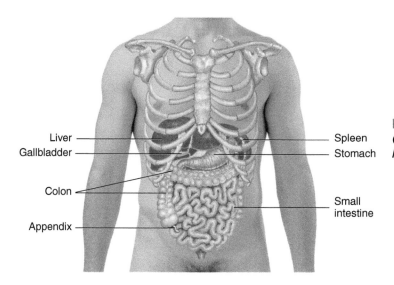

Figure 3-1 Surface anatomy of the gastrointestinal system. (From Wilson SF, Giddens JF. *Health Assessment for Nursing Practice.* 2nd ed. St Louis: Mosby; 2001 [p. 479, Figure 20-1].)

Liver
Gallblader
Colon
Appendix

Spleen
Stomach
Small intestine

diaphragm posterior to the midaxillary line, deep to the ninth, tenth, and eleventh ribs (12 cm in length and 7 cm in width). The normal spleen does not extend beyond the costal margin and is usually not palpable. Like the liver, it moves inferiorly with inspiration.

GLOSSARY OF SIGNS AND SYMPTOMS

- **Constipation** is the difficult or infrequent evacuation of feces.
- **Diarrhea** is abnormally frequent passage of poorly formed or watery stool. A quantified amount is the passage of >300 mL of liquid feces in a 24-hour period.
- **Dysphagia** is difficulty swallowing, a sense that food or liquid is sticking in the throat. The sensation of a lump in the throat that is not associated with swallowing **(globus hystericus)** is not true dysphagia.
- **Flatus** is the expulsion of gastrointestinal (GI) air through the anus. The presence of flatus is rarely pathologic, although patients with malabsorption syndromes, such as lactose intolerance, may pass excessive amounts of gas.
- **Halitosis** is foul-smelling breath. Although it is unpleasant, it does not generally reflect GI disease.
- **Hematemesis** is the vomiting of blood from the upper GI tract, proximal to the ligament of Treitz. It generally reflects brisk bleeding. **Coffee-ground emesis** also reflects upper GI bleeding (or swallowed blood, as in epistaxis), but it is generally slower, having had time for the gastric acid to convert hemoglobin (which is red) into hematin (which is brown). Hematemesis should be carefully differentiated from hemoptysis, which is the *coughing up* of blood from the respiratory tract.
- **Hematochezia** is the passage of bloody stools. Although hematochezia generally reflects lower GI bleeding (distal to the ligament of Treitz), it may also reflect brisk upper GI bleeding with rapid transit.
- **Jaundice** refers to the yellowish staining of skin and other tissues with bile pigment. The presence of jaundice is reliably correlated with hyperbilirubinemia. Bilirubin is normally taken up by liver cells and excreted in the bile. Mechanisms underlying jaundice include increased production of bilirubin, decreased uptake by liver cells, decreased ability to conjugate bilirubin, and decreased excretion. Unconjugated bilirubin binds with albumin; therefore, jaundice is observed clinically in tissues rich in albumin, such as skin and eyes **(scleral icterus).** Jaundice occurs with bilirubin concentrations of 40 to 45 μmol/L. It is best observed in natural light.

- **Melena** is the passage of dark, tarry, malodorous stools. It typically results from upper GI bleeding, although blood in the small bowel or right colon may appear as melena with prolonged transit times. Tests of melena stools for occult blood yield positive results. Tests of black stools caused by foods and substances, such as iron and bismuth, should yield negative results for occult blood.
- **Obstipation** is the absence of both flatus and of the passage of bowel movements, a symptom of intestinal obstruction.
- **Steatorrhea** is the passage of fatty stools. The stools are pale, soft, greasy, malodorous, and difficult to flush away. It is caused by malabsorption of fat, which occurs in such conditions as pancreatic insufficiency or celiac disease. Some patients in whom steatorrhea is documented by measurement of fecal fat do not have symptoms.

Abdominal Pain

- **Visceral pain** originates in the abdominal organs and is caused by forceful contracations or distension of hollow organs. The pain tends to be midline and poorly localized (Figure 3-2). It is described as gnawing, burning, crampy, or achy and is often associated with nausea and vomiting.
- **Parietal pain** originates in the parietal peritoneum and is usually caused by inflammation. It may be described as a steady aching pain or a sharp intermittent pain that is aggravated by movement and coughing. Parietal pain is well localized over the involved structure.
- **Referred pain** is felt at a location remote from the involved structure. The pain is felt at the level of somatic innervation (dermatome) to which the sympathetic pain carrying nerves innervate. It tends to radiate from the original site and is well localized. Pain may be referred from abdominal to nonabdominal sites (e.g., cholecystitis may cause pain in the right shoulder because of involvement of the phrenic nerve).
- **Rebound tenderness** is abdominal tenderness that occurs when pressure is suddenly released. The classical method of detection is to slowly press over the painful area and then quickly withdraw. However, this painful examination is probably unnecessary if the patient reports localized abdominal pain with coughing and rocking the pelvis back and forth (or shaking the bed). Rebound tenderness is considered a sign of peritoneal irritation.

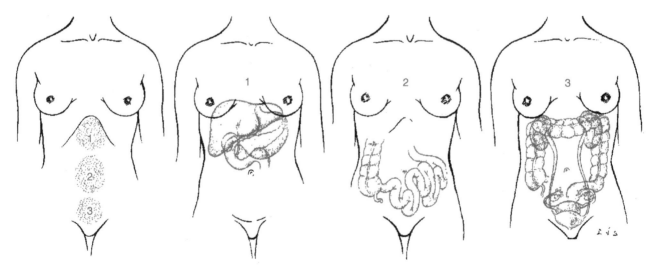

Figure 3-2 Localization of visceral pain. (From Feldman M, Sleisenger MH, Scharschmidt BF. *Sleisenger & Fordtran's Gastrointestinal and Liver Disease.* 6th ed. Philadelphia: Saunders; 1998 [p. 82].)

ESSENTIAL SKILLS

APPROACH TO HISTORY OF ABDOMINAL PAIN

- **ID:** Age, sex
- Use the acronym **ChLORIDE FPP** to ask the patient about the presenting concern:
  - **Character:** "What is the pain like?"
    - Sharp
    - Crampy
    - Dull
  - **Location:** "Where does the pain originate?" (Figure 3-3)
    - RUQ
    - Right lower quadrant (RLQ)
    - LUQ
    - Left lower quadrant (LLQ)
    - Suprapubic
    - Epigastric
    - Flank
  - **Onset:** "When did the pain start? How did it come on (sudden versus gradual)?"
  - **Radiation:** "Does the pain move anywhere?"
  - **Intensity:** "How severe is the pain on a scale of 1 to 10, with 1 being mild pain and 10 being the worst?"
    - "How does the pain affect your activities of daily living?"
    - "Is the pain getting better, getting worse, or staying the same?"
  - **Duration:** "How long has the pain been there (acute versus chronic)?"
  - **Events associated:**
    - "Have you had fever or chills?"
    - "Have you experienced nausea or vomiting, reflux, or hematemesis?"
    - "Have you experienced hematuria, change in color of urine, dysuria, polyuria, urinary frequency, nocturia, or anuria?"
    - "How is your appetite? Have you lost or gained weight?"
    - "Have you experienced diarrhea, steatorrhea, constipation, melena, or hematochezia?"
    - "Have you had jaundice?"
    - If the patient is female: "When was your most recent menstrual period? Are you pregnant? Have you had vaginal discharge or irritation?"

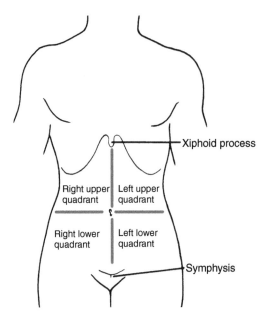

Figure 3-3 Division of the abdomen into quadrants. (From Wilkins RL, Sheldon RL, Krider SJ. *Clinical Assessment in Respiratory Care.* 4th ed. St. Louis: Mosby; 2000 [p. 90, Figure 4-26].)

- Frequency: "Have you ever had this pain before? How often does the pain come (intermittent versus constant)?"
- Palliative factors: "Does anything make the pain better? If so, what?"
  - Lying in one position
  - Analgesic medication
  - Abstaining from food; abstaining from particular foods
- Provocative factors: "Does anything make the pain worse? If so, what?"
  - Movement
  - Eating (in general), eating particular foods
- **Past medical history (PMH)/past surgical history (PSH):**
  - Previous surgeries
  - Malignancy
  - Hepatitis, previous blood transfusions
  - Inflammatory bowel disease (IBD), irritable bowel syndrome (IBS)
  - Other medical problems
- **Medications (MEDS):** Antacids, laxatives
- **Allergies and sensitivities**
- **Social history (SH):** Smoking, use of alcohol (EtOH), use of street drugs, and sexual history (sexual practices, number of sexual partners in the last 6 to 12 months, use of condoms)
- **Family history (FH):** IBD, hemochromatosis

Evidence

- According to a Cochrane Database review, the use of analgesia in patients with abdominal pain improves patient comfort but causes no significant changes in the findings of the physical examination or in assignment of an incorrect diagnosis.[1]
- A phase 1 emergency department study[2] was conducted to identify features of the history, physical examination, laboratory tests, and imaging in patients with nonspecific abdominal pain that were useful for predicting the need for an urgent intervention, which was defined as a condition necessitating "surgical or medical treatment to prevent death or major morbidity." Through statistical modeling, the investigators found that the most useful finding in the history and physical examination was an initial temperature of more than 37.7° C (99.9° F) with a positive likelihood ratio (+LR) of 3.17 (sensitivity 25%; specificity 92%). The aspects of the history and physical examination included in this study are listed in Table 3-1.
- Although the absence of a "gold standard" is problematic, internists were able to reliably ($\kappa = 0.95$) differentiate organic from nonorganic causes of abdominal pain through clinical assessment (+LR 3.97 for "probable" diagnoses; 95% confidence interval [CI] 1.55 to 10.21; the sensitivity and specificity were 100% for "undoubted" diagnosis).[3] Another study identified several independent historical predictors of organic abdominal complaints: male sex, greater age, epigastric pain, no specific character to pain (pain that is *not* described as "burning," "cutting," "terrible," "feeling of pressure," "dull," or "boring"), pain affecting sleep, history of blood in stool, and no pain relief after defecation.[4] None of these symptoms was characterized by both high sensitivity and high specificity, and all odds ratios were less than 2.0.

Pearl

- It is important to manage pain. If the patient is in a great deal of pain, it should be addressed early in the encounter. Getting the patient's pain under control facilitates history taking and examination.

APPROACH TO THE GASTROINTESTINAL EXAMINATION

Patient Positioning

- The patient should initially be placed in a supine position with the arms relaxed at the sides and the legs uncrossed. Patient position will change for particular examination maneuvers.

Table 3-1	Guideline for Abdominal Pain in the ED Setting (GAPEDS): Clinical Predictor Variables

History	**Physical Examination**
Age	Pulse rate, initial
Sex	Systolic blood pressure, initial
Pain, diffuse or localized?	Respiratory rate, initial
Pain location, if localized	Temperature, initial
Pain, sudden or gradual onset?	Bowel sounds present?
Does pain radiate?	Rebound tenderness?
Nausea in past 24 hours?	McBurney's point tenderness?
Vomiting in past 24 hours?	Murphy's sign present?
Anorexia in past 24 hours?	Rovsing's sign present?
Diarrhea in past 24 hours?	Costovertebral angle tenderness present?
Flatus in past 24 hours?	Stool grossly bloody?
Melena in past 24 hours?	Stool heme positive?
Hematochezia in past 24 hours?	Does examination change during ED visit?
Hematemesis in past 24 hours?	
Does pain resolve during ED visit?	
Does patient vomit during ED visit?	

From Gerhardt RT, Nelson BK, Keenan S, et al. Derivation of a clinical guideline for the assessment of nonspecific abdominal pain: The Guideline for Abdominal Pain in the ED Setting (GAPEDS) phase 1 study. *Am J Emerg Med.* 2005;23:709-717.
ED, Emergency department.

Inspection

- **Skin:** Look for scars, striae, dilated veins (caput medusae, spider nevi), excoriations, jaundice, and ulcerations.
- **Umbilicus:** Check contour and location, and look for obvious herniation.
- **Contour:** Check for flat, protuberant, scaphoid, or bulging flanks; symmetry; and visible organs or masses.
- **Peristalsis:** This may be seen in thin patients (increased in obstruction).
- **Pulsations:** Check for normal aortic pulsation in epigastrium (increased with abdominal aortic aneurysm [AAA])
- **Abdominal wall movement:** This is visible with respiration.

Auscultation

- **Bowel sounds:** Clicks, gurgles, and borborygmi (loud prolonged gurgles of hyperperistalsis). Before you decide that bowel sounds are absent, listen in each quadrant for 2 to 3 minutes.
- **Friction rubs:** Listen over liver and spleen (inflammation of peritoneal surface of organ).

Palpation

- Before you palpate, ask the patient to cough and point to the most tender area with one finger. Palpate the most tender area last.
  - **Light palpation:** Gently palpate each quadrant to identify tenderness, muscular resistance, and superficial masses. Distinguish between voluntary guarding and involuntary muscular spasm. Voluntary guarding decreases when the patient is relaxed. To optimize relaxation, position the patient supine with arms at the side, and ask the patient to breathe through the mouth with the jaw open. Involuntary rigidity that persists despite relaxation may indicate peritoneal inflammation.

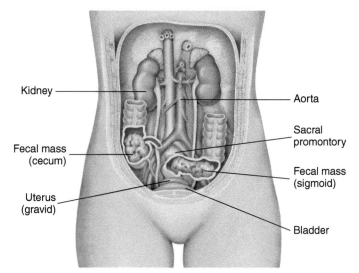

Figure 3-4 Structures commonly palpated as abdominal masses. (From Seidel HM, Ball JW, Dains JE, et al. *Mosby's Guide to Physical Examination.* 5th ed. St. Louis: Mosby; 2003 [p. 548, Figure 16-18].)

- **Deep palpation:** Palpate all four quadrants, using the volar surface of your fingers. Identify any masses, and describe the size, shape, consistency, tenderness, and mobility (Figure 3-4). Pinpoint pain as accurately as possible.
- **Rebound tenderness:** Press your fingers in firmly and slowly, then quickly withdraw them. Watch and listen to the patient for signs of pain. Pain on withdrawal constitutes rebound tenderness. You can assess this indirectly by asking the patient to cough, by shaking the bed, or by percussion. Increased, localized pain with these maneuvers is suggestive of peritoneal irritation or inflammation.

Percussion
- Percuss lightly in all four quadrants. Tympany usually dominates, but scattered areas of dullness are normal (representative of feces/fluid). Note amount and distribution of gas. Identify possible masses. Estimate the size of the liver by percussing from above and below the costal margins. Percuss Traube space and for Castell sign. Test for shifting dullness to identify the presence of ascites.

Other Pertinent Examinations
- A pelvic examination in female patients may be necessary to assess pelvic structures, e.g., ovarian cyst, ovarian torsion, ectopic pregnancy, or pelvic inflammatory disease (PID) (see Chapter 11, p. 310). In male patients, examine the groin and genitalia for hernias (see pp. 92-93). Perform a digital rectal examination (DRE) (see pp. 93-94). Examine the liver and spleen (see pp. 89-92).

Specific Signs
- **McBurney's point:** This spot is one-third the distance between the anterior superior iliac spine and the umbilicus. Tenderness at McBurney point is a "classic" sign of appendicitis.
- **Psoas sign:** Ask the patient to raise the right thigh against resistance, or ask the patient to lie on his or her left side and extend the right leg at the hip. Increased abdominal pain is suggestive of irritation of the psoas muscle.
- **Obturator sign:** Flex the right thigh at the hip with the knee bent. Rotate the leg internally at the hip. Right hypogastric pain is suggestive of irritation of the obturator muscle.
- **Murphy's sign:** Hook your fingers under the right costal margin, and ask the patient to take a deep breath. A sharp increase in tenderness or sudden stop in inspiratory effort is suggestive of acute cholecystitis.
- **Rovsing's sign:** Pain in the RLQ during left-sided pressure or deep palpation is suggestive of localized peritoneal irritation, as in appendicitis.

Evidence

- In the physical examination of patients with abdominal pain, interrater variation among residents, physicians, and attending physicians is surprisingly high in an emergency department setting. Although agreement about the presence of masses was "almost perfect" ($\kappa = 0.82$; 95% CI 0.56 to 1.00), agreement about the presence of guarding, distension, and tenderness was only moderate. The level of agreement on the location of tenderness was even more variable, ranging from "fair" for LUQ tenderness ($\kappa = 0.39$; 95% CI 0.16 to 0.62) to "substantial" for epigastric tenderness ($\kappa = 0.69$; 95% CI 0.54 to 0.84). Senior residents agreed more consistently with attending physicians than did junior residents, which suggests that experience and expertise may affect the quality of the abdominal examination.[5]

LIVER: EXAMINATION

Patient Positioning

- The patient should be positioned supine with the arms relaxed at the sides and the legs uncrossed.

Inspection

- **Extrahepatic stigmata** of liver disease: Look for dilated veins, jaundice, excoriations, and other extrahepatic signs of liver disease (see pp. 100-102).
- **Skin:** Check for scars, striae, rashes, and other lesions.
- **Umbilicus:** Check location and contour, and look for herniation.
- **Abdomen:** Check contour (flat, protuberant, scaphoid, or bulging flanks) and symmetry, and look for visible masses. Ask the patient to take a deep breath, and observe the hepatic area.

Auscultation

- Use the diaphragm of the stethoscope to auscultate the RUQ for a venous hum or **Cruveilhier's sign,** a humming noise indicative of increased collateral circulation between the portal and systemic circulation. Note any hepatic bruits (which may occur in liver cancer and alcoholic hepatitis) or friction rubs (indicative of inflammation of the peritoneal surface of the liver). A venous hum should be continuous and softer than an arterial bruit.
- If the abdomen is distended or the abdominal muscles are tense, a "scratch test" may be useful for determining the lower border of the liver. Place the diaphragm of the stethoscope over the liver, and with the finger of your other hand, scratch the abdominal surface lightly, moving toward the border of the liver. When you encounter the liver, the sound you hear in the stethoscope is magnified.

Percussion

- Start percussing in an area of tympany below the umbilicus in the RLQ, and percuss upward to the lower border of the liver dullness in the midclavicular line (MCL). Failure to correctly identify the MCL will lead to an imprecise measurement because of the shape of the liver (Figure 3-5). Mark the area of transition from tympany to dullness with a skin marker. Next, percuss in an area of lung resonance down toward the liver in the MCL. Again, mark the area of transition from resonance to dullness. Measure the span between the two marks. The normal liver spans 6 to 12 cm at the right MCL and 4 to 8 cm in the midsternal line and varies with patient. Measuring by means of percussion typically underestimates the size of the liver.

Palpation

- **Light palpation:** Use a light, gentle dipping motion in the area around the liver. Look at the patient's face for expressions of pain or increased resistance to palpation.
- **Bimanual palpation:** Place your left hand behind the patient, parallel to and supporting the eleventh and twelfth ribs. Remind the patient to relax on your hand.

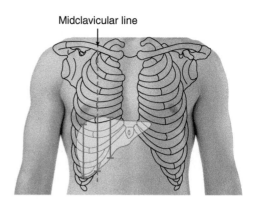

Figure 3-5 Variation in estimated liver span according to deviation from the midclavicular line (MCL). (Based on Naylor CD. Physical examination of the liver. *JAMA*. 1994;271:1859-1865, [Figure 2].)

Press your left hand anteriorly. Place your right hand on the patient's right abdomen, with your fingertips well below the lower border of the liver, oblique or parallel to the right costal margin. Ask the patient to take a deep breath, and press gently posteriorly and cranially to palpate the liver edge as it descends to meet your fingers. If palpable, the edge of a normal liver is soft, well-defined, and regular; its surface is smooth. Try to trace the liver edge laterally and medially. Note any nodules, tenderness, and irregularity.

Evidence

- In one study, investigators used both percussion and palpation to estimate liver size; in comparison with ultrasonographic assessment, these techniques did not enable examiners to reliably detect hepatomegaly. They used a liver percussion span of ≥10 cm or an ultrasonographic span of ≥13 cm as indicative of hepatomegaly in a mixed population of medical inpatients with an average body mass index of 20. The confidence intervals for +LR for percussion included 1 (i.e., not useful), whereas the +LR for palpation was slightly better, ranging from 2.2 to 3.0, for which the 95% CIs did not include 1.[6]
- Palpability of the liver edge increases the probability of hepatomegaly slightly (+LR 2.5; 95% CI 2.2 to 2.8).[7]

Pearls

- Use indirect **fist percussion** to check for liver tenderness when the liver is not palpable. Place the palm of your left hand over the lower right rib cage. Gently strike the dorsal surface of your left hand with your right fist. Compare the sensation in the LUQ and RUQ of the abdomen. The healthy liver is not tender to percussion.
- A pulsatile liver edge may be associated with tricuspid valvular disease or constrictive pericarditis.

SPLEEN: EXAMINATION

Patient Positioning

- The patient should initially be positioned supine with the arms relaxed at the sides and the legs uncrossed. The patient is asked to roll onto the right side (right lateral decubitus position) for Nixon's method of percussion and as part of splenic palpation.

Inspection

- **Skin:** Look for scars, striae, dilated veins, rashes, and other lesions.
- **Umbilicus:** Check location and contour, and look for herniation.
- **Abdomen:** Check contour (flat, protuberant, scaphoid, bulging flanks) and symmetry, and look for visible masses. Ask the patient to take a deep breath, and observe the splenic area.

Auscultation

- Place the diaphragm of the stethoscope in the LUQ, tenth intercostal space. Listen for a splenic friction rub, as in inflammation of the peritoneal surface of the spleen (e.g., splenic infarct).

Percussion

- The spleen enlarges anteriorly, caudally, and medially toward the right iliac fossa. When the spleen is enlarged, the tympany of the colon and stomach is replaced by the dullness of a solid organ. Percuss for the spleen, beginning in the right iliac fossa toward the left costal margin.
- **Castell's sign:** Percuss the lowest intercostal space in the left anterior axillary line; this area is usually tympanitic. Ask the patient to take a deep breath, and percuss again. The percussion note should remain tympanitic if the spleen is of normal size. A change in percussion note from tympany to dullness constitutes a positive Castell's sign and is suggestive of splenic enlargement.
- **Traube's space:** Percuss along Traube's space (lower left anterior chest wall between the area of lung resonance above and the costal margin below). Note the lateral extent of tympany, which marks the splenic border (midaxillary line). Traube's space may also be defined as the space bordered by the left anterior sixth rib, midaxillary line, and costal margin. Dullness in Traube's space is suggestive of splenic enlargement.
- **Nixon's method:** With the patient in the right lateral decubitus position, begin to percuss at the midpoint of the left costal margin, and proceed in the perpendicular plane toward the axillary region. A span of dullness exceeding 8 cm is indicative of splenomegaly (Figure 3-6).

Palpation

- The normal spleen is usually not palpable.
- **Light palpation:** Gently palpate, using a light dipping motion, in the LUQ. Increased resistance to palpation and changes in facial expression such as grimacing are suggestive of tenderness.
- **Bimanual palpation:** Use your left hand to reach over the patient and support his or her lower left rib cage. Starting in the right iliac fossa, use your right hand to palpate across the midline toward the region below the left costal margin. Ask the patient to take a deep breath. Try to palpate the tip or edge of the spleen as it comes down to meet your fingertips. Attempt to palpate the splenic notch. Note any tenderness. Assess the splenic contour, and measure the distance between the spleen's lowest

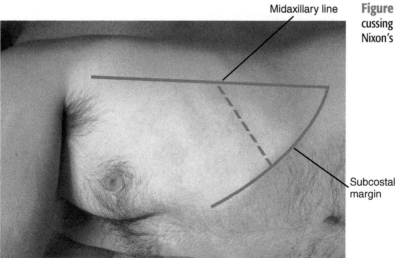

Midaxillary line

Subcostal margin

Figure 3-6 Area for percussing the spleen according to Nixon's method.

Table 3-2 Usefulness of Percussion in Detecting Splenomegaly		
Percussion Technique	**+LR**	**−LR**
To elicit Castell's sign	4.8	0.2
Percussion in Traube's space	2.2	0.5
Nixon's method	**9.8**	0.4

Modified from Grover SA, Barkun AN, Sackett DL. The rational clinical examination: does this patient have splenomegaly? *JAMA.* 1993;270:2218-2221.
−LR, Negative likelihood ratio; +LR, positive likelihood ratio.
Boldface represents findings associated with positive likelihood ratios ≥5 or with negative likelihood ratios ≤0.2. These are said to be moderate- to high-impact items.

point and the left costal margin. Repeat with the patient lying on the right side with the legs slightly flexed at the hips and knees. In this position, gravity may render the spleen more easily palpable.

Evidence

- Bedside examination of the spleen is of limited usefulness when the clinical suspicion of splenomegaly is less than 10%. If clinical suspicion is higher (>10%), imaging may be required because clinical examination is not sensitive and specific enough to confidently exclude splenomegaly (Table 3-2). Palpation for splenomegaly has a +LR of 7.3 and a −LR of 0.5. The presence of both percussion dullness and a palpable spleen likely confirms splenomegaly.[8]

HERNIAS: EXAMINATION

- A **hernia** is the protrusion of a structure or viscus through the tissues that normally contain it. The most common type of hernia is an inguinal hernia.
- An **indirect inguinal hernia** passes through the internal inguinal ring, lateral to the inferior epigastric artery, into the inguinal canal. Indirect inguinal hernias are the most common type of hernia and often occur in younger patients. With a patent processus vaginalis, this hernia can extend into the scrotum or labia majora.
- A **direct inguinal hernia** protrudes through the abdominal wall, medial to the inferior epigastric artery, and usually emerges near the superficial inguinal ring. Direct inguinal hernias are often the result of weakness in the transversalis fascia and are associated with increased age and thinning musculature.
- In a **femoral hernia,** the viscus passes through the femoral ring into the femoral canal. The hernia is palpable just inferior to the inguinal ligament. Femoral hernias occur almost exclusively in women. Because of the small space through which a femoral hernia protrudes, it is at high risk for strangulation.
- Hernias may also develop at the umbilicus **(umbilical hernia)** or at the site of a surgical incision **(incisional hernia).**
- **Spigelian hernias** are rare. These occur when a viscus protrudes through the linea semilunaris at the lateral edge of the rectus sheath.

Patient Positioning

- The examination for a hernia may start with the patient supine and be repeated with the patient in a standing position. If the mass is notable and can be characterized while the patient is supine, the patient need not stand.

Inspection

- Inspect the anterior abdominal wall, groin, and external genitalia for skin changes, lumps, bulges, scars, venous engorgement, and asymmetry.
- Describe the shape and location of any masses.

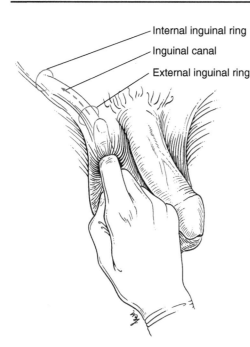

Internal inguinal ring
Inguinal canal
External inguinal ring

Figure 3-7 Examination for inguinal hernia. (From Swartz M. *Textbook of Physical Diagnosis: History and Examination.* 6th ed. Philadelphia: Saunders; 2010 [p. 539, Figure 18-33].)

- Ask the patient to cough or bear down. Inspect the anterior abdominal wall and inguinal wall for any changes in contour. A groin mass with a transmitted cough impulse is most likely to represent a hernia.
- Use a small light source to transilluminate a scrotal mass. A hernia or tumor cannot be transilluminated.

Auscultation
- If a bulge is identified in the groin or genitalia, it may be auscultated with the diaphragm of the stethoscope. Listen for any bowel sounds (presence of bowel within the mass).

Palpation
- Palpate any identified masses. Note the size and consistency of the mass and whether it is reducible. Note any tenderness.
- **Inguinal hernias** (Figure 3-7): Place your index finger on the scrotal skin above the testicle. Gently invaginate the skin, and follow the spermatic cord into the inguinal canal. In this position, ask the patient to cough or bear down. If a hernia is present, you will feel a transmitted cough impulse against your finger with this maneuver (performing the examination with the patient standing may facilitate hernia identification). An impulse that strikes the tip of the finger is likely to represent an indirect hernia, whereas an impulse that strikes the pad of the finger or the side of the finger is more consistent with a direct inguinal hernia. Look at the patient's face for indications of pain during the examination.

DIGITAL RECTAL EXAMINATION: EXAMINATION

- The DRE is part of many clinical assessments such as GI bleeding, abdominal pain, major trauma, and cancer surveillance. It can also be part of a therapeutic approach to stool impaction.

Patient Positioning
- The patient may be positioned in a number of ways for the DRE. Consider the patient's comfort during this sensitive examination. Ask the patient to lie on his or her left side and to flex the knees, bringing them toward the chest. Alternatively, the

patient can be examined standing, bent over the examination table. The lithotomy position (supine at the end of the examining table with knees flexed and feet in stirrups) is also useful.

Inspection
- Spread the buttocks, and inspect the anus and perianal area for inflammation, bleeding, fistulas, fissures, or hemorrhoids. Asking the patient to strain may accentuate hemorrhoids.

Palpation
- Begin by palpating any abnormal areas detected on inspection of the anus and perianal area, noting any tenderness or induration.
- Now explain the rectal examination to the patient, and warn him or her about the coolness of the lubricant.
- Use your gloved, index finger to apply gentle, steady pressure at the anus. Ask the patient to take a deep breath, and insert your finger into the patient's rectum (Figure 3-8).
- Note **sphincter tone.** This is especially important in evaluating for neurologic injury.
- Palpate the **rectal walls** for polyps or masses. Ensure that you fully palpate the anterior, posterior, and lateral walls of the rectum. The sensation of external compression on the rectum or a rectal shelf is known as **Blumer's shelf** and is associated with malignancy.
- In a male patient, palpate the **prostate** gland, which lies anterior to the anterior rectal wall in men. Note any tenderness and the size, symmetry, consistency, and nodularity of the prostate gland. Tenderness is suggestive of prostatitis. In cases of trauma, a "high-riding" prostate is associated with urethral disruption.
- After the examination is complete, inspect your gloved finger for blood, and note the color of the stool. Use a guaiac test to check the stool for the presence of occult blood.

Evidence
- It is said that the DRE should be omitted only "if the patient does not have an anus or the examiner does not have fingers." However, the evidence suggests that the DRE may not contribute much diagnostically with regard to trauma and patients with RLQ pain. For example, a British study of patients with RLQ pain revealed that right-sided tenderness on the DRE had a +LR of 1.2 (95% CI 1.0 to 1.5) and a −LR of 0.9 (95% CI 0.8 to 1.0) for the diagnosis of appendicitis.[9]

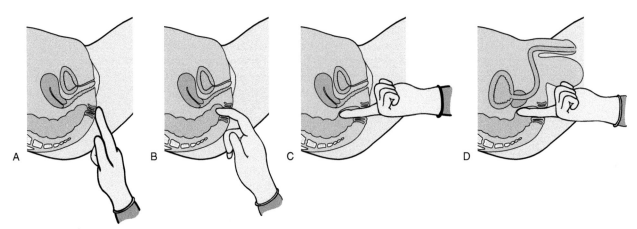

Figure 3-8 Technique for digital rectal examination. **A,** Applying pressure to the rectum. **B,** Insertion of examiner's finger into patient's rectum. **C,** Anatomic considerations for rectal examination in a woman. **D,** Anatomic considerations for rectal examination in a man. (From Munro JF, Campbell IW, eds. *Macleod's Clinical Examination.* 10th ed. Edinburgh: Churchill Livingstone; 2000 [p. 175, Figure 5.22].)

ASCITES: EXAMINATION

- **Ascites** is the effusion and accumulation of fluid in the peritoneal cavity. It is clinically detectable when >500 mL has accumulated. The patient may notice increased abdominal girth or weight gain. Massive ascites may cause shortness of breath because the ascitic abdomen prevents movement of the diaphragm and lung expansion.

Patient Positioning
- The patient should be positioned supine with the arms relaxed at the sides and the legs uncrossed.

Inspection
- Observe the shape of the abdomen and flanks. Suspect ascites in patients with bulging flanks, a protuberant abdomen, and a protruding umbilicus.

Palpation
- **Fluid wave** (Figure 3-9): Ask the patient or an assistant to press the hypothenar aspect of one or both hands firmly down the midline of the patient's abdomen. This stops transmission of a wave through fat. Tap one flank sharply with your fingertips, and palpate on the opposite flank for an impulse transmitted through fluid. An easily detected fluid wave is suggestive of ascites. This test result is often not positive until ascites is obvious and is sometimes positive in patients without ascites.

Percussion
- Ascitic fluid characteristically sinks with gravity, whereas gas-filled loops of bowel float to the top. Thus, percussion produces a dull note in dependent areas of the ascitic abdomen. In a supine patient, look for dullness of the flanks by percussing outward in several directions from the central area of tympany. Using a skin marker, map the border between tympany and dullness.
- **Shifting dullness** (Figure 3-10): Ask the patient to turn onto one side. Wait 20 to 25 seconds. Percuss from an area of tympany (upper side) to dullness (dependent

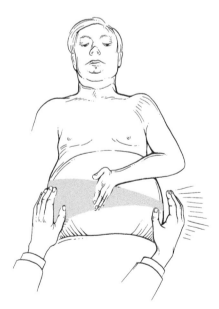

Figure 3-9 Testing for a fluid wave. (From Swartz M. *Textbook of Physical Diagnosis: History and Examination*. 6th ed. Philadelphia: Saunders; 2010 [p. 497, Figure 17-19].)

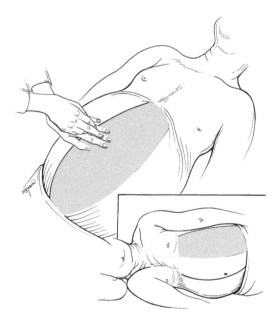

Figure 3-10 Testing for shifting dullness. *Shaded areas* represent areas where dullness transitions to tympany. Note the shift to dependent areas in accordance with changes in patient position. (From Swartz M. *Textbook of Physical Diagnosis: History and Examination*. 6th ed. Philadelphia: Saunders; 2010 [p. 497, Figure 17-18].)

side) in several places to map the border between tympany and dullness. In a normal patient, the borders between tympany and dullness are relatively constant. In an ascitic abdomen, the dullness will shift to the dependent portion of the abdomen.

DYSPHAGIA: HISTORY

> **INSTRUCTIONS TO CANDIDATE: A 57-year-old man presents to his family physician, complaining of "trouble swallowing." He is losing weight because he is unable to eat. Obtain a detailed history, exploring possible causes.**

DD$_X$: VITAMINS C
- Traumatic: Ingestion of a caustic substance
- Autoimmune/allergic: Collagen vascular disease (e.g., scleroderma)
- Metabolic: Iron-deficiency anemia (Plummer-Vinson syndrome)
- Idiopathic/iatrogenic: Benign esophageal stricture, achalasia, and neurogenic disorders (e.g., stroke, Parkinson disease, bulbar palsy, Guillain-Barré syndrome, amyotrophic lateral sclerosis [Lou Gehrig disease])
- Neoplastic: Esophageal, pharyngeal, mediastinal (e.g., lung, lymphoma)
- Congenital/genetic: Pharyngeal pouch

History
- Ask the patient the following:
  - Character: "Describe your difficulty with swallowing."
    - "Do you have difficulty initiating swallowing or making swallowing movements (indicative of neuromuscular disease)? Any aspiration?"
    - "Does food or liquid ever come out your nose (indicative of pharyngeal pouch)?"
    - "Do you have trouble swallowing solids, liquids, or both?"
  - Location: "Where does the food get stuck: In your chest? In your throat?"
  - Onset: "When did it start? How has it progressed (e.g., initial difficulty with solids and then liquids)? Is it getting worse? How quickly? Has the pattern changed? If so, how?"
  - Radiation: "Is swallowing painful? Any pain elsewhere?"
  - Intensity: If pain is a salient feature: "Describe the type of pain (sharp, burning, squeezing, or cramping). How severe is the pain on a scale of 1 to 10, with 1 being mild pain and 10 being the worst? How does your swallowing difficulty affect your daily life?"
  - Duration: "How long does the pain last? Do you experience difficulty swallowing every time you have a meal or drink something?"
  - Events associated:
    - "Do you have nausea or vomiting? Reflux? Nasal or oral regurgitation? What do the regurgitated contents look like?"
    - "Do you have wheezing (compression of airway by a mass)? Hoarseness? Hemoptysis?"
    - Neurogenic: "Are you experiencing weakness? Tremor? Diplopia?"
    - Diet: "What are you eating?"
    - Constitutional symptoms: "Are you experiencing fever, chills, night sweats, weight loss, anorexia, or asthenia?"
  - Frequency: "How often does the pain happen? Is it intermittent or constant?"
  - Palliative factors: "Does anything make the pain better? If so, what?"
  - Provocative factors: "Does anything make the pain worse? If so, what?"
- **PMH/PSH:** Nasogastric tube, gastroesophageal reflux disease, Barrett esophagus, esophageal cancer, neuromuscular disorders, collagen vascular disease, ischemic heart disease/angina, diabetes mellitus, iron deficiency, or ingestion of caustic agent

- **MEDS:** Previous radiation therapy, taking pills without water, ingestion of antacids, iron supplementation
- **SH:** Smoking, use of EtOH, and use of street drugs
- **FH:** Esophageal cancer, neuromuscular disease

Evidence

- Patients who have malnutrition that is severe, as measured by the Subjective Global Assessment tool, are more likely to experience postoperative complications (+LR 4.4).[10] This assessment tool classifies patients as well nourished, moderately or suspected to be malnourished, or severely malnourished, by focusing on the following characteristics[10]:
  - Weight loss in the previous 6 months: <5% is insignificant, 5% to 10% is potentially significant, >10% is definitely significant
  - Dietary intake in relation to the patient's usual intake: normal or decreased
  - Significant GI symptoms such as anorexia, nausea, vomiting, and diarrhea that are present nearly daily for 2 or more weeks
  - Functional capacity: full capacity or decreased function
  - Physical findings of malnutrition:
    - Loss of subcutaneous fat (triceps muscle, costal margin, interossei of the hand, deltoid muscle)
    - Muscle wasting (deltoid, quadriceps muscles)
    - Ankle edema
    - Sacral edema
    - Ascites
- The Patient Generated Subjective Global Assessment tool is useful in hospitalized patients with cancer; it can be used to predict the classification of malnutrition on the basis of the Subjective Global Assessment score (+LR 5.6; 95% CI 2.0 to 15.5; −LR 0.02; 95% CI 0.003 to 0.16).[11]

HEMATEMESIS: HISTORY

> **INSTRUCTIONS TO CANDIDATE: A 42-year-old homeless woman well known to the emergency department presents, complaining of vomiting for 2 days. She now notes blood in her emesis. Obtain a detailed history, exploring possible causes.**

DD$_X$: VITAMINS C

- **V**ascular: Esophageal varices, angiodysplasia, and aortoenteric fistula
- **T**raumatic: Mallory-Weiss tear, nose bleed (swallowed blood)
- **M**etabolic: Coagulopathy
- **I**diopathic/**i**atrogenic: Esophagitis, gastritis, and peptic ulcer disease (PUD)
- **S**ubstance abuse and **p**sychiatric
- **First evaluate airway, breathing, and circulation (ABCs).** It may be necessary to perform an immediate intervention, such as administering supplemental O_2, establishing intravenous access, or initiating airway management.
  - Is the patient able to talk? Swallow? Cough?
  - Are both lungs ventilated? Is the patient oxygenating (check mentation, pulse oximetry)?
  - Are vital signs abnormal? Is the peripheral circulation (pulses, capillary refill) abnormal?
  - If no immediate interventions are required, proceed to obtain the history.

History

- Ask the patient the following:
  - **Character:** "Describe the bleeding. Have you noticed bright red blood or coffee grounds in your vomit? Did you begin to vomit before the bleeding began

(indicative of protracted retching and vomiting as in a Mallory-Weiss tear), or did you vomit blood from the outset?"

- Location: "Where is the blood coming from? Are you coughing up blood, vomiting blood, or swallowing blood from a nosebleed, for example?"
- Onset: "When was the first time this bleeding happened? How has it progressed (sudden versus insidious)?"
- Radiation: "Any other bleeding (bleeding from another location)? Nosebleed? Lower GI bleeding?"
- Intensity: "How severe is the bleeding? Has it gotten worse? How much blood have you vomited (quantify)?"
- Duration: "How long has the bleeding been going on (acute versus chronic)"?
- Events associated:
  - "Have you had abdominal pain? What is your stool like (melena, hematochezia)?"
  - "Have you experienced weakness/fatigue (indicative of anemia)? Chest pain?"
  - "Have you experienced palpitations or shortness of breath? Lightheadedness or fainting?"
  - "Have you noticed easy bruising? Prolonged bleeding from cuts or dental work?"
  - "Was your bleeding preceded by protracted retching or vomiting (indicative of Mallory-Weiss tear)?"
  - "Have you been taking nonsteroidal anti-inflammatory drugs (NSAIDs) or drinking a lot of alcohol?" The use of NSAIDs or EtOH is sometimes associated with gastritis, which is often painless.
  - "Have you had periodic epigastric pain lasting weeks or longer, which may have been relieved by food or antacids? Have you been waking at night with epigastric pain?" Such a history may be indicative of PUD.
  - "Have you had fever, chills, night sweats, weight loss, anorexia, or asthenia (constitutional symptoms)?"
- Frequency: "Has this blood with vomiting happened before? How often does the bleeding happen (intermittent versus constant)?"
- Palliative factors: "Does anything make the vomiting and bleeding better? If so, what?"
- Provocative factors: "Does anything make the vomiting and bleeding worse? If so, what?"
- **Previous investigations:** Upper GI series, endoscopy, or previous requirement for transfusions
- **PMH/PSH:** PUD, liver disease, coagulopathy, esophageal varices, previous GI bleeding, previous GI surgery, or AAA repair (aortoenteric fistula)
- **MEDS:** NSAIDs/acetylsalicylic acid (ASA), anticoagulants, or corticosteroids
- **SH:** Smoking, use of EtOH, use of street drugs
- **FH:** Coagulopathy

DIARRHEA: HISTORY

INSTRUCTIONS TO CANDIDATE: A 33-year-old man presents to the emergency department with a 6-day history of diarrhea and intermittent vomiting. He vomits twice in the triage center. Obtain a detailed history, exploring possible causes.

DD$_X$: VITAMINS C
- Vascular: Ischemic colitis
- Infectious: Bacterial, parasitic, or viral gastroenteritis; pseudomembranous colitis
- Autoimmune/allergic: Celiac disease, Whipple disease
- Metabolic: Drug reactions, carcinoid syndrome, hyperthyroidism
- Idiopathic/iatrogenic: IBD, IBS, malabsorption, runner's diarrhea
- Congenital/genetic: Cystic fibrosis, lactose intolerance

Table 3-3 Pinpointing the Source of Diarrhea

Small Bowel	Large Bowel
Large-volume stools	Frequent, small-volume stools
Gross blood is infrequent	Gross blood may be present
Foul-smelling liquid stools ± undigested food (malabsorption caused by sloughed villi)	Tenesmus

History
- Ask the patient the following:
  - Character: "Describe your bowel movements" (Table 3-3).
    - "Are the stools frequent, voluminous, and poorly formed (diarrhea)?"
    - "Are the stools large, oily, malodorous but somewhat formed (steatorrhea)?"
    - "Are the stools frequent and formed but small?"
    - "Is any blood, pus, or mucus in the stool? Describe the color of your stool."
    - "Does diarrhea persist even after you fast?"
    - "Do you experience nocturnal diarrhea or fecal incontinence?"
    - "Have your bowel habits changed in any way? Describe your usual bowel movements."
    - "Describe the emesis. Does it have the appearance of blood or coffee grounds?"
  - Location: "Where were you when the vomiting and diarrhea started? Have you traveled recently?"
  - Onset: "When did the diarrhea start (sudden versus insidious)? When did the vomiting start?"
  - Intensity: "How severe are the diarrhea and vomiting? What is the number of stools per day, and what is the approximate volume of stool? Has it gotten worse? What is the number of episodes of vomiting per day? Has it gotten worse? Are you able to keep down any fluids?"
  - Duration: "How long has the diarrhea been going on (acute versus chronic)? How long have you been vomiting?"
  - Events associated:
    - "Have you had fever or chills? Abdominal pain? How is your appetite? Have you experienced orthostatic presyncope or syncope?"
    - "Have you consumed dairy or meat products in preceding 72 hours (undercooked hamburger or chicken, shellfish; ask about lactose intolerance)? Have you eaten excessive cereal, prunes, or roughage?"
    - "Have you had periods of constipation (which occur in IBS)?"
    - "Have you traveled to tropical or subtropical regions? Have you had infectious contacts? Could you have ingested contaminated water?"
    - "What are your sexual practices (check for anal penetration)? Do you have an increased urge to defecate (tenesmus)?"
    - IBD: "Have you had chronic diarrhea, abdominal pain, tenesmus, weight loss, or extraintestinal manifestations (e.g., uveitis, erythema nodosum, and peripheral arthritis)?"
    - Constitutional symptoms: "Have you had fever, chills, night sweats, weight loss, anorexia, or asthenia?"
  - Frequency: "Has this ever happened to you before? Is every bowel movement like diarrhea (intermittent versus constant)?"
  - Palliative factors: "Does anything make these symptoms better? If so, what?"
    - Fasting
    - Oral rehydration therapy
    - Antiemetics; antidiarrheal agents

■ Provocative factors: "Does anything make it worse? If so, what?
  ◆ Dairy products
  ◆ Solid foods
- **Previous investigations:** Stool analysis, endoscopy
- **PMH/PSH:** IBD, celiac disease, hyperthyroidism, previous GI surgery, cystic fibrosis, human immunodeficiency virus (HIV) infection/acquired immune deficiency syndrome (AIDS), or malignancy
- **MEDS:** Laxatives, antidiarrheal agents, antibiotics (pseudomembranous colitis), corticosteroids, quinidine, or antihypertensive agents
- **SH:** Smoking, use of EtOH, diet, and sexual practices (anal penetration)
- **FH:** IBD, cystic fibrosis, GI malignancy, or celiac disease

EXTRAHEPATIC MANIFESTATIONS OF LIVER DISEASE: PHYSICAL EXAMINATION

> **INSTRUCTIONS TO CANDIDATE: A 27-year-old man with chronic viral hepatitis presents with jaundice. Perform a focused physical examination for extrahepatic manifestations of liver disease (Figure 3-11).**

Vital Signs
- Heart rate (HR), blood pressure (BP), respiratory rate (RR), and temperature
- Fever (may be noted in acute viral hepatitis, alcoholic hepatitis, or infection such as spontaneous bacterial peritonitis)

General
- **Fetor hepaticus (liver breath):** Caused by volatile sulfur compounds produced by intestinal bacteria that accumulate in the blood and urine as a result of defective hepatic metabolism
- **Cirrhotic habitus:** Wasted extremities with protuberant belly
- **Muscle wasting:** Temporalis muscle, first digiti interosseous muscle
- **Vitamin deficiency:** Beefy tongue, angular cheilosis, and koilonychia

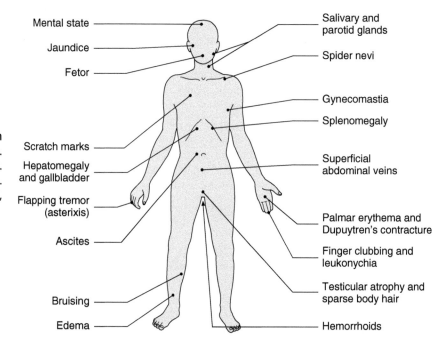

Figure 3-11 Areas for focused examination and clinical features of advanced liver disease. (Adapted from Munro JF, Campbell IW, eds. *Macleod's Clinical Examination.* 10th ed. Edinburgh: Churchill Livingstone; 2000 [p. 67, Figure 5.14].)

Skin

- Xanthelasma, tendon xanthomas
- Jaundice, excoriations
- Spider nevi: Arterioles in the skin with radiating capillary branches that resemble the legs of a spider. It blanches with diascopy (use of a transparent microscope slide to apply pressure over a lesion and observe its behavior).
- Caput medusae: Dilated cutaneous veins radiating from the umbilicus
- Petechiae, ecchymosis
- Edema caused by hypoalbuminemia
- **Hands:**
  - **Dupuytren contracture:** thickening and shortening of the fibrous bands in palmar fascia
  - Palmar erythema
  - **Leukonychia:** Pale nails, caused by hypoalbuminemia
  - Clubbing

Head, Eyes, Ears, Nose, and Throat (HEENT)

- Parotid gland hypertrophy
- Scleral icterus
- Virchow node: A firm, palpable left infraclavicular lymph node. Its presence is presumptive evidence of visceral malignancy, generally intra-abdominal.

Abdomen

- Examine the spleen and liver for enlargement, noting the consistency and any tenderness (see pp. 89-92).
- Examine for ascites (see pp. 95-96).
- Pale stools caused by malabsorption (biliary obstruction)

Genitourinary System

- **Hypogonadism:** Testicular atrophy, impotence, and loss of pubic hair (especially axillary)
- Gynecomastia (caused by impaired estrogen conjugation)
- Dark urine (caused by hyperbilirubinemia)

Neurologic System

- Personality changes
- Confusion, altered level of consciousness caused by toxic nitrogenous substances in systemic circulation
- **Asterixis:** Involuntary jerking movements, especially in the hands, caused by the arrhythmic lapses of sustained posture. It is best elicited by asking the patient to extend his or her arms, extend the wrists, and spread the fingers.
- Constructional apraxia (e.g., difficulty drawing five-point star)
- Ataxia

Findings Associated with Other Hepatic Disease

- **Kayser-Fleischer ring:** Green-yellow pigmented ring around cornea, caused by copper deposited in Descemet membrane, in association with Wilson disease
- **Tanned skin appearance:** Deposition of iron in skin in association with hemochromatosis

Evidence

- Table 3-4 shows sensitivities and specificities derived from a meta-analysis of studies of the use of clinical examination to diagnose histologically confirmed cirrhosis. The patients were highly selected on the basis of suspicion of liver disease (e.g., elevated liver enzyme levels) and referral for liver biopsy; in other words, the study groups had a high pretest probability.[12]

Table 3-4 Usefulness of Clinical Examination in Diagnosis of Cirrhosis

Clinical Feature	Sensitivity (95% CI)	Specificity (95% CI)
Ascites	34% (22%–49%)	95% (89%–98%)
Collateral circulation	42% (26%–61%)	94% (71%–99%)
Encephalopathy	15% (6%–33%)	98% (97%–99%)
Firm liver	68% (55%–79%)	75% (62%–85%)
Jaundice	36% (25%–48%)	85% (80%–89%)
Spider angiomata	50% (39%–61%)	88% (75%–95%)

From de Bruyn G, Graviss EA. A systematic review of the diagnostic accuracy of physical examination for the detection of cirrhosis. *BMC Med Inform Decis Mak.* 2001;1:8 (Table 3). CI, Confidence interval.

Pearl
- Portal hypertension is associated with clinical manifestations at areas of portal-systemic anastomosis: esophageal veins (esophageal varices), rectal veins (hemorrhoids), and paraumbilical veins (caput medusae).

RIGHT LOWER QUADRANT PAIN: HISTORY AND PHYSICAL EXAMINATION

INSTRUCTIONS TO CANDIDATE: An 18-year-old woman presents to the emergency department with RLQ pain and loss of appetite since yesterday. Obtain a focused history, and perform a focused physical examination, exploring possible causes.

DD$_X$: VITAMINS C
- Infectious: PID/tubo-ovarian abscess, psoas abscess
- Traumatic: Musculoskeletal injury
- Idiopathic/iatrogenic: Appendicitis, mesenteric adenitis, ascending diverticulitis, incarcerated hernia, Crohn disease, ruptured ectopic pregnancy, ovarian torsion, and renal colic

History
- Ask the patient the following:
  - Character: "What is the pain like: sharp and localized? Crampy? Dull?"
  - Location: "Where does the pain originate?"
  - Onset: "When did the pain start? How did it come on (sudden versus gradual)?"
  - Radiation: "Does the pain move anywhere?"
  - Intensity: "How severe is the pain on a scale of 1 to 10, with 1 being mild pain and 10 being the worst?"
    - "Is the pain getting better, getting worse, or staying the same?"
  - Duration: "How long does the pain last (intermittent versus constant)?"
  - Events associated:
    - Appendicitis: "Have you had fever, nausea or vomiting, loss of appetite, or initial dull central abdominal pain that later localized to the RLQ?"
    - Pregnancy: "When was your most recent menstrual period? Have you had any vaginal bleeding?"
    - PID: "Have you had fever, foul vaginal discharge, or intermenstrual bleeding?"
    - Renal colic: "Have you had blood in your urine? Have you passed any stones or gritty urine?"
    - Intestinal obstruction/incarcerated hernia: "When did you last pass a bowel movement or flatus? Have you been vomiting?"
    - Crohn disease: "Have you had chronic diarrhea, weight loss, or extraintestinal manifestations (e.g., uveitis, erythema nodosum, and peripheral arthritis)?"

- Frequency: "Have you ever had this pain before? How often does the pain come?"
- Palliative factors: "Does anything make the pain better? If so, what (e.g., lying in a particular position)?"
- Provocative factors: "Does anything make the pain worse? If so, what (e.g., movement)?"
- **PMH/PSH:** Previous surgeries, malignancy, IBD, IBS, PID, sexually transmitted infection, ectopic pregnancy, or renal colic
- **MEDS:** Analgesics
- **SH:** Smoking, use of EtOH, use of street drugs, and sexual history (sexual practices, number of sexual partners in the last 6-12 months, use of condoms)
- **FH:** IBD, renal colic

Physical Examination
- **Vital signs (Vitals):** Measure HR, BP, RR, and temperature.
  - Low-grade fever and mild tachycardia may be noted in appendicitis.
- **General:** Document apprehension and flushed appearance. Check capillary refill. Note patient's position on the stretcher and whether she is lying still or moving about. Note any apparent distress.
- **HEENT:** Look at the mucous membranes to gauge hydration. Inspect the sclerae.
- **Respiratory system (Resp):** Check chest expansion (symmetry), and auscultate the lungs (breath sounds, adventitious sounds).
- **Cardiovascular system (CVS):** Palpate peripheral pulses. Note pulse volume, contour, and rhythm. Auscultate the heart, listening for extra heart sounds or flow murmurs associated with hyperdynamic circulation.
- **Abdomen:** Inspect the abdomen. Auscultate for bowel sounds (which may be decreased in peritonitis). Before you decide that bowel sounds are absent, listen in each quadrant for 2 to 3 minutes. Percuss lightly in all four quadrants. Percussion produces pain in a patient with appendicitis or peritonitis. Before you palpate, ask the patient to cough and to point to the most tender area with one finger. Palpate the most tender area last. Perform light and deep palpation, and identify any masses or areas of tenderness. Check for rebound tenderness. Examine the liver and spleen. Perform a DRE. A retrocecal appendix may produce tenderness on palpation of the rectal walls.
- **Genitourinary:** It is important to perform a pelvic examination (see p. 310). Note any discharge, inflammation of the cervix, cervical motion tenderness, adnexal tenderness, or pelvic masses. Note uterine size.

Evidence
- Table 3-5 shows how parts of the clinical examination may help to diagnose acute appendicitis.

Pearls
- In acute appendicitis, rebound tenderness is referred to as **McBurney's point.**
- A patient with appendicitis may have positive **psoas, obturator,** and **Rovsing's signs.**

Table 3-5	Usefulness of Clinical Examination in Diagnosis of Acute Appendicitis	
Clinical Feature	**+LR (95% CI)**	**−LR (95% CI)**
Migration of pain to RLQ*	3.2 (2.4–4.2)	0.5 (0.4–0.6)
Anorexia*	1.3 (1.1–1.4)	0.6 (0.5–0.8)
Temperature >37.2° C†	1.3 (0.97–1.7)	0.8 (0.65–1.0)
"Fever"*	1.9 (1.6–2.3)	0.58 (0.51–0.67)
Tenderness in RLQ‡	1.2 (1.1–1.2)	0.2 (0.1–0.4)
Guarding‡	1.6 (1.5–1.8)	0.5 (0.46–0.6)
Rebound tenderness‡	1.8 (1.6–2.0)	0.5 (0.46–0.6)
Rigidity*	3.8 (2.96–4.8)	0.8 (0.79–0.85)
Psoas sign*	2.4 (1.2–4.7)	0.9 (0.83–0.98)
DRE‡	1.2 (1.0–1.5)	0.9 (0.8–1.0)

*Data from Wagner JM, McKinney WP, Carpenter JL. Does this patient have appendicitis? *JAMA*. 1996;276:1589-1594.

†Data from Cardall T, Glasser J, Guss DA. Clinical value of the total white blood cell count and temperature in the evaluation of patients with suspected appendicitis. *Acad Emerg Med*. 2004;11:1021-1027.

‡Data from Dixon JM, Elton RA, Rainey JB, et al. Rectal examination in patients with pain in the right lower quadrant of the abdomen. *BMJ*. 1991;302:386-388.

CI, Confidence interval; DRE, digital rectal examination; −LR, negative likelihood ratio; +LR, positive likelihood ratio; RLQ, right lower quadrant.

RIGHT UPPER QUADRANT PAIN AND JAUNDICE: HISTORY AND PHYSICAL EXAMINATION

INSTRUCTIONS TO CANDIDATE: A 40-year-old woman presents to the emergency department with severe RUQ pain for 8 hours. She is also worried because her friend told her she looked yellow. Obtain a focused history, and perform a focused physical examination.

DD$_X$: VITAMINS C (Jaundice)
- **I**nfectious: Viral hepatitis
- **T**raumatic: Resorption of a large hematoma
- **A**utoimmune/**a**llergic: Autoimmune hepatitis
- **M**etabolic: Hemolysis
- **I**diopathic/**i**atrogenic: Biliary obstruction (stone/stricture)
- **N**eoplastic: Obstructing biliary lesion
- **S**ubstance abuse and **p**sychiatric: Alcoholic or toxic hepatitis
- **C**ongenital/genetic: Gilbert syndrome

DD$_X$: VITAMINS C (RUQ Pain)
- **V**ascular: Right-sided heart failure (congestive hepatomegaly)
- **I**nfectious: Acute pyelonephritis, right-sided pneumonia, and viral hepatitis
- **T**raumatic: Musculoskeletal injury
- **A**utoimmune/**a**llergic: Autoimmune hepatitis
- **I**diopathic/**i**atrogenic: Acute cholecystitis, duodenal ulcer/PUD

History

- Ask the patient the following:
  - **Character:** "What is the pain like? Sharp and localized? Crampy? Dull? Describe your current color."
  - **Location:** "Where does the pain originate?"
  - **Onset:** "When did the pain start? How did it come on (sudden versus gradual)? When did you first notice a change in your skin color?"
  - **Radiation:** "Does the pain move anywhere?"
  - **Intensity:** "How severe is the pain on a scale of 1 to 10, with 1 being mild pain and 10 being the worst? Is the pain or jaundice getting better, getting worse, or staying the same?"
  - **Duration:** "How long does the pain last (intermittent versus constant)? How long have you had jaundice (acute versus chronic)?"
  - **Events associated:**
    - "Have you had fever or chills? Nausea or vomiting? How is your appetite?"
    - "When was your most recent bowel movement? Are you passing flatus? Have you had diarrhea?"
    - "Have you been injured recently?"
    - **Cholelithiasis:** "Do you tolerate fatty meals? Do you have episodic RUQ pain?"
    - **Hepatitis:** "Have you had a recent infection or malaise? Do you have an aversion to smoking? Have you traveled recently? Have you been exposed to persons with hepatitis? Have you had multiple sexual partners? Have you used intravenous drugs? Have you received blood transfusions?"
    - **Biliary obstruction:** "Do you have pale stools, dark urine, or itching (pruritus)?"
    - **Constitutional symptoms:** "Have you had fever, chills, night sweats, weight loss, anorexia, or asthenia?"
  - **Frequency:** "Have you ever had this pain before? How often does the pain come (intermittent versus constant)? Have you ever had jaundice before?"
  - **Palliative factors:** "Does anything make the pain better? If so, what?"
  - **Provocative factors:** "Does anything make the pain worse? If so, what?"
- **PMH/PSH:** Cholelithiasis, hepatitis, cirrhosis, malignancy, hemolytic disorders, or Gilbert syndrome
- **MEDS:** Hepatotoxic drugs (e.g., ASA, isoniazid, methotrexate, anticonvulsants, antipsychotics, oral contraceptive pill, selected herbal preparations)
- **SH:** Smoking, use of EtOH, use of street drugs, use of intravenous drugs, and sexual history
- **Immunizations:** Hepatitis
- **FH:** Wilson disease, hemochromatosis, or Gilbert syndrome

Physical Examination

- **Vitals:** Measure HR, BP, RR, and temperature.
- **General:** Check capillary refill. Note any icterus, and observe the patient's position on the stretcher and whether she is lying still or moving about. Note any apparent distress.
- **HEENT:** Look at the mucous membranes to gauge hydration. Inspect the sclerae.
- **Resp:** Check chest expansion (symmetry), and auscultate the lungs (breath sounds, adventitious sounds).
- **CVS:** Palpate peripheral pulses. Note pulse volume, contour, and rhythm. Auscultate the heart, listening for extra heart sounds or flow murmurs associated with hyperdynamic circulation.
- **Abdomen:** Inspect the abdomen. Auscultate for bowel sounds (which may be decreased in peritonitis). Before you decide that bowel sounds are absent, listen in each quadrant for 2 or 3 minutes. Percuss lightly in all four quadrants. Percussion produces pain in a patient with peritoneal irritation. Before you palpate, ask the patient to cough and to point to the most tender area with one finger. Palpate the most tender area or areas last. Perform light and deep palpation, and identify any

Table 3-6 Usefulness of Clinical Examination in Diagnosis of Acute Cholecystitis

Clinical Feature	No. of Patients	+LR (95% CI)	−LR (95% CI)
Emesis*	1338	1.5 (1.1–2.1)	0.6 (0.3–0.9)
Fever (<35° C)*	1292	1.5 (1.0–2.3)	0.9 (0.8–1.0)
Jaundice on examination†	88	0.9‡	1.0‡
Murphy's sign*	565	2.8 (0.8–8.6)	0.5 (0.2–1.0)
RUQ tenderness*	1001	1.6 (1.0–2.5)	0.4 (0.2–1.1)
Rebound tenderness*	1381	1.0 (0.6–1.7)	1.0 (0.8–1.4)

*Data from Trowbridge RL, Rutkowski NK, Shojania KG. Does this patient have acute cholecystitis? *JAMA.* 2003;289:80-86.
†Data from Singer AJ, McCracken G, Henry MC, et al. Correlation among clinical, laboratory, and hepatobiliary scanning findings in patients with suspected acute cholecystitis. *Ann Emerg Med.* 1996;28:267-272.
‡Confidence interval (CI) not available.
−LR, Negative likelihood ratio; +LR, positive likelihood ratio; RUQ, right upper quadrant.

masses or areas of tenderness. Check for rebound tenderness. Examine the liver and spleen. Note any hepatomegaly or tenderness. Perform a DRE.
- **Murphy's sign:** Slide your fingers under the right costal margin, and ask the patient to take a deep breath. A sharp increase in tenderness or sudden stop in inspiratory effort is suggestive of acute cholecystitis.
- **Neurologic system (Neuro):** Check the patient's mental status (orientation to person, place, and time).

Evidence
- Table 3-6 shows how parts of the clinical examination help diagnose acute cholecystitis.

Pearls
- Charcot triad for cholecystitis: fever, jaundice, and RUQ pain
- Reynold's pentad for ascending cholangitis: Charcot triad plus altered mental status and hypotension
- Courvoisier's sign is a palpable, nontender gallbladder in the setting of jaundice and is often associated with malignancy

EPIGASTRIC PAIN: HISTORY AND PHYSICAL EXAMINATION

INSTRUCTIONS TO CANDIDATE: A 70-year-old man presents to the emergency department with excruciating epigastric pain and vomiting. He has been living alone since his wife died 2 years ago and admits to drinking a "flask daily." Obtain a focused history, and perform a focused physical examination.

DD$_X$: VITAMINS C
- **V**ascular: Leaking/ruptured AAA, myocardial infarction, aortic dissection, and right-sided heart failure (congestive hepatomegaly)
- **I**nfectious: Viral hepatitis, pneumonia
- **T**raumatic: Musculoskeletal injury
- **A**utoimmune/allergic: Autoimmune hepatitis
- **I**diopathic/iatrogenic: Perforated viscus, acute cholecystitis, pancreatitis (e.g., biliary stones), duodenal ulcer/PUD
- **S**ubstance abuse and psychiatric: Alcoholic pancreatitis, alcoholic/toxic hepatitis

- **First evaluate ABCs.** It may be necessary to perform an immediate intervention, such as administering supplemental O_2, establishing intravenous access, or initiating airway management.
  - Is the patient able to talk? Swallow? Cough?
  - Are both lungs ventilated? Is the patient oxygenating (check mentation, pulse oximetry)?
  - Are vital signs abnormal? Is the peripheral circulation (pulses, capillary refill) abnormal?
  - If no immediate interventions are required, proceed to obtain the history, and perform the physical examination.

History
- Ask the patient the following:
  - **Character:** "What is the pain like: sharp and localized? Crampy? Dull? Describe the vomitus. Does it appear to contain any blood or coffee grounds?"
  - **Location:** "Where does the pain originate?"
  - **Onset:** "When did the pain start? How did it come on (sudden versus gradual)? When did the vomiting start?"
  - **Radiation:** "Does the pain move anywhere?"
  - **Intensity:** "How severe is the pain on a scale of 1 to 10, with 1 being mild pain and 10 being the worst? Is it getting better, getting worse, or staying the same? How many episodes of vomiting per day? Has it gotten worse? Are you able to keep down any fluids?"
  - **Duration:** "How long does it last (intermittent versus constant)? How long have you been vomiting?"
  - **Events associated:**
    - "Have you been injured recently? Any falls?"
    - Myocardial infarction: "Have you experienced diaphoresis, shortness of breath, or radiation of pain down your arm or to your jaw?"
    - Pancreatitis: "Have you had central abdominal pain or radiation of pain to the back?"
    - PUD: "Have you had periodic epigastric pain (lasting weeks or longer), relieved by food or antacids? Have you been waking at night with epigastric pain?"
    - Renal colic: "Have you had blood in your urine? Have you passed stones or gritty urine?"
    - Intestinal obstruction/incarcerated hernia: "When did you last pass a bowel movement or flatus? Have you been vomiting?"
    - Constitutional symptoms: "Have you had fever, chills, night sweats, weight loss, anorexia, or asthenia?"
  - **Frequency:** "Have you ever had this pain before? How often does the pain come (intermittent versus constant)?"
  - **Palliative factors:** "Does anything make the pain better? If so, what?"
    - Lying in one position
  - **Provocative factors:** "Does anything make the pain worse? If so, what?"
    - Movement
- **PMH/PSH:** Previous surgery, malignancy, cardiovascular disease (CVD), PUD, biliary colic, renal colic
- **MEDS:** Analgesics, antibiotics, anticoagulants, cardiac medications (e.g., β-blockers would suppress HR)
- **SH:** Smoking, EtOH, street drugs, and sexual history
- **FH:** IBD, renal colic

Physical Examination
- **Vitals:** Measure HR, BP, RR, and temperature.
- **General:** Check capillary refill. Observe the patient's position on the stretcher and whether he is lying still or moving about. Note any apparent distress.

- **Skin:** Note any painful nodules in the extremities (fat necrosis).
- **HEENT:** Look at the mucous membranes to gauge hydration. Inspect the sclerae.
- **Resp:** Check chest expansion (symmetry). Auscultate the lungs, and describe the breath sounds and adventitious sounds. You may note inspiratory crackles in pulmonary edema.
- **CVS:** Measure the jugular venous pressure (JVP), and assess for hepatojugular reflux (increased venous pressure in congestive heart failure [CHF]). Palpate peripheral pulses. Note pulse volume, contour, and rhythm. Inspect and palpate the apical impulse. Palpate for thrills and heaves. Auscultate the heart, listening for an S_3, an S_4, or a murmur. Auscultate for abdominal bruits.
- **Abdomen:** Inspect the abdomen. Blue or green ecchymosis in the flank from extravasation of hemolyzed blood **(Grey Turner's sign)** and bluish discoloration at the umbilicus **(Cullen's sign)** are associated with pancreatitis. Auscultate for bowel sounds (may be decreased in pancreatitis). Percuss lightly in all four quadrants. Percussion produces pain in a patient with peritoneal irritation. Before you palpate, ask the patient to cough and to point to the most tender area with one finger. Palpate the most tender area last. Perform light and deep palpation. Identify any masses (pulsatile or nonpulsatile) or areas of tenderness. Check for rebound tenderness. Examine the liver and spleen. Perform a DRE.

LEFT LOWER QUADRANT PAIN: HISTORY AND PHYSICAL EXAMINATION

INSTRUCTIONS TO CANDIDATE: A 58-year-old woman presents to the emergency department with sharp LLQ pain, worsening over 2 days. She has had one similar episode, which occurred last year and resolved spontaneously over several days. Obtain a focused history, and perform a focused physical examination.

DD$_X$: VITAMINS C
- **V**ascular: Leaking/ruptured AAA, aortic dissection
- **I**nfectious: PID/tubo-ovarian abscess
- **T**raumatic: Musculoskeletal injury
- **I**diopathic/**i**atrogenic: Sigmoid diverticulitis, incarcerated hernia, perforated viscus, Crohn disease, ulcerative colitis, ruptured ectopic pregnancy, ovarian torsion, and renal colic

History
- Ask the patient the following:
  - **Character:** "What is the pain like? Sharp and localized? Crampy? Dull?"
  - **Location:** "Where does the pain originate?"
  - **Onset:** "When did the pain start? How did it come on (sudden versus gradual)?"
  - **Radiation:** "Does the pain move anywhere?"
  - **Intensity:** "How severe is the pain on a scale of 1 to 10, with 1 being mild pain and 10 being the worst? Is it getting better, getting worse, or staying the same?"
  - **Duration:** "How long does the pain last (intermittent versus constant)?"
  - **Events associated:**
    - "Have you had fever or chills? Nausea or vomiting? How is your appetite? Have you experienced a change in bowel habit? When was your most recent bowel movement?"
    - "Have you been injured recently?"
    - Pregnancy: "When was your most recent menstrual period? Have you had vaginal bleeding?"
    - PID: "Have you had fever, foul vaginal discharge, or intermenstrual bleeding?"

- ◆ Renal colic: "Have you had blood in your urine? Have you passed stones or gritty urine?"
- ◆ Intestinal obstruction/incarcerated hernia: "When did you last pass stool or flatus? Have you been vomiting?"
- ◆ IBD: "Have you had chronic diarrhea, tenesmus, abdominal pain, weight loss, or extraintestinal manifestations (e.g., uveitis, erythema nodosum, and peripheral arthritis)?"
- ◆ Constitutional symptoms: "Have you had fever, chills, night sweats, weight loss, anorexia, or asthenia?"
- ▪ Frequency: "Have you ever had this pain before? How often does the pain come (intermittent versus constant)?"
- ▪ Palliative factors: "Does anything make the pain better? If so, what?"
  - ◆ Lying in one position
- ▪ Provocative factors: "Does anything make the pain worse? If so, what?"
  - ◆ Movement
- **PMH/PSH:** Diverticular disease, previous surgeries, malignancy, IBD, IBS, PID, sexually transmitted infections, ectopic pregnancy, or renal colic
- **MEDS:** Analgesics, antibiotics
- **SH:** Smoking, use of EtOH, use of street drugs, and sexual history
- **FH:** IBD, renal colic

Physical Examination
- **Vitals:** Measure HR, BP, RR, and temperature.
- **General:** Check capillary refill. Observe the patient's position on the stretcher and whether she is lying still or moving about. Note any apparent distress.
- **HEENT:** Look at the mucous membranes to gauge hydration. Inspect the sclerae.
- **Resp:** Check chest expansion (symmetry), and auscultate the lungs (breath sounds, adventitious sounds).
- **CVS:** Measure the JVP. Although it is not a reliable indicator of hydration status, the JVP is a useful clinical finding. Palpate peripheral pulses. Note pulse volume, contour, and rhythm. Auscultate the heart, listening for extra heart sounds or flow murmurs associated with hyperdynamic circulation.
- **Abdomen:** Inspect the abdomen. Auscultate for bowel sounds (may be decreased in peritonitis). Before you decide that bowel sounds are absent, listen in each quadrant for 2 to 3 minutes. Percuss lightly in all four quadrants. Percussion produces pain in a patient with peritoneal irritation. Before you palpate, ask the patient to cough and to point to the most tender area with one finger. Palpate the most tender area or areas last. Perform light and deep palpation, and identify any masses or areas of tenderness. Check for rebound tenderness. Examine the liver and spleen. Perform a DRE, and note the presence of any blood.
- **Genitourinary system:** It is important to perform a pelvic examination (see p. 310). Note any discharge, inflammation of the cervix, cervical motion tenderness, adnexal tenderness, or pelvic masses. Note uterine size.

Evidence
- In a study of 1287 patients, of whom 11% had a diagnosis of diverticulitis at 1 year of follow-up, patients with diverticulitis were more likely to be older; to experience isolated left-sided tenderness, rebound tenderness, and rectal tenderness; to have a history of constipation; and to have had previous episodes of similar pain.[13]

LOWER GASTROINTESTINAL BLEEDING: HISTORY AND PHYSICAL EXAMINATION

> **INSTRUCTIONS TO CANDIDATE:** A 77-year-old woman presents to the emergency department, complaining of passing bright red blood with her bowel movements. Obtain a detailed history, exploring possible causes, and perform a focused physical examination.

DD$_X$: VITAMINS C

- **Vascular:** Esophageal varices, aortoenteric fistula, angiodysplasia, and ischemic colitis
- **Infectious:** Invasive diarrhea (e.g., enteroinvasive *Escherichia coli*)
- **Traumatic:** Mallory-Weiss tear, anorectal trauma (consider possibility of elder abuse), and anal fissures
- **Metabolic:** Coagulopathy
- **Idiopathic/iatrogenic:** Diverticular disease, IBD, and proctitis
- **Neoplasm**
- **First evaluate ABCs.** It may be necessary to perform an immediate intervention, such as administering supplemental O_2, establishing intravenous access, or initiating airway management.
  - Is the patient able to talk? Swallow? Cough?
  - Are both lungs ventilated? Is the patient oxygenating (check mentation, pulse oximetry)?
  - Are vital signs abnormal? Is the peripheral circulation (pulses, capillary refill) abnormal?
  - If no immediate interventions are required, proceed to obtain the history, and perform the physical examination.

History

- Ask the patient the following:
  - **Character:** "Describe the bleeding."
    - Color of the stools (black or tarlike versus bright red blood)
    - Blood mixed throughout stool versus streaking on the surface of the stool or toilet paper versus in the toilet water
    - Stool form (diarrhea/loose/watery stool versus well-formed/solid stool)
  - **Location:** "Where is the blood coming from (rectal versus vaginal versus urinary tract)?"
  - **Onset:** "When did the bleeding start (sudden versus insidious)?"
  - **Radiation:** "Have you noticed any other bleeding (bleeding from another location)?"
  - **Intensity:** "How severe is the bleeding (quantify)? Has it gotten worse?"
  - **Duration:** "How long has the bleeding been going on (acute versus chronic)?"
  - **Events associated:**
    - "Have you experienced syncope? Chest pain? Shortness of breath?"
    - "Have you eaten suspect food (undercooked hamburger or chicken, shellfish)?"
    - "Does your diet include beets (which would produce red stools) or iron or bismuth (which would produce black stools)?"
    - "Did you experience any abdominal pain in the days leading up to the onset of bleeding?" This may be a prodrome of ischemic colitis.
    - Malignancy: "Have you noticed any reduction in stool caliber ('pencil stools'), weight loss, or constitutional symptoms?"
    - Anal fissure: "Do you have pain on defecation or perianal itching?"
    - IBD: "Do you have chronic diarrhea, tenesmus, abdominal pain, weight loss, or extraintestinal manifestations (e.g., uveitis, erythema nodosum, and peripheral arthritis)?"

- ◆ Abuse: "Are you safe at home? Are you experiencing any physical or sexual abuse? Are you being threatened?" (See Chapter 11, pp. 312-313, for checklist on abuse.)
  - ▪ Frequency: "How often does the bleeding happen (intermittent versus constant)?"
  - ▪ Palliative factors: "Does anything make the bleeding better? If so, what?"
  - ▪ Provocative factors: "Does anything make the bleeding worse? If so, what?"
- **Previous investigations:** Endoscopy (colonoscopy, sigmoidoscopy, anoscopy), barium enema
- **PMH/PSH:** Hemorrhoids, diverticulosis, IBD, malignancy, intestinal polyps, PUD, esophageal varices, alcoholism, or coagulopathy
- **MEDS:** NSAIDs/ASA, anticoagulants, antibiotics and gastric acid suppressants (pseudomembranous colitis), or corticosteroids
- **SH:** Smoking, use of EtOH, foreign travel (enteric infection), sexual history (e.g., anal penetration)
- **FH:** Malignancy (particularly GI malignancy), intestinal polyps, IBD, or coagulopathy

Physical Examination
- **Vitals:** Measure HR, BP, RR, and temperature.
  - ▪ Be alert for signs of circulatory shock: hypotension, tachycardia, thready pulses, decreased capillary refill, and tachypnea.
- **General:** Document apprehension, diaphoresis, pallor, and apparent distress.
- **HEENT:** Inspect the sclerae.
- **Resp:** Check chest expansion (symmetry), and auscultate the lungs (breath sounds, adventitious sounds).
- **CVS:** Measure the JVP. Although it is not a reliable indicator of hydration status, the JVP is a useful clinical finding. Palpate peripheral pulses. Note pulse volume, contour, and rhythm. Auscultate the heart, listening for extra heart sounds or murmurs.
- **Abdomen:** Inspect the abdomen. Auscultate for bowel sounds. Percuss lightly in all four quadrants. Percussion produces pain in a patient with peritoneal irritation. Before you palpate, ask the patient to cough and to point to the most tender area with one finger. Palpate the most tender area or areas last. Perform light and deep palpation, and identify any masses or areas of tenderness. Check for rebound tenderness. Examine the liver and spleen. Inspect the perianal area, looking for fissures, hemorrhoids, or signs of trauma. Perform a DRE, noting any masses or fresh blood. Perform a test for occult blood in the stool.
- **Neuro:** Check mental status (orientation to person, place, and time).

SAMPLE CHECKLISTS

Liver: Examination

INSTRUCTIONS TO CANDIDATE: Demonstrate examination of the liver, and describe your actions.

Key Points	Satisfactorily Completed
Introduces self to the patient	❏
Determines how the patient wishes to be addressed	❏
Washes hands	❏
Explains nature of the examination to the patient	❏
Examines the patient in a logical manner	❏
Inspection:	
• Looks for fullness/masses in RUQ	❏
• Asks the patient to take a deep breath, and observes the RUQ	❏
Percussion:	
• From resonance to dullness	❏
• From below and above costal margin	❏
Palpation:	
• From RLQ toward the RUQ	❏
• On inspiration	❏
• Describes the quality of the liver edge, if palpable	❏
• Indicates direction of hepatic movement on inspiration	❏
Auscultation:	
• Notes any venous hum, bruit, or friction rub	❏
Drapes the patient appropriately	❏
Makes appropriate closing remarks	❏

Splenomegaly: Examination

INSTRUCTIONS TO CANDIDATE: Demonstrate a focused physical examination for splenomegaly.

Key Points	Satisfactorily Completed
Introduces self to the patient	❏
Determines how the patient wishes to be addressed	❏
Washes hands	❏
Explains nature of the examination to the patient	❏
Examines the patient in a logical manner	❏
Inspection:	
• Notes visible signs of splenomegaly	❏
• Asks patient to take a deep breath, and observes splenic area	❏
Percussion:	
• Lower border of spleen	❏
• Traube's space	❏
• Castell's sign	❏

Key Points	Satisfactorily Completed
Palpation:	
• Uses hand to support patient's left rib cage	❏
• Starts palpation with right hand in RLQ toward the LUQ	❏
• Attempts to palpate splenic tip as patient inspires	❏
• Turns patient to right lateral decubitus position and palpates as above	❏
• Indicates direction of splenic movement on inspiration	❏
Indicates direction of splenic enlargement	❏
Differentiates enlarged spleen from enlarged kidney	❏
Auscultation:	
• Notes any venous hum, bruit, or friction rub	❏
Drapes the patient appropriately	❏
Makes appropriate closing remarks	❏

Ascites: Examination

INSTRUCTIONS TO CANDIDATE: Perform a focused physical examination for ascites, and describe your findings.

Key Points	Satisfactorily Completed
Introduces self to the patient	❏
Determines how the patient wishes to be addressed	❏
Washes hands	❏
Explains nature of the examination to the patient	❏
Examines the patient in a logical manner	❏
Inspection:	
• Looks for protuberant abdomen	❏
• Looks for bulging flanks	❏
• Looks for herniated umbilicus	❏
Percussion:	
• Tests for shifting dullness	❏
Palpates for fluid wave or thrill:	
• Uses one or both hands of the patient or assistant in patient's midline	❏
• Palpates with one hand while tapping with the other	❏
Drapes the patient appropriately	❏
Makes appropriate closing remarks	❏

Visible Extrahepatic Manifestations of Liver Disease: Examination

INSTRUCTIONS TO CANDIDATE: Inspect for visible extrahepatic stigmata of liver disease, and describe your findings.

Key Points	Satisfactorily Completed
Introduces self to the patient	❏
Determines how the patient wishes to be addressed	❏
Washes hands	❏
Explains nature of the examination to the patient	❏

Continued

Key Points	Satisfactorily Completed
Examines the patient in a logical manner	❑
Examines the face:	
• Scleral icterus	❑
• Kayser-Fleischer rings	❑
• Xanthelasma	❑
• Parotid enlargement	❑
Examines the hands:	
• Clubbing	❑
• Leukonychia	❑
• Palmar erythema	❑
• Dupuytren contracture	❑
• Tendinous xanthoma	❑
Examines the chest (in men):	
• Gynecomastia	❑
• Axillary hair loss	❑
Examines the abdomen:	
• Caput medusae	❑
• Distension (ascites)	❑
Looks for signs of wasting:	
• Arms and legs	❑
• First interosseous muscle in the hand	❑
• Temporalis muscle	❑
Looks for other abnormalities:	
• Excoriations	❑
• Bruising	❑
• Spider nevi	❑
• Peripheral edema	❑
• Testicular atrophy	❑
Drapes the patient appropriately	❑
Makes appropriate closing remarks	❑

Right Lower Quadrant Pain: History and Physical Examination

INSTRUCTIONS TO CANDIDATE: A 16-year-old boy presents to his family doctor with a 2-day history of RLQ pain. Obtain a focused history, and perform a focused physical examination.

Key Points	Satisfactorily Completed
Introduces self to the patient	❑
Determines how the patient wishes to be addressed	❑
Washes hands	❑
Establishes the purpose of the encounter	❑
Establishes the presenting concern in the patient's own words	❑
History of abdominal pain:	
• Characterizes the pain	❑
• Establishes the location of pain	❑
• Ascertains whether pain radiates or has migrated	❑
• Establishes the onset and pattern of the pain, including the frequency	❑
• Asks about previous episodes of similar pain	❑

Key Points	Satisfactorily Completed
• Asks about the severity of the pain on a scale	❏
• Asks about palliative and provocative factors	❏
Inquires about associated symptoms:	
• Fever	❏
• Change in bowel habit (diarrhea, constipation)	❏
• Nausea, vomiting, or both	❏
• Lumps or bulges in groin or scrotum	❏
• Testicular pain or swelling	❏
Performs relevant review of systems:	
• Weight loss	❏
• Skin changes	❏
• Joint pain	❏
• Eye problems: vision change, eye pain, eye redness	❏
• Hematuria	❏
Asks about relevant social history:	
• Smoking	❏
• Alcohol use	❏
Asks about past medical and surgical history:	
• IBD	❏
Asks about medications:	
• Prescription drugs	❏
• Over-the-counter drugs	❏
Explains nature of the examination to the patient	❏
Examines the patient in a logical manner	❏
Vital signs:	
• Requests a complete set of vital sign measurements	❏
• Notes any abnormalities such as tachycardia and fever	❏
• Palpates peripheral pulses, noting volume, contour, and rhythm	❏
Inspection:	
• Checks abdominal contour	❏
• Looks for scars	❏
• Looks for inguinal bulges	❏
• Looks for scrotal enlargement	❏
• Transilluminates a scrotal mass if such a mass is present	❏
Auscultation:	
• Auscultates in each quadrant of the abdomen (bowel sounds may be decreased in areas of peritoneal irritation)	❏
Percussion:	
• Lightly percusses abdomen, noting any localized or referred tenderness	❏
• Percusses the liver span	❏
• Percusses for splenomegaly (Castell's sign and Traube's space)	❏
Palpation:	
• Lightly palpates, noting areas of tenderness	❏
• Palpates deeper, noting tenderness and masses	❏
• Palpates for liver edge and spleen tip	❏
• Palpates for inguinal hernias, including transmitted cough impulse	❏
Performs DRE, noting masses and, in particular, right-sided tenderness	❏
Drapes the patient appropriately	❏
Makes appropriate closing remarks	❏

ADVANCED SKILLS

CONSTIPATION: HISTORY

> **INSTRUCTIONS TO CANDIDATE:** A 64-year-old man presents to his family doctor, requesting a laxative because he is always "blocked up." Obtain a detailed history, exploring possible causes.

DD$_X$: VITAMINS C
- **V**ascular: Stroke (atonic colon)
- **T**raumatic: Spinal cord injury (atonic colon), anal fissure
- **M**etabolic: Hypothyroidism, hypercalcemia, drugs (e.g., chronic laxative use), and diet
- **I**diopathic/**i**atrogenic: IBS, fecal impaction, bowel obstruction (e.g., adhesions), and rectal stricture
- **N**eoplastic: Bowel tumor (benign or malignant)
- **C**ongenital/genetic: Hirschsprung disease

History
- Ask the patient the following:
  - Character: "Describe your current bowel movements."
    - "Is your stool too hard? Is defecation painful (fissures or perianal disease)? How frequently do you defecate?"
    - "Describe the color and shape of your stool."
    - "Has there been any change in your bowel habit? Describe your usual bowel movements."
    - "Has there been any change in the caliber of your stools ('pencil stools')?"
    - "When was your last bowel movement?"
  - Onset: "When did the constipation start (sudden versus insidious)?"
  - Intensity: "How severe is the constipation? How many stools do you have per day and per week? Has it gotten worse?"
  - Duration: "How long has the constipation been going on (acute versus chronic)?"
  - Events associated:
    - "Have you noticed a change in bowel habits or caliber of stool? Abdominal pain?"
    - Diet: "Have you decreased your fiber or roughage intake? Have you decreased your fluid intake?"
    - IBS: "Do you have periods of diarrhea alternating with periods of constipation?"
    - Intestinal obstruction: "When did you last pass stool or flatus? Have you been vomiting?"
    - Hypothyroidism: "Have you noticed cold intolerance or weight gain?"
    - Hyperparathyroidism: "Have you had bone pain or fractures, renal stones, abdominal pain, or anxiety or depression?"
    - Constitutional symptoms: "Have you had fever, chills, night sweats, weight loss, anorexia, or asthenia?"
  - Frequency: "Has this 'blocking up' happened to you before? How often does the constipation happen (intermittent versus constant)?"
  - Palliative factors: "Does anything make it better? If so, what?"
    - "Have you made any dietary modifications?"
  - Provocative factors: "Does anything make it worse? If so, what?"
- **PMH/PSH:** IBS, stroke, GI malignancy, rectal stricture, perianal disease, hyperparathyroidism, hypothyroidism, or diabetes mellitus

- **MEDS:** Opioids, atropine, tricyclic antidepressants, long-term use of cathartics, or use of enemas
- **SH:** Smoking, use of EtOH, and diet
- **FH:** GI malignancy, hypothyroidism

STEATORRHEA: HISTORY

> **INSTRUCTIONS TO CANDIDATE: A 22-year-old woman presents to her family physician, complaining of "greasy," foul-smelling stools. She also notes weight loss. Obtain a detailed history, exploring possible causes.**

DD$_X$: VITAMINS C
- Infectious: *Giardia lamblia,* postinfectious malabsorption (villous sloughing)
- Autoimmune/allergic: Celiac disease, Whipple disease
- Idiopathic/iatrogenic: Chronic pancreatitis, biliary obstruction
- Congenital/genetic: Cystic fibrosis

History
- Ask the patient the following:
  - Character: "Describe your bowel movements."
    - "Are the stools large, oily, and malodorous but somewhat formed?"
    - "Is there any blood, pus, or mucus in the stool? Describe the color of your stool."
    - "Have you noticed a change in your bowel habits? Describe your usual bowel movements."
  - Onset: "When did the greasy stools start (sudden versus insidious)?"
  - Intensity: "How many stools do you have per day, and what is the approximate volume of stool? Has the number of episodes gotten worse?"
  - Duration: "How long have you been passing fatty stools (acute versus chronic)?"
  - Events associated:
    - "How is your appetite? How much weight have you lost? Do you have nausea or vomiting?"
    - "Do you have abdominal pain?" (This may be indicative of pancreatitis.)
    - "Have you experienced abdominal distension or bloating? Flatulence?"
    - "Have you noticed edema?" (This may be indicative of hypoalbuminemia.)
    - "Have you noticed easy bruising (which may reflect vitamin K deficiency)? Bone pain (which may reflect vitamin D malabsorption)?"
  - Frequency: "How often do you pass greasy stools? Is every stool greasy (intermittent versus constant)?"
  - Palliative factors: "Does anything make it better? If so, what?"
    - Fasting
  - Provocative factors: "Does anything make it worse? If so, what?"
    - Fatty foods
    - Dairy products
    - Gluten
- **Previous investigations:** Stool analysis, endoscopy, or biopsy
- **PMH/PSH:** Pancreatitis, diabetes mellitus, cystic fibrosis, IBD, Whipple disease, chronic liver failure, jaundice, celiac disease, or GI surgery
- **MEDS:** Cholesterol-reducing drugs, "diet" drugs, or herbal medicines
- **SH:** Smoking; use of EtOH, travel history, camping, use of a well (ingestion of contaminated water [*Giardia* species or "beaver fever"])
- **FH:** IBD, cystic fibrosis, or celiac disease

SAMPLE CHECKLIST

Small Bowel Obstruction: Radiographic Interpretation and Physical Examination

INSTRUCTIONS TO CANDIDATE: Assess the following labeled radiographs, and then state your interpretation and appropriate differential diagnosis (Figure 3-12). Perform a focused examination on the patient, describing your actions.

Key Points	Satisfactorily Completed
Radiograph:	
• Multiple air-fluid levels and small bowel dilatation	❑
• Assessment: small bowel obstruction	❑
Differential diagnosis:	
• Intestinal adhesions	❑
• Cecal or small bowel (e.g., lymphoma) neoplasm	❑
• Incarcerated hernia	❑
• IBD	❑
Examines the patient in a logical manner	❑
Vital signs:	
• Requests a complete set of vital sign measurements	❑
• Notes any abnormalities such as tachycardia or hypotension	❑
• Palpates peripheral pulses, noting volume, contour, and rhythm	❑
Percussion:	
• Lightly percusses abdomen, noting any localized or referred tenderness (often tympanitic in small bowel obstruction)	❑
• Percusses the liver span	❑
• Percusses for splenomegaly (Castell's sign and Traube's space)	❑
Inspection:	
• Looks for peristaltic waves	
• Notes any abdominal distension	
Palpation	
States the need to perform DRE	
Drapes the patient appropriately	❑
Makes appropriate closing remarks	❑

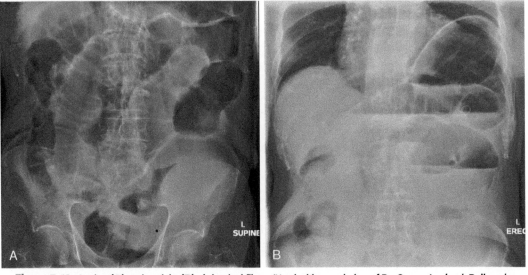

Figure 3-12 Supine **(A)** and upright **(B)** abdominal films. (Used with permission of Dr. Osama Loubani, Dalhousie University, Halifax, Nova Scotia.)

Evidence

- Table 3-7 shows how parts of the clinical examination help diagnose bowel obstruction.

Table 3-7	Usefulness of Clinical Examination in Diagnosis of Bowel Obstruction	

Clinical Feature	+LR	−LR
Visible peristalsis	**21**	0.9
Distended abdomen	**5.8**	0.4
Generalized tenderness	**5.1**	0.7
Increased bowel sounds	3.5	0.7
Reduced bowel sounds	3.2	0.8
Rigidity	2.7	0.9
Abdominal mass	2.2	0.9
Previous abdominal surgery	2.7	0.4

From Böhner H, Yang Q, Franke C, et al. Simple data from history and physical examination help to exclude bowel obstruction and to avoid radiographic studies in patients with acute abdominal pain. *Eur J Surg.* 1998;164:777-784.

−LR, Negative likelihood ratio; +LR, positive likelihood ratio.

Boldface represents findings associated with positive likelihood ratios ≥5 or with negative likelihood ratios ≤0.2. These are said to be moderate- to high-impact items.

REFERENCES

1. Manterola C, Astudillo P, Losada H, et al. Analgesia in patients with acute abdominal pain. *Cochrane Database Syst Rev.* 2007;3:CD005660.
2. Gerhardt RT, Nelson BK, Keenan S, et al. Derivation of a clinical guideline for the assessment of nonspecific abdominal pain: the Guideline for Abdominal Pain in the ED Setting (GAPEDS) phase 1 study. *Am J Emerg Med.* 2005;23:709-717.
3. Martina B, Bucheli B, Stotz M, et al. First clinical judgment by primary care physicians distinguishes well between nonorganic and organic causes of abdominal or chest pain. *J Gen Intern Med.* 1997;12:459-465.
4. Muris JW, Starmans R, Fijten GH, et al. Non-acute abdominal complaints in general practice: diagnostic value of signs and symptoms. *Br J Gen Pract.* 1995;45:313-316.
5. Pines J, Uscher Pines L, Hall A, et al. The interrater variation of ED abdominal examination findings in patients with acute abdominal pain. *Am J Emerg Med.* 2005;23:483-487.
6. Joshi R, Singh A, Jajoo N, et al. Accuracy and reliability of palpation and percussion for detecting hepatomegaly: a rural hospital-based study. *Indian J Gastroenterol.* 2004;23:171-174.
7. Naylor CD. Physical examination of the liver. *JAMA.* 1994;271:1859-1865.
8. Grover SA, Barkun AN, Sackett DL. The rational clinical examination: does this patient have splenomegaly? *JAMA.* 1993;270:2218-2221.
9. Dixon JM, Elton RA, Rainey JB, et al. Rectal examination in patients with pain in the right lower quadrant of the abdomen. *BMJ.* 1991;302:386-388.
10. Detsky AS, Smalley PS, Chang J. The rational clinical examination: is this patient malnourished? *JAMA.* 1994;271:54-58.
11. Bauer J, Capra S, Ferguson M. Use of the scored Patient-Generated Subjective Global Assessment (PG-SGA) as a nutrition assessment tool in patients with cancer. *Eur J Clin Nutr.* 2002;56:779-785.
12. de Bruyn G, Graviss EA. A systematic review of the diagnostic accuracy of physical examination for the detection of cirrhosis. *BMC Med Inform Decis Mak.* 2001;1:6.
13. Laurell H, Hansson LE, Gunnarsson U. Acute diverticulitis—clinical presentation and differential diagnostics. *Colorectal Dis.* 2007;9:496-501; discussion. *Colorectal Dis.* 2007;9:501-502.

Genitourinary System

ANATOMY

- The **kidneys** are retroperitoneal organs that are often impalpable in normal adults (Figure 4-1). Because of the presence of the liver on the right side, the right kidney is positioned more caudally than the left kidney. The twelfth rib protects the superior poles of the kidneys.
- The **urinary bladder** is a distensible, muscular, pelvic organ that functions to store urine until it can be voided. When full, the bladder can extend out of the pelvis and may be palpated in the abdomen as high as the level of the umbilicus. *An overly distended bladder may be mistaken for an abdominal mass.*
- The **prostate** is a walnut-sized gland that is inferior to the urinary bladder and encapsulates part of the male urethra (Figure 4-2). Its relationship with the urethra accounts for the changes in urinary function that accompany prostatic enlargement. Because of its proximity to the anterior rectal wall, the prostate can be palpated on digital rectal examination (DRE).
- The **scrotum** is a sac that encases the testicles, divided in such a way that each testicle has its own pouch. The lymphatic drainage of the scrotum differs from that of the testes: The scrotal lymph vessels drain to the superficial inguinal lymph nodes, whereas the testicular lymph vessels drain to the retroperitoneum.

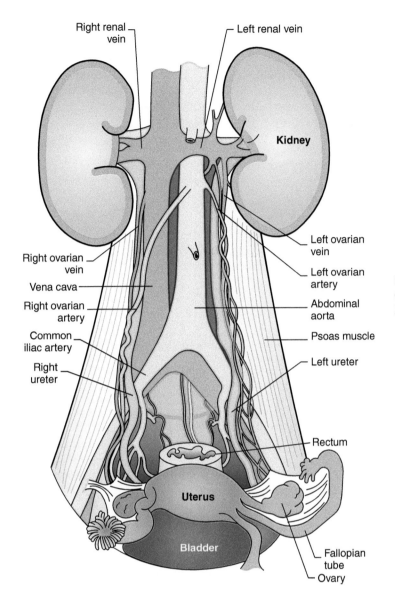

Figure 4-1 Genitourinary anatomy. (Adapted from DiSaia PJ, Creasman WT. *Clinical Gynecologic Oncology.* 6th ed. St. Louis: Mosby; 2002 [p. 73, Figure 3-18].)

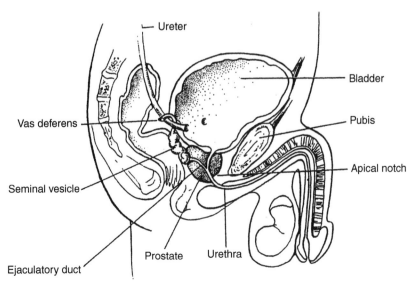

Figure 4-2 Cross-sectional anatomy of the male pelvis. (From Lepor H. *Prostatic Diseases.* Philadelphia: Saunders; 2000 [p. 18, Figure 2-2].)

- The **testicles** are suspended by the spermatic cord in the scrotum. The **epididymis** lies on the superior pole of the testicle. The venous drainage of the testicles has particular clinical relevance. The right testicular vein drains directly into the inferior vena cava (IVC), whereas the left testicular vein drains into the left renal vein. Varicoceles appear almost exclusively on the left side. An isolated varicocele on the right side should prompt investigation as to a retroperitoneal or intra-abdominal cause.
- Relevant female genital anatomy is discussed in Chapter 11.

GLOSSARY OF SIGNS AND SYMPTOMS

- **Dysuria** is pain or other difficulty in urination.
- **Hematuria** is blood in the urine. It is classified as microscopic (grossly normal) or macroscopic (red to brown discoloration). The dipstick reagents are sensitive to hemoglobin and myoglobin. A positive dipstick result with no red blood cells (RBCs) on microscopic study is suggestive of myoglobinuria. On microscopic study, 2 to 3 RBCs per high-powered field is considered to be within normal limits.
- **Hesitancy** is an involuntary delay in starting the urinary stream. Difficulty "making urine" may refer to hesitancy, to increased force necessary to pass urine, or to the inability to empty the bladder completely.
- **Strangury** is the difficult passage of small amounts of urine that is accompanied by pain and an urgency to void.

Incontinence

- **Urinary incontinence** is involuntary leakage of urine. Continence depends on a normal urinary bladder and competent sphincters (voluntary and involuntary). Urinary incontinence occurs in both men and women but is more common among women.
- **Stress incontinence** is the leakage of urine associated with increased intra-abdominal pressure, such as that caused by coughing, laughing, lifting, or increased activity. This leakage typically results from sphincter insufficiency (pelvic floor laxity).
- **Urge incontinence** is the loss of urine accompanied by a sudden, strong desire to void. This typically results from detrusor overactivity that arises from conditions such as cystitis, bladder cancer, bladder calculi, or neurogenic bladder.
- **Mixed incontinence** is a combination of stress and urge incontinence.
- **Overflow incontinence** occurs in the chronically distended bladder. When pressure inside the bladder exceeds sphincteric resistance, leakage occurs. This is usually associated with urinary obstruction, chronic anticholinergic therapy, or spinal cord injury.
- **Functional incontinence** arises in people with cognitive or mobility difficulties.

ESSENTIAL SKILLS

KIDNEY: EXAMINATION

- A normal kidney in a normal person is not palpable. A normal right kidney may be palpable in an especially thin person with poor abdominal musculature. A normal left kidney is rarely palpable. Causes of kidney enlargement include tumors, cysts, and hydronephrosis.

Palpation

- **Right kidney:** Place your left hand under the patient parallel to the twelfth rib, with your fingertips just reaching the costovertebral angle (CVA). Lift your left hand to displace the kidney anteriorly. Place your right hand on the right upper quadrant

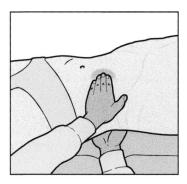

Figure 4-3 Bimanual palpation of the left kidney. (From Munro JF, Campbell IW, eds. *Macleod's Clinical Examination.* 10th ed. Edinburgh: Churchill Livingstone; 2000 [p. 166, Figure 5-13, *A*].)

(RUQ) lateral and parallel to the rectus muscle. Ask the patient to take a deep breath. At the peak of inspiration, place your right hand deep into the RUQ to "catch" the right kidney between your hands. Ask the patient to exhale and to stop breathing briefly. Release the pressure of your right hand, and feel the kidney slide back into its expiratory position. Note the size, shape, contour, consistency, and any tenderness. The lower pole of the kidney is rounded, whereas the liver edge is sharper, extends further medially and laterally, and cannot be "captured."

- **Left kidney** (Figure 4-3): Move to the patient's left side. Use your right hand to lift from below at the twelfth rib. Use your left hand to feel deep in the left upper quadrant (LUQ), and proceed in the same way as for the RUQ. Because the left kidney is more superior in its position than the right kidney, it is less often palpable.

Fist Percussion
- Ask the patient to sit up. Place your left hand in the CVA, and strike your hand with the hypothenar aspect of your right fist (Figure 4-4). Use enough force to produce a painless but audible thud. CVA tenderness is suggestive of pyelonephritis or a musculoskeletal problem.

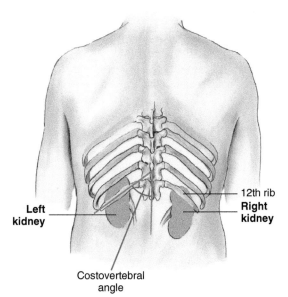

Left kidney

12th rib
Right kidney

Costovertebral angle

Figure 4-4 Costovertebral angle. (From Jarvis C. *Physical Examination and Health Assessment.* 3rd ed. Philadelphia: Saunders; 1996 [p. 602, Figure 19-5].)

DIFFERENTIATING SPLENOMEGALY FROM AN ENLARGED KIDNEY: EXAMINATION

Border
- The spleen has a notched medial border; the kidney does not.

Extension
- The spleen enlarges inferiorly and anteriorly toward the right lower quadrant (RLQ) and may extend beyond the midline of the abdomen. The kidney enlarges inferiorly and does not cross the midline.

Movement during Respiration
- Like the liver, the spleen moves with respiration. The kidney is retroperitoneal and should not move substantially during respirations.

Palpation
- In splenomegaly, you can palpate deep to the medial and lower borders of the mass but not between the mass and the costal margin. With an enlarged kidney, you should be able to palpate between the mass and the costal margin but not deep to its medial and lower borders.

Percussion
- In splenomegaly, the LUQ is dull to percussion; with an enlarged kidney, it is tympanitic because of the interposing bowel.

Evidence
- Bedside examination of the spleen is of limited usefulness when the clinical suspicion of splenomegaly is less than 10%. If clinical suspicion is higher (>10%), imaging may be required because clinical examination is not sensitive and specific enough to confidently exclude splenomegaly. However, the presence of both percussion dullness and a palpable spleen likely confirms splenomegaly.[1]

PROSTATE: EXAMINATION

Patient Positioning
- The patient may be positioned in a number of ways for the DRE. Consider the patient's comfort during this sensitive examination. Ask the patient to lie on his left side and flex the knees, bringing them toward the chest. Alternatively, the patient can be examined standing, bent over the examination table. The lithotomy position (supine at the end of the examining table with knees flexed and feet in stirrups) is also useful.

Palpation
- Explain the rectal examination to the patient, and warn him about the coolness of the lubricant.
- Use your gloved index finger to apply gentle, steady pressure at the anus. Ask the patient to take a deep breath, and insert your finger into the rectum (Figure 4-5).
- Note **sphincter tone.** The state of sphincter tone is especially important in evaluating for neurologic injury.
- Palpate the **rectal walls** for polyps or masses. Ensure that you fully palpate the anterior, posterior, and lateral walls of the rectum. The sensation of external compression on the rectum or a rectal shelf is known as **Blumer's shelf** and is associated with malignancy.
- Palpate the **prostate** gland, which lies anterior to the anterior rectal wall in boys and men. Note any tenderness and the size, symmetry, consistency, and nodularity of the prostate gland. Tenderness is suggestive of prostatitis. In cases of major trauma, a "high-riding" prostate is associated with urethral disruption.
- After the examination is complete, inspect your gloved finger for blood, and note the color of the stool. Use a guaiac test to check the stool for the presence of occult blood.

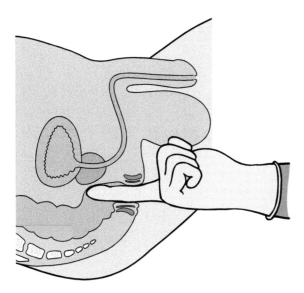

Figure 4-5 Technique for digital prostate examination. (From Munro JF, Campbell IW, eds. *Macleod's Clinical Examination*. 10th ed. Edinburgh: Churchill Livingstone; 2000 [p. 175, Figure 5.22.D].)

TESTICLE: EXAMINATION

Patient Positioning
- The patient may be positioned supine or standing for the examination of the testicle. Consider the patient comfort's during this sensitive examination.

Inspection
- The scrotum is best inspected with the patient standing. Observe the lie of the testicles within the scrotum. The left testicle is often lower than the right testicle, although the opposite is true in many men. Note any asymmetry or masses (Figure 4-6). Use a small light source to transilluminate a scrotal mass. A hernia or tumor cannot be transilluminated, whereas a hydrocele can be transilluminated clearly. Inspect the skin for excoriations, rashes, ulcerations, or other abnormality.
- Cremasteric reflex: Elicit the cremasteric reflex by stroking the upper medial thigh firmly either up or down. The resulting contraction of the cremasteric muscle causes a rise of the ipsilateral hemiscrotum. Absence of the cremasteric reflex is common before the age of 30 months[2] (Figure 4-7).

Auscultation
- Masses in the scrotum may be auscultated with the diaphragm of the stethoscope. Listen for any bowel sounds indicative of bowel within the mass, as in an indirect inguinal hernia.

Palpation
- Begin by confirming the presence of two testicles within the scrotum. Palpate each testicle separately.

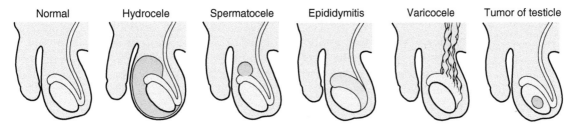

Figure 4-6 Causes of scrotal asymmetry. (From Munro JF, Campbell IW, eds. *Macleod's Clinical Examination*. 10th ed. Edinburgh: Churchill Livingstone; 2000 [p. 1729, Figure 5.19].)

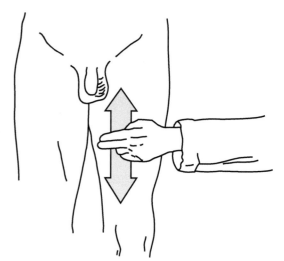

Figure 4-7 Elicitation of the cremasteric reflex.

- Use your gloved index finger and thumb to gently grasp the anterior and posterior aspects of the testicle. Use your other gloved hand to similarly grasp the superior and inferior poles of the testicle.
- Note the size, shape, contour, and consistency of each testicle, and any tenderness in each one. Note any asymmetry.
- Palpate the epididymis at the superior pole of each testicle, and follow the spermatic cord into the inguinal canal. Palpate both spermatic cords simultaneously by rolling the scrotal skin between the thumb and index finger of each hand, superior to the testicles. Again, note any asymmetry, masses, or tenderness.

URINARY INCONTINENCE: HISTORY

INSTRUCTIONS TO CANDIDATE: A 56-year-old woman presents to her family doctor with a history of leaking urine. This problem limits her activities outside of the home. Obtain a detailed history, exploring possible causes.

DD$_X$
- Stress incontinence
- Urge incontinence
- Mixed incontinence
- Overflow incontinence

History
- Ask the patient the following:
  - Character: "Describe the trouble you are having with urine leakage."
    - "Does the leakage occur with coughing, laughing, sneezing, or lifting?"
    - "Do you experience a strong and sudden urge to void (i.e., urinary urgency)?"
    - "Do you have a sensation of incomplete emptying? Do you have a continued urge to void even when urinary flow has stopped?"
  - Onset: "When did this trouble start? Has it come about suddenly or gradually?"
  - Intensity: "Do you lose small amounts of urine (dribbling) or large quantities? Is the problem getting better, getting worse, or staying the same? Do you need to wear an incontinence pad or diaper? How often must you change it? How does wearing one affect your daily life?"
  - Duration: "How long has this problem been going on (acute versus chronic)?"

- Events associated:
  - "Do you have pain (abdominal, flank, groin)?"
  - "Do you have pain with urination, a sense of urgency, or frequent urination (irritative symptoms)?"
  - "Do you have urinary hesitancy, increased force needed to urinate, or a sense of incomplete emptying (obstructive symptoms)?"
- Frequency: "Have you ever had this trouble before? Do you have it every day (intermittent versus constant)?"
- Palliative factors: "Does anything make it better? If so, what?"
  - Frequent voiding
  - Decreased fluid intake
  - Kegel's exercises
- Provocative factors: "Does anything make it worse? If so, what?
  - Exercise
  - Lifting
  - Laughing
  - Coughing or sneezing
  - Increased fluid intake
- **Past medical history (PMH)/past surgical history (PSH):** Diabetes, malignancy, pelvic radiation, neurologic disease (stroke, multiple sclerosis, spinal cord injury, Parkinson disease), previous surgery on the genitourinary (GU) tract (urethropexy, vaginal repair, resection of malignancy), GU trauma, or pregnancy (method of delivery and complications such as urethral injury)
- **Medications (MEDS):** Anticholinergics, diuretics
- **Social history (SH):** Smoking, use of alcohol (EtOH), use of street drugs, and sexual history

Evidence

- If the patient reports occurrence of urinary incontinence with coughing, sneezing, lifting, walking, or running, stress incontinence is likely to be the diagnosis (positive likelihood ratio [+LR] 2.2; 95% confidence interval [CI] 1.6 to 3.2), whereas the absence of patient-reported urinary incontinence in these settings decreases the likelihood of stress incontinence (−LR 0.39; 95% CI 0.25 to 0.61).[3]
- If the patient reports urinary urgency, the likelihood of urge incontinence is significantly increased (+LR 4.2; 95% CI 2.3 to 7.6). The absence of patient-reported urinary urgency decreases the probability of urge incontinence (−LR 0.48; 95% CI 0.36 to 0.62).[3]

PAINLESS HEMATURIA: HISTORY

> **INSTRUCTIONS TO CANDIDATE: A 69-year-old man presents to his family doctor, complaining of blood in his "water." Obtain a focused history, exploring possible causes.**

DD$_X$: VITAMINS C (Painless Hematuria)

- **I**nfectious: Urinary tract infection (UTI)
- **A**utoimmune/**a**llergic: Wegener granulomatosis, Goodpasture syndrome
- **M**etabolic: Sickle cell anemia, coagulopathy, and drugs
- **I**diopathic/**i**atrogenic: Glomerulonephritis, stones (bladder, renal)
- **N**eoplastic: Bladder or kidney tumor

History

- Ask the patient the following:
  - **Character:** "Describe the color of your urine. Are any clots present?"
  - **Location:** "Do you notice blood at the beginning, middle, or end of the stream?"

- Onset: "When did you first notice blood in your urine? How did this start (sudden versus insidious)?"
- Intensity: "How much blood is there? Is it getting better, getting worse, or staying the same?"
- Duration: "How long has this been going on (acute versus chronic)?"
- Events associated:
  - "Have you been injured recently? Have you had any urinary procedures recently such as urinary catheterization, endoscopy of the bladder, or transurethral resection of the prostate (TURP)?"
  - "Do you have pain (abdominal, flank, penile)?"
  - Stones: "Do you have grit or stones in the urine?
  - UTI: "Have you experienced painful urination, frequent urination, or loss of bladder control?"
  - Renal-pulmonary syndrome: "Have you coughed up blood or been short of breath on exertion (SOBOE)?"
  - Constitutional symptoms: "Have you had fever, chills, night sweats, weight loss, anorexia, or asthenia?"
- Frequency: "How often do you see blood in the urine? Do you see blood every time you urinate (intermittent versus constant)?"
- Palliative factors: "Does anything make it better? If so, what?"
  - Increased fluid intake
- Provocative factors: "Does anything make it worse? If so, what?"
- **PMH/PSH:** Bladder/kidney cancer, stones, sickle cell anemia, bleeding diathesis, Goodpasture syndrome, or Wegener granulomatosis
- **MEDS:** Chemotherapy (hemorrhagic cystitis), rifampin (discolors urine), or anticoagulation
- **SH:** Smoking, use of EtOH, use of street drugs, and occupational or recreational exposures such as industrial dyes and solvents that increase risk of bladder cancer
- **Family history (FH):** Sickle cell anemia, coagulopathy

FLANK PAIN AND HEMATURIA: HISTORY AND PHYSICAL EXAMINATION

INSTRUCTIONS TO CANDIDATE: A 48-year-old woman presents to the emergency department with the "worst pain" she has ever had. It radiates into her groin. The triage nurse asks her for a urine sample. Much to the patient's alarm, she passes "bloody" urine into the sample bottle. Obtain a focused history, and perform a focused physical examination.

DD$_X$: VITAMINS C
- **V**ascular: Ruptured/leaking abdominal aortic aneurysm (AAA)
- **I**nfectious: UTI
- **M**etabolic: Coagulopathy, sickle cell crisis
- **I**diopathic/**i**atrogenic: Renal colic, hemorrhagic cystitis, incarcerated/strangulated hernia, appendicitis, and diverticulitis

History
- Ask the patient the following:
  - **C**haracter: "What is the pain like? Sharp and localized? Crampy? Dull? What color is the urine? Bright red? Have you seen any clots?"
  - **L**ocation: "Where does the pain originate?"
  - **O**nset: "When did the pain start? How did it come on (sudden versus gradual)? When did you first notice blood in your urine?"
  - **R**adiation: "Does the pain move anywhere? To the groin? Do you have any pain with urination? Any other bleeding?"
  - **I**ntensity: "How severe is the pain on a scale of 1 to 10, with 1 being mild pain and 10 being the worst? Is it getting better, getting worse, or staying the same?"

- Duration: "How long does the pain last (intermittent versus constant)?"
- Events associated:
  - ♦ "Have you seen any grit or stones in your urine? Do you have painful urination?"
  - ♦ "Do you have nausea or vomiting? Fever or chills?"
  - ♦ "Do you have abdominal pain? Have you noticed a change in bowel habit?"
- Frequency: "Have you ever had this pain before? How often does the pain come? Have you had any previous episodes of hematuria?"
- Palliative factors: "Does anything make the pain better? If so, what?"
  - ♦ Analgesic medications
  - ♦ Particular position
- Provocative factors: "Does anything make the pain worse? If so, what?"
  - ♦ Movement
- **PMH/PSH:** Renal colic, sickle cell anemia, AAA, previous surgery
- **MEDS:** Analgesics, anticoagulants, or chemotherapy (hemorrhagic cystitis)
- **SH:** Smoking, use of EtOH, and use of street drugs
- **FH:** Sickle cell anemia, renal colic, AAA

Physical Examination
- **Vital signs (Vitals):** Evaluate heart rate (HR), blood pressure (BP), respiratory rate (RR), and temperature.
- **General:** Check capillary refill. Note the patient's position on the stretcher and whether she is lying still or moving about. Note any apparent distress, pallor, or diaphoresis.
- **Respiratory system (Resp):** Check chest expansion (symmetry), and auscultate the lungs (breath sounds, adventitious sounds).
- **Cardiovascular system (CVS):** Measure the jugular venous pressure (JVP). Palpate peripheral pulses. Note pulse volume, contour, and rhythm. Auscultate the heart, listening for extra heart sounds or flow murmurs associated with hyperdynamic circulation. Auscultate for abdominal bruits.
- **Abdomen:** Inspect the abdomen. Note any bulges or obvious hernias. Auscultate for bowel sounds. Percuss lightly in all four quadrants. Before you palpate, ask the patient to cough and to point to the most tender area with one finger. Palpate the most tender area or areas last. Perform light and deep palpation, and identify any masses (pulsatile or nonpulsatile) or areas of tenderness. Check for rebound tenderness. Examine for hernias (see pp. 92-93). Examine the liver and spleen. Perform a DRE. A retrocecal appendix may produce tenderness on palpation of the rectal walls.
- **GU:** Percuss the CVA for tenderness (see Figure 4-4). Palpate the kidneys. Note any asymmetry. Examine the external genitalia for signs of trauma, ulceration, or other abnormality.

Pearls
- Rebound tenderness is referred to as **McBurney's point** in appendicitis.
- A patient with appendicitis may have positive **psoas, obturator,** and **Rovsing's signs.**

URINARY TRACT INFECTION: HISTORY AND PHYSICAL EXAMINATION

> **INSTRUCTIONS TO CANDIDATE:** A 22-year-old woman presents to the emergency department because of a burning sensation with urination. She is concerned that she may have an infection. Obtain a focused history, and perform a focused physical examination.

DD$_X$: VITAMINS C
- Infectious: UTI, sexually transmitted infection (STI), vaginitis
- Traumatic: Passage of a stone (trauma to the urethra)
- Idiopathic/iatrogenic: Urethral syndrome

History

- Ask the patient the following:
  - **Character:** "Describe the pain. Is there any change in the quality of your urine (color, odor, quantity)?"
  - **Location:** "Where is the pain? Does pain occur at the beginning, middle, or end of the stream or throughout the stream?"
  - **Onset:** "How did the pain start? Was the onset sudden or gradual?"
  - **Radiation:** "Does the pain move anywhere? Where: to the groin? To the back?"
  - **Intensity:** "How bad is the pain on a scale of 1 to 10, with 1 being mild pain and 10 being the worst? Is it getting better, getting worse, or staying the same?"
  - **Duration:** "How long has the pain been going on (acute versus chronic)?"
  - **Events associated:**
    - "Have you had fever or chills?"
    - "Have you had nausea or vomiting?"
    - "Are you pregnant?"
    - "Do you have pain (suprapubic, flank, groin, external genitalia)?"
    - "Do you have genital ulcers or sores?"
    - "Have you noticed vaginal discharge?"
    - "Have you seen any grit or stones in your urine?"
    - UTI: "Have you experienced frequent urination, painful urination, blood in the urine, urinary urgency, loss of bladder control, or flank pain?" (Risk factors for UTI: Female gender [short urethra], pregnancy, urinary obstruction, GU malformation, and neurogenic bladder.)
  - **Frequency:** "Have you ever experienced this sensation before? If so, when was the last time? Does it hurt every time you urinate (intermittent versus constant)?"
  - **Palliative factors:** "Does anything make it better? If so, what?"
    - Analgesic medications
    - Increased fluid intake
  - **Provocative factors:** "Does anything make it worse? If so, what?"
    - Sexual activity
    - Type of clothing
- **Risk factors for acute UTI in young women:** recent sexual intercourse, use of spermicide during sexual intercourse, history of UTI
- **PMH/PSH:** STIs, UTI, GU malformations, nephrolithiasis, or diabetes mellitus
- **MEDS:** Antibiotics, analgesics, or antivirals (for herpes)
- **SH:** Smoking, use of EtOH, use of street drugs, and sexual history (number of sexual partners in the previous 6 to 12 months, use of condoms)

Physical Examination

- **Vitals:** Evaluate HR, BP, RR, and temperature.
- **Resp:** Auscultate the lungs (breath sounds, adventitious sounds).
- **CVS:** Palpate peripheral pulses. Note pulse volume, contour, and rhythm. Auscultate the heart, listening for extra heart sounds or murmurs.
- **Abdomen:** Inspect the abdomen. Auscultate for bowel sounds. Percuss lightly in all four quadrants. Before you palpate, ask the patient to cough and to point to the most tender area with one finger. Palpate the most tender area or areas last. Perform light and deep palpation, and identify any masses or areas of tenderness. Check for rebound tenderness. Palpate the liver and spleen.
- **GU:** Percuss the CVA for tenderness. Palpate the kidneys. Inspect the external genitalia and urethral meatus for ulcerations. Depending on the history, you may wish to perform a pelvic examination. Note any discharge, inflammation of the cervix, cervical motion tenderness, adnexal tenderness, or pelvic masses. Note uterine size.

Evidence

- The probability that a urine culture will yield positive results in an asymptomatic woman is about 5%. The probability of positive urine culture results in a symptomatic woman who presents to a clinician is about 50%.[4]

- Women with recurrent UTI can often self-diagnose the condition (+LR 4.0; 95% CI 2.9 to 5.5).[4,5]
- Symptoms that increase the probability of UTI[4]:
  - Dysuria (+LR 1.5; 95% CI 1.2 to 2.0)
  - Urinary frequency (+LR 1.8; 95% CI 1.1 to 3.0)
  - Hematuria (+LR 2.0; 95% CI 1.3 to 2.9)
  - Back pain (+LR 1.6; CI 95% 1.2 to 2.1)
- Symptoms that decrease the probability of UTI[4]:
  - Absence of dysuria (−LR 0.5; 95% CI 0.3 to 0.7)
  - History of vaginal discharge (+LR 0.3; 95% CI 0.1 to 0.9)
  - History of vaginal irritation (+LR 0.2; 95% CI 0.1 to 0.9)
- Flank pain, abdominal pain, and fever were not found to be informative in the diagnosis of acute UTI in young women; that is, the 95% confidence intervals for the likelihood ratios included 1.0.[4]
- In a systematic review, Hurlbut and Littenberg[6] found that the combination of nitrite-positive and leukocyte esterase–positive results of urine dipstick testing was most accurate, with 75% sensitivity and 82% specificity. The calculated +LR is 4.2, and the −LR is 0.3. Using a Fagan nomogram, you will find that symptomatic patients with a "positive" dipstick result have a high probability of UTI (80%), whereas patients with a "negative" dipstick result still have a significant probability of UTI (20% to 30%).

Pearls
- UTIs can be described according to the anatomic location of infection as urethritis, cystitis, or pyelonephritis. The "gold-standard" for diagnosing a UTI is a urine culture from a clean urine specimen, with consideration given to bacterial load and the number and type of organisms involved.
- **Urethral syndrome** is characterized by urinary urgency, frequency, and dysuria in the absence of an identifiable cause such as infection or obstruction.

TESTICULAR PAIN: HISTORY AND PHYSICAL EXAMINATION

> **INSTRUCTIONS TO CANDIDATE: An 18-year-old man presents to the emergency department with pain in the left testicle. Obtain a focused history, and perform a focused physical examination.**

DD$_X$: VITAMINS C (Testicular Pain)
- Vascular: Hemorrhage into testicular tumor
- Infectious: Epididymitis, orchitis, cellulitis or fasciitis (Fournier gangrene)
- Traumatic: Acute injury
- Idiopathic/iatrogenic: Incarcerated/strangulated inguinal hernia, torsion of testicular appendages
- Neoplastic: Testicular tumor
- Congenital/genetic: Testicular torsion (bell-clapper deformity)

History
- Ask the patient the following:
  - **Character:** "What is the pain like?"
  - **Location:** "Where does the pain originate?"
  - **Onset:** "When did the pain start? How did it come on (sudden versus gradual)? What were you doing when the pain started?"
  - **Radiation:** "Does the pain move anywhere? Groin? Penis? Contralateral testicle?"
  - **Intensity:** "How severe is the pain on a scale of 1 to 10, with 1 being mild pain and 10 being the worst? Is it getting better, getting worse, or staying the same?"
  - **Duration:** "How long has the pain been present? Is it constantly present or intermittent?"

- Events associated:
  - "Do you have nausea or vomiting?"
  - "Do you have urinary symptoms? Urethral discharge?"
  - "Have you sustained a recent injury?"
  - "Have you had fever or chills?"
  - "Have you experienced abdominal pain? Change in bowel habit?"
  - Frequency: "Have you ever had this pain before? If so, when and under what circumstances did it resolve?"
  - Palliative factors: "Does anything make the pain better? If so, what?"
    - Analgesic medications
    - Particular position
  - Provocative factors: "Does anything make the pain worse? If so, what?"
    - Movement
- **PMH/PSH:** Manipulation or instrumentation of the urinary tract, STIs, inguinal hernia, testicular malignancy
- **MEDS:** Analgesics
- **SH:** Sexual history, including new partners and the use of condoms

Physical Examination
- **Vitals:** Evaluate HR, BP, RR, and temperature.
- **General:** Check capillary refill. Note the patient's position on the stretcher. Note any apparent distress, pallor, or diaphoresis.
- **Resp:** Auscultate the lungs (breath sounds, adventitious sounds).
- **CVS:** Palpate peripheral pulses. Note pulse volume, contour, and rhythm. Auscultate the heart.
- **Abdomen:** Inspect the abdomen. Note any bulges or obvious hernias. Auscultate for bowel sounds. Percuss lightly in all four quadrants. Before you palpate, ask the patient to cough and to point to the most tender area with one finger. Palpate the most tender area or areas last. Perform light and deep palpation, and identify any masses (pulsatile or nonpulsatile) or areas of tenderness. Check for rebound tenderness. Examine for hernias (see pp. 92-93). Perform a DRE.
- **GU:** Percuss the CVA for tenderness (see Figure 4-4). Palpate the kidneys, noting any asymmetry. Examine the external genitalia for signs of trauma, excoriations, ulcerations, or other abnormality. Observe and describe the lie of the testicles within the scrotum. Note any swelling or deformity of the scrotum (see Figure 4-6). Using a small light source, transilluminate any scrotal masses. Torsion of a testicular appendage may appear as a small blue or black dot. Assess the cremasteric reflex (see Figure 4-7). Masses in the scrotum may be auscultated with the diaphragm of the stethoscope. Use your gloved index finger and thumb to gently grasp the anterior and posterior aspects of the testicle. Use your other gloved hand to similarly grasp the superior and inferior poles of the testicle. Note the size, shape, contour, and consistency of each testicle, and any tenderness in it. Note any asymmetry. Palpate the epididymis at the superior pole of each testicle, and follow the spermatic cord into the inguinal canal.

Evidence
- No physical sign can reliably rule out testicular torsion. However, the ipsilateral absence of the cremasteric reflex and the presence of an abnormal testicular lie significantly increase the likelihood that testicular torsion is present.[7]

Pearls
- Many patients with testicular torsion report a similar episode of pain in the past that spontaneously resolved.
- The so-called **bell-clapper deformity** is a congenital, often bilateral abnormality whereby the testicles are mobile, dangling within the scrotum from a redundant spermatic cord.

SAMPLE CHECKLISTS

Kidney and Differentiation from Spleen: Examination

INSTRUCTIONS TO CANDIDATE: Demonstrate an examination of this patient's left kidney. Explain how to clinically differentiate an enlarged kidney from splenomegaly.

Key Points	Satisfactorily Completed
Introduces self to the patient	❑
Determines how the patient wishes to be addressed	❑
Washes hands	❑
Explains nature of the examination to the patient	❑
Examines the patient in a logical manner	❑
Inspection:	
• Looks for signs of fullness (posteriorly)	❑
Auscultation:	
• Listens for abdominal bruits	❑
Palpation:	
• Uses bimanual technique	❑
• Palpates upper border	❑
• Palpates lower border	❑
• Asks patient to inhale during palpation	❑
Differentiates between an enlarged kidney and splenomegaly:	
• Direction of enlargement	❑
• Palpation of upper border of kidney	❑
• Splenic notch	❑
• Presence of splenic hum	❑
Drapes the patient appropriately	❑
Makes appropriate closing remarks	❑

Scrotal Swelling: Examination

INSTRUCTIONS TO CANDIDATE: Demonstrate a GU examination in a 27-year-old man with scrotal swelling.

Key Points	Satisfactorily Completed
Introduces self to the patient	❑
Determines how the patient wishes to be addressed	❑
Washes hands	❑
Explains nature of the examination to the patient	❑
Examines the patient in a logical manner	❑
Inspection:	
• Looks for signs of trauma	❑
• Inspects external genitalia, noting skin integrity, discoloration, and the presence of any skin lesions	❑
• Observes and describes the lie of the testicles within the scrotum	❑

Continued

Key Points	Satisfactorily Completed
• Transilluminates the scrotal mass	❏
• Assesses the cremasteric reflexes	❏
Auscultation:	
• Listens for bowel sounds within the scrotal mass	❏
Palpation:	
• Uses bimanual technique	❏
• Palpates superior and inferior aspects of the testicles	❏
• Palpates anterior and posterior aspects of the testicles	❏
• Palpates the epididymis and spermatic cords	❏
• Palpates inguinal region for the presence of hernias	❏
• Palpates regional lymph nodes	❏
Differentiates testicular from nontesticular causes:	
• Attempts to "get above" the swelling	❏
• Determines whether mass lesion is separate from the testicle	❏
• Differentiates solid from cystic lesions by using transillumination and palpation	❏
Drapes the patient appropriately	❏
Makes appropriate closing remarks	❏

ADVANCED SKILLS

URINARY HESITANCY: HISTORY AND PHYSICAL EXAMINATION

> **INSTRUCTIONS TO CANDIDATE: A 70-year-old man presents with difficulty "making his water." Obtain a focused history, and perform a focused physical examination.**

DD$_X$: VITAMINS C
- Infectious: UTI
- Traumatic: Posttraumatic urethral stricture
- Idiopathic/iatrogenic: Bladder calculi
- Neoplastic: Prostatic enlargement (benign prostatic hypertrophy or malignancy), bladder tumor
- Congenital/genetic: Urethral stricture (may also be a result of scarring)

History
- Ask the patient the following:
  - Character: "Describe your difficulty with 'making your water.'"
    - "Do you have difficulty initiating the stream despite the urge to void? Do you need increased force to pass urine?"
    - "Do you have a sensation of incomplete emptying? Do you have a continued urge to void even when urinary flow has stopped?"
    - "Have you noticed changes in the caliber of the stream (e.g., dribbling)?"
  - Location: "In what setting do you notice this problem? At home? In public places (psychological component)?"
  - Onset: "When did this trouble begin? How did it come about (sudden versus gradual)?"
  - Intensity: "How severe is this trouble? Is it getting better, getting worse, or staying the same? Does it cause constant discomfort (full bladder)? Incontinence?"
  - Duration: "How long has this been going on?"
  - Events associated:
    - "Have you experienced urinary frequency at night (nocturia)? Urinary urgency?"
    - "Have you experienced abdominal distension or fullness? Incontinence (overflow from distended bladder)?"
    - "Do you pass small amounts of urine, accompanied by pain and urgency (bladder calculi)?"
    - "Do you have pain (abdominal, flank, groin)"
    - "Do you see blood in your urine?"
    - "Do you have fever or chills?"
    - "Have you ever passed a kidney stone (hematuria, flank pain, gritty urine)?"
  - Frequency: "Have you ever had this trouble before? If so, when? Does it happen every time you try to urinate (intermittent versus constant)?"
  - Palliative factors: "Does anything make the pain better? If so, what?"
    - Pressing on the abdomen while urinating
  - Provocative factors: "Does anything make the pain worse? If so, what?"
    - Increased fluid intake
- **PMH/PSH:** Malignancy, benign prostatic hypertrophy, renal colic, previous surgery
- **MEDS:** Anticholinergics
- **SH:** Smoking, use of EtOH, use of street drugs, and sexual history
- **FH:** Prostate cancer, renal colic

Physical Examination

- **Vitals:** Evaluate HR, BP, RR, and temperature.
- **General:** Note cachexia, the patient's position on the stretcher, and any apparent distress.
- **Resp:** Auscultate the lungs (breath sounds, adventitious sounds).
- **CVS:** Palpate peripheral pulses. Note pulse volume, contour, and rhythm. Auscultate the heart, listening for extra heart sounds or murmurs.
- **Abdomen:** Inspect the abdomen. Auscultate for bowel sounds. Percuss lightly in all four quadrants. If the urinary bladder is distended, there may be dullness in the suprapubic area to percussion that extends as far as the umbilicus. Before you palpate, ask the patient to cough and to point to the most tender area with one finger. Palpate the most tender area or areas last. Perform light and deep palpation, and identify any masses or areas of tenderness. Check for rebound tenderness. Examine the liver and spleen.
- **GU:** Percuss the CVA for tenderness. Palpate the kidneys. Examine the prostate gland by DRE (see pp. 124-125). Use your gloved index finger to apply gentle, steady pressure at the anus. Ask the patient to take a deep breath, and insert your examining finger into the patient's rectum. Palpate the prostate gland, which lies anterior to the anterior rectal wall (see Figure 4-2). Note any tenderness and the size, symmetry, consistency, and nodularity of the prostate gland.

Evidence

- A Cochrane Database review on prostate cancer screening[8] concluded that evidence was insufficient to support or refute routine prostate cancer screening for reducing rates of mortality from prostate cancer. The review included two large, randomized clinical trials with notable methodologic weakness. The pooled data demonstrated no significant difference in rates of mortality from prostate cancer between patients who were screened and those who were not screened.
- Two large studies were published in 2009. The European Randomized Study of Screening for Prostate Cancer included 162,243 men between 55 and 69 years of age. Of these patients, 72,952 were randomly assigned to be screened for prostate cancer with a prostate-specific antigen (PSA) test about once every 4 years. This study revealed that 1410 men would need to be screened and 48 additional cases of prostate cancer would need to be treated to prevent one prostate cancer death.[9] The Prostate, Lung, Colorectal, and Ovarian (PLCO) Cancer Screening Trial included 76,693 men between the ages of 55 and 74 years; 38,343 patients were randomly assigned to be screened with an annual PSA test and DRE. The rates of death from prostate cancer were low in both the control and screening groups and were not significantly different between the groups.[10]

PENILE ULCER: HISTORY AND PHYSICAL EXAMINATION

INSTRUCTIONS TO CANDIDATE: A 24-year-old man presents to his family doctor with an ulcer on his penis. Obtain a focused history, and perform a focused physical examination.

DD$_X$: VITAMINS C

- **Infectious:** Syphilis, herpes, chancroid, granuloma inguinale, lymphogranuloma venereum
- **Traumatic:** Repetitive trauma
- **Autoimmune/allergic:** Behçet disease
- **Neoplastic:** Malignancy

History

- Ask the patient the following:
  - **Character:** "What does the ulcer look like?"
  - **Location:** "Where is the ulcer located? Are you circumcised or uncircumcised?"
  - **Onset:** "How did you first come to notice this ulcer on your penis? When you first noticed it, what did it look like?"
  - **Radiation:** "Are there any ulcers on your scrotum or in the surrounding area? Are there any ulcers in your mouth or elsewhere on your body?"
  - **Intensity:** "How large is the ulcer? Has it changed in size or shape since you first noticed it? Is it getting better, getting worse, or staying the same?"
  - **Duration:** "When did you first notice the ulcer? How long has it been present?"
  - **Events associated:**
    - "Have you had fever or chills? Malaise?"
    - "Have you noticed bleeding from the ulcer?"
    - "Have you noticed penile discharge?"
    - "Do you have urinary symptoms (dysuria, urinary frequency)?"
    - "Do you have groin pain? Groin mass?"
    - "Do you have any rash?"
    - "Do you have any eye concerns (redness, pain) or joint problems?"
  - **Frequency:** "Have you ever had an ulcer like this before? If so, how often?"
  - **Palliative factors:** "Does anything make the ulcer better? If so, what?"
    - Topical agents
  - **Provocative factors:** "Does anything make the ulcer worse? If so, what?"
    - Sexual intercourse, masturbation
- **PMH/PSH:** Human immunodeficiency virus (HIV) infection, STIs, autoimmune disease (e.g., vasculitis)
- **MEDS:** Topical agents, antibiotics, antivirals, antiretrovirals
- **SH:** Sexual history, including new partners and use of condoms; smoking, use of EtOH, and use of street drugs
- **FH:** Behçet disease, vasculitis

Physical Examination

- **Vitals:** Evaluate HR, BP, RR, and temperature.
- **General:** Note any apparent distress, pallor, or diaphoresis.
- **Skin:** Perform a complete dermatologic examination, including inspection of all hair-bearing and non–hair-bearing cutaneous surfaces, hair, mucous membranes, and nails.
- **Lymphatic system:** Examine regional lymph nodes in relation to skin findings, particularly in the groin (note size, shape, mobility, consistency, tenderness, warmth, and number of enlarged nodes).
- **Resp:** Auscultate the lungs (breath sounds, adventitious sounds).
- **CVS:** Palpate peripheral pulses. Note pulse volume, contour, and rhythm. Auscultate the heart, listening for extra heart sounds or murmurs.
- **Abdomen:** Inspect the abdomen. Note any bulges or obvious hernias. Auscultate for bowel sounds. Percuss lightly in all four quadrants. Perform light and deep palpation, and identify any masses (pulsatile or nonpulsatile) or areas of tenderness. Examine for hernias (see pp. 92-93). Perform a DRE.
- **GU:** Examine the external genitalia for signs of trauma, excoriations, ulcerations, or other abnormality. Be sure to retract the foreskin, if present, and inspect the glans penis. Describe any skin lesions using the terminology outlined in Chapter 7 (pp. 224-225). Note any discharge from the urethral meatus. Observe and describe the lie of the testicles within the scrotum. Note any swelling or deformity of the scrotum (see Figure 4-6). Using a small light source, transilluminate any scrotal masses. Masses in the scrotum may be auscultated with the diaphragm of the stethoscope. Use your gloved index finger and thumb to gently grasp the anterior and posterior aspects of the patient's testicle. Use your other gloved hand to similarly grasp the

superior and inferior poles of the testicle. Note the size, shape, contour, and consistency of each testicle, and any tenderness in it. Note any asymmetry. Palpate the epididymis at the superior pole of each testicle, and follow the spermatic cord into the inguinal canal.

Pearls
- Table 4-1 lists the differential diagnosis of penile ulcers.
- The most common infectious causes of genital ulcers in the developed world are primary syphilis, genital herpes, and chancroid.[11]
- Clinical characteristics—including location of ulcer, size and number of lesions, induration and depth of the ulcer, duration of the ulceration, and regional lymph node enlargement—are not accurately predictive of the cause of genital ulcers.[12]

Table 4-1   Differential Diagnosis of Penile Ulcers

Generally Painful	Generally Painless
Chancroid	Granuloma inguinale
Herpes	Lymphogranuloma venereum
Behçet disease	Primary syphilis
	Penile carcinoma
	Traumatic

REFERENCES

1. Grover SA, Barkun AN, Sackett DL. The rational clinical examination: does this patient have splenomegaly? *JAMA*. 1993;270:2218-2221.
2. Caesar RE, Kaplan GW. The incidence of the cremasteric reflex in normal boys. *J Urol*. 1994;152(2 Pt 2):779-780.
3. Holroyd-Leduc JM, Tannenbaum C, Thorpe KE, et al. What type of urinary incontinence does this woman have? *JAMA*. 2008;299:1446-1456.
4. Bent S, Nallamothu BK, Simel DL, et al. Does this woman have an acute uncomplicated urinary tract infection? *JAMA*. 2002;287:2701-2710.
5. Gupta K, Hooton TM, Roberts PL, et al. Patient-initiated treatment of uncomplicated recurrent urinary tract infections in young women. *Ann Intern Med*. 2001;135:9-16.
6. Hurlbut T, Littenberg B. The diagnostic accuracy of rapid dipstick tests to predict urinary tract infection. *Am J Clin Pathol*. 1991;96:582-588.
7. Schmitz D, Safranek S. Clinical inquiries. How useful is a physical exam in diagnosing testicular torsion? *J Fam Pract*. 2009;58:433-434.
8. Ilic D, O'Connor D, Green S, et al. Screening for prostate cancer. *Cochrane Database Syst Rev*. 2006;3:CD004720.
9. Schröder FH, Hugosson J, Roobol MJ, et al. Screening and prostate-cancer mortality in a randomized European study. *N Engl J Med*. 2009;360:1320-1328.
10. Andriole GL, Crawford ED, Grubb RL 3rd, et al. Mortality results from a randomized prostate-cancer screening trial. *N Engl J Med*. 2009;360:1310-1319.
11. Centers for Disease Control and Prevention, Workowski KA, Berman SM. Sexually transmitted diseases treatment guidelines, 2006. *MMWR Recomm Rep*. 2006;55(RR-11):1-94.
12. Hope-Rapp E, Anyfantakis V, Fouéré S, et al. Etiology of genital ulcer disease: a prospective study of 278 cases seen in an STD clinic in Paris. *Sex Transm Dis*. 2010;37:153-158.

CHAPTER 5

Nervous System

Rose P. Mengual, ACP, MD

ANATOMY

- The **central nervous system** is composed of the brain and spinal cord. The remainder of the nervous system that resides outside the brain and spinal cord is collectively referred to as the **peripheral nervous system.** The peripheral nervous system is further subdivided into the somatic and autonomic nervous systems. This chapter concentrates on the assessment of the somatic nervous system.

Brain

- The brain, or **cerebrum,** is divided into the right and left cerebral hemispheres. The surface of the cerebrum is marked by elevations (**gyri**) and grooves (**sulci**). Several major sulci further subdivide the brain into four lobes: (1) frontal, (2) temporal,

(3) parietal, and (4) occipital lobes (Figure 5-1). The **central sulcus** is a key landmark that separates the **primary somatosensory cortex** (postcentral gyrus) from the **primary motor cortex** (precentral gyrus).

- The different areas of the body are topographically mapped onto these cortices and known as the somatosensory and motor **homunculi,** respectively (Figure 5-2).

Spinal Cord

- Incoming **(afferent)** sensory signals enter the spinal cord and ascend to the thalamus and appropriate sensory cortex (Figure 5-3). Sensations of vibration, proprioception, and light touch ascend the spinal cord via the **posterior (dorsal) columns**. Sensations of pain, temperature, and crude touch ascend the spinal cord via the **anterolateral pathways (spinothalamic tract).**

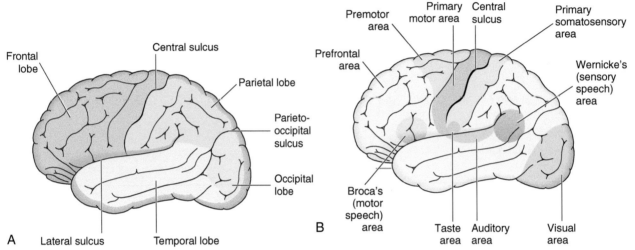

Figure 5-1 The lobes and principal sulci of the cerebrum **(A),** and the main sensory and motor areas **(B).** (From Waugh A, Grant A. *Ross and Wilson Anatomy and Physiology in Health and Illness.* 10th ed. Philadelphia: Elsevier; 2006 [**A,** p. 151, Figure 7.14; **B,** p. 152, Figure 7.16].)

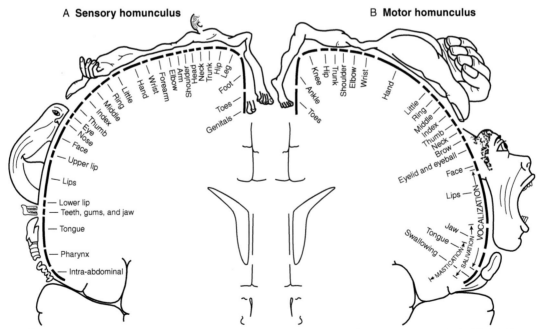

Figure 5-2 The sensory and motor homunculi. (Redrawn from Fix JD. *High-Yield Neuroanatomy.* 2nd ed. Philadelphia: Lippincott Williams & Wilkins; 2000 [p. 123].)

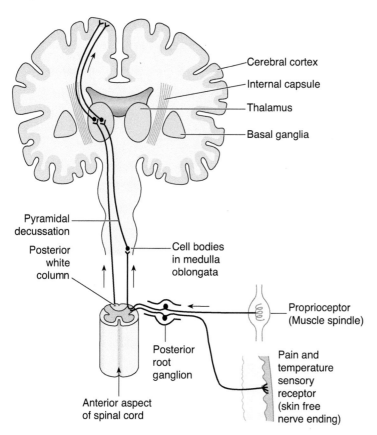

Figure 5-3 Sensory (afferent) pathways. Pain and temperature via anterolateral pathway (spinothalamic tract) and proprioception and vibration via posterior (dorsal) column. (Adapted from Waugh A, Grant A. *Ross and Wilson Anatomy and Physiology in Health and Illness.* 10th ed. Philadelphia: Elsevier; 2006 [p. 159, Figure 7.25].)

- Outgoing **(efferent)** motor signals are carried by **upper motor neurons** that originate in the primary motor cortex and descend toward the spinal cord. The upper motor neurons decussate at the level of the junction of the medulla and spinal cord (pyramidal decussation) and continue to descend the spinal cord until they synapse with **lower motor neurons** just before exiting the anterior horn (Figure 5-4).
- A total of 31 spinal nerves exit the spinal cord. The spinal cord extends to the level of L1 or L2 and terminates as the **conus medullaris,** which is anchored to the coccyx by the **filum terminale.** Below the level of L1, the spinal nerves descend within the spinal canal as the **cauda equina** (Figure 5-5).
- A **dermatome** is a territory of skin supplied with sensory innervation by a specific spinal nerve. A **myotome** is a muscle group supplied with motor innervation by a specific spinal nerve.

Brainstem and Cranial Nerves
- Of the 12 **cranial nerves,** most originate in the brainstem (Figure 5-6). The majority of the cranial nerves have both motor and sensory components, and several are responsible for specialized sensory function.
- The brainstem houses several essential areas, including the reticular activating system and the cardiac and respiratory centers.

Reflex Arc (Figure 5-7)
- Specialized stretch receptors are activated and transmit afferent signals to the spinal cord via the dorsal root. Within the spinal cord, a direct synapse is formed with lower motor neurons through which an efferent motor signal is conveyed. Additional synapses with inhibitory interneurons aid in modulating the reflex response.

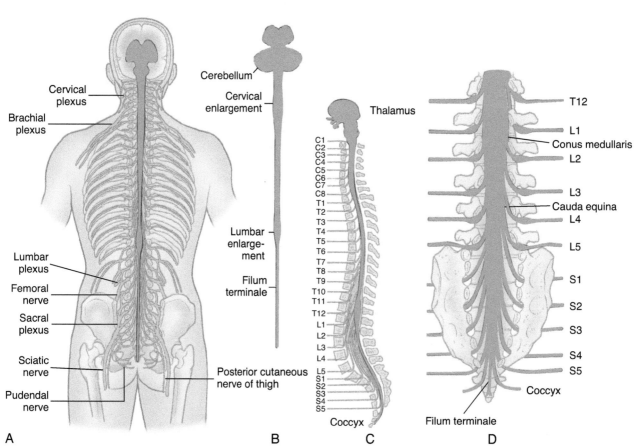

Figure 5-4 Motor (efferent) pathways. Upper motor neuron originates in cerebral cortex and reaches synapse with lower motor neuron in the anterior horn of spinal cord. (From Waugh A, Grant A. *Ross and Wilson Anatomy and Physiology in Health and Illness.* 10th ed. Philadelphia: Elsevier; 2006 [p. 153, Figure 7.17].)

Figure 5-5 Location of spinal cord, spinal nerves, and cauda equina in relation to the vertebral column. **A,** Posterior view. **B,** Anterior view of brainstem and spinal cord. **C,** Lateral view, showing relationship of spinal cord to vertebrae. **D,** Enlargement of caudal area with group of nerve fibers composing the cauda equina. (From Seidel HM, Ball JW, Dains JE, et al. *Mosby's Guide to Physical Examination.* 6th ed. St. Louis: Mosby; 2006 [p. 767, Figure 22-7].)

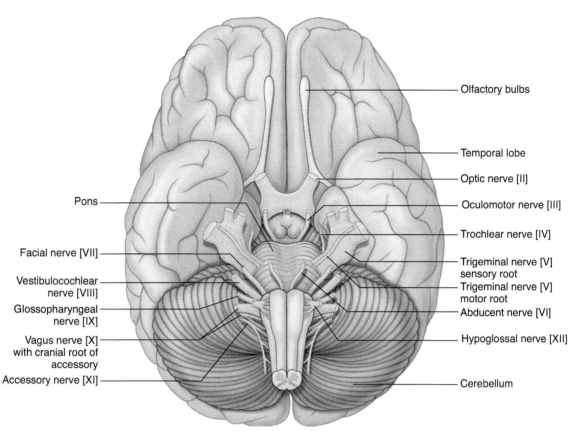

Figure 5-6 Origins of the cranial nerves. (From Drake RL, Vogl AW, Mitchell AWM, et al. *Gray's Anatomy for Students.* 2nd ed. Philadelphia: Elsevier; 2010 [Figure 8.49].)

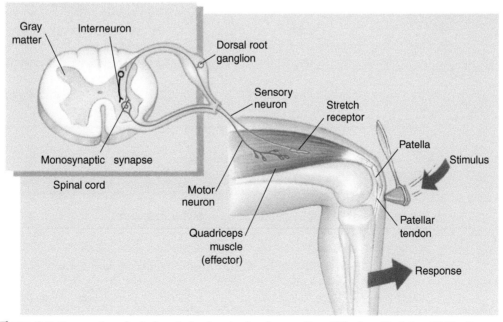

Figure 5-7 Cross-section of spinal cord, showing simple reflex arc. (From Thibodeau GA, Patton KT. *The Human Body in Health & Disease.* 4th ed. St. Louis: Elsevier; 2005 [Figure 9-7].)

GLOSSARY OF SIGNS AND SYMPTOMS

Altered Level of Consciousness
- **Confusion** is an alteration in memory, awareness, alertness, or attention.
- **Delirium** is an acute confusional state characterized by fluctuating attention and level of alertness. It most commonly has an acute organic or structural cause that is reversible. Features suggestive of delirium include abnormal vital signs, abrupt onset, multiple medical comorbid conditions, or multiple medications.
- **Depressed level of consciousness** represents a continuum that ranges from mild obtundation to somnolence and ultimately coma. Coma is a state of unconsciousness.
- The **AVPU scale** is an objective and easily understood classification system used to describe level of consciousness and responsiveness (**a**lert, **v**erbal, **p**ain, and **u**nresponsive) (Table 5-1).
- The **Glasgow Coma Scale** (GCS) is a numeric scale derived for use with trauma patients to describe level of consciousness; it is also useful for determining prognosis and evaluating progress of patients with brain injury. Three domains are evaluated: eye opening, verbal response, and motor response. The lowest score obtainable in each domain is 1, and the GCS score ranges from 3, for an unconscious patient, to 15, for the patient with a normal level of consciousness (Table 5-2).

Headache
- **Tension headaches** are the most common cause of headache and are thought to result from muscular tension of the head, neck, or jaw. Tension headaches are classically described as feeling "tight" or "like a vise" and may be chronic or intermittent in nature.

Table 5-1 AVPU Scale for Level of Responsiveness

Acronym Initial	Level of Responsiveness	Description
A	Alert	Awake and alert; spontaneously attends to examiner
V	Verbal	Awakens or responds only with verbal stimulation
P	Pain	Awakens or responds only to painful or physical stimulation
U	Unresponsive	Does not awaken or respond with verbal or painful stimulation

Table 5-2 Glasgow Coma Scale

Eye Opening	Verbal Response	Motor Response	Points
None	None	None	1
To pain	Incomprehensible sounds	Decerebrate posture (abnormal extension)	2
To voice	Inappropriate words	Decorticate posture (abnormal flexion)	3
Spontaneous	Confused	Withdrawal	4
	Alert, appropriate	Localizes	5
		Obeys commands	6

- **Migraine headaches** are thought to result from neurovascular instability. Migraines may be preceded by a recognizable aura and are classically described as intermittent, severe, unilateral, and pulsating. Migraine headache is often accompanied by nausea, vomiting, photophobia, or phonophobia, or a combination of these. Uncommon neurologic symptoms, including visual or cognitive change, numbness, or paresis, may result.
- **Subarachnoid hemorrhage** is a life-threatening cause of headache that most commonly results from a ruptured cerebral aneurysm. The classic presentation of subarachnoid hemorrhage is a sudden, severe headache in which the pain is maximal at onset. It may be accompanied by sudden loss of consciousness, nausea, vomiting, and meningeal irritation.

Seizure
- **Seizure** is an abnormal discharge of neurons of the cerebral cortex that results in a variety of clinical manifestations, depending on the region of the brain involved.
- A **generalized seizure** affects both cerebral cortices, resulting in loss of consciousness and usually a tonic phase of sustained muscle contraction, followed by a clonic phase of rhythmic muscle contraction and relaxation.
- **Partial seizures** are localized to one cerebral hemisphere, and the clinical manifestation is specific to the particular region of the brain involved.
- **Epilepsy** is a condition of recurring intermittent seizure activity without an identifiable secondary cause. The most common causes of seizure recurrence are nonadherence to an antiseizure medication regimen, illness or infection, sleep deprivation, and drug interactions.

Tremor
- **Tremor** is a rhythmic involuntary movement disorder that most commonly involves the hands but can also involve the face, neck, trunk, and lower limbs.
- **Action tremor** is a tremor that is accentuated during particular movements or postures that involve voluntary muscle groups.
- **Rest tremors** persist in the absence of movements or actions. The pill-rolling tremor of Parkinson disease is an example of a rest tremor.

Vertigo
- **Vertigo** is an abnormal perception of movement or spinning that is usually accompanied by loss of balance and by nausea and vomiting. Vertigo may be classified as central and peripheral; the former is more likely to be of pathologic origin and thereby necessitates more urgent evaluation.
- **Peripheral vertigo** is caused by a problem involving the inner ear and is characterized by sudden, severe, short-lived vertigo usually triggered by repositioning of the head without accompanying neurologic symptoms. The three most common diagnoses assigned to patients with peripheral vertigo are benign paroxysmal positional vertigo, acute otitis media, and vestibular neuronitis.
- **Central vertigo** is caused by a central nervous system process or mass lesion. Its onset may be gradual or sudden. It is characterized by milder symptoms lasting from days to months, and it is apparently not triggered by head position or movement. Central vertigo is often accompanied by other neurologic findings determined by the underlying cause and area of the brain affected. Common causes of central vertigo include brain tumor, infection, and concussion.

Hearing Loss
- **Conductive** hearing loss results from impairment in the sound wave transmission through the auditory canal, tympanic membrane, or middle ear. Causes of conductive hearing loss include canal occlusion by cerumen or foreign body, acute otitis media, middle ear effusion, cholesteatoma, and otosclerosis.

- **Sensorineural** hearing loss results from impairment in the neural transmission of sound signals from the inner ear to the auditory cortex via neural pathways. Causes of sensorineural hearing loss include noise exposure, congenital syndromes, Ménière disease, and autoimmune disease.

Head Injury
- Head injuries range in severity from minor to major. The severity of head injury can be predicted by historical and physical findings and categorized on the basis of the GCS score.
- **Concussion** is a temporary interruption in neurologic function as a result of head injury that may or may not involve a loss of consciousness. Symptoms may range from brief altered consciousness to brief loss of consciousness, amnesia, headache, or confusion.

Neuropathic Pain
- **Neuropathic pain** is debilitating and usually chronic pain resulting from injury, inflammation, degeneration, erosion, or compression of the spinal cord, one or more spinal nerves, or one or more peripheral nerves. Neuropathic pain is typically described as burning, shooting, or like an electric shock.

ESSENTIAL SKILLS

APPROACH TO HEADACHE: HISTORY

- Headache is a common presenting concern in emergency and primary care settings. In many cases, the cause is benign, but it is important to consider several life- or function-threatening diagnoses in all patients presenting with headache (Table 5-3).

DD$_X$: VITAMINS C
- **V**ascular: Migraine, subarachnoid hemorrhage, temporal arteritis
- **I**nfectious: Cerebral abscess, meningitis, sinusitis
- **T**raumatic: Head injury, concussion, intracranial hemorrhage (subdural hematoma, epidural hematoma (Figure 5-8)
- **I**diopathic/iatrogenic: Post–lumbar puncture headache
- **N**eoplastic: Brain tumor (Figure 5-9)
- **S**ubstance abuse and psychiatric: Carbon monoxide poisoning

DD$_X$: Other
- Tension headache, cluster headache, acute angle closure glaucoma, occipital neuralgia

Table 5-3   Life- or Function-Threatening Causes of Headache

1. Subarachnoid hemorrhage
2. Cerebral venous sinus thrombosis
3. Meningitis
4. Acute angle closure glaucoma
5. Temporal arteritis
6. Space-occupying lesion
7. Raised intracranial pressure
8. Carbon monoxide poisoning

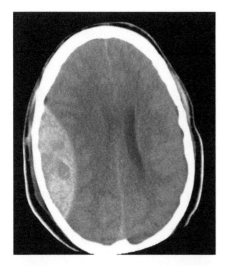

Figure 5-8 Computed tomogram showing epidural hematoma secondary to blunt force trauma to right temporal region. (Courtesy of Dr. Osama Loubani, Dalhousie University, Halifax, Nova Scotia.)

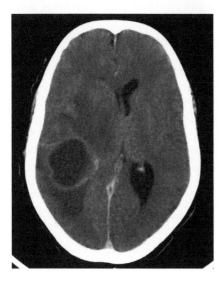

Figure 5-9 Computed tomogram showing glioblastoma multiforme. A malignant right parietal mass with surrounding vasogenic edema, ventricular compression, and midline shift. (Courtesy of Dr. Osama Loubani, Dalhousie University, Halifax, Nova Scotia.)

History

- Ask the patient the following:
  - **Ch**aracter: "Describe the pain."
    - Pulsating or throbbing (migraine)
    - Tightness or vise-like (tension headache)
    - Worst headache of the patient's life (subarachnoid hemorrhage)
    - Ache
    - Sharp
  - **L**ocation: "Where do you feel the headache? Does one spot hurt more than any other?"
    - Unilateral (migraine, cluster)
    - Bilateral (tension)
    - Occiput (occipital neuralgia)
    - Neck (cluster, meningitis, subarachnoid hemorrhage)
    - One or both eyes or orbital region (cluster, glaucoma, temporal arteritis)
  - **O**nset: "When did the pain start? How did it come on (sudden versus gradual)? If it occurred suddenly, what were you doing at the time?"
  - **R**adiation: "Does the pain radiate to other areas?"
    - Neck (cluster, meningitis, subarachnoid hemorrhage)
    - One or both eyes or periorbital region (cluster, glaucoma, temporal arteritis)
    - Teeth (cluster, sinusitis)

- Intensity: "How severe is the pain on a scale of 1 to 10, with 1 being mild pain and 10 being the worst? Is it getting better, getting worse, or staying the same?"
  - Compare intensity at time of assessment with intensity at onset.
  - Determine whether pain was maximal at onset. If it was not, determine time to reach maximal intensity.
- Duration: "Does the pain occur at certain times? How long does it last? Has it been constant or intermittent?"
- Events associated:
  - "Have you experienced nausea, vomiting, or fainting (possibly indicative of subarachnoid hemorrhage)?"
  - "Have you experienced decreased vision, jaw pain with chewing (claudication), joint pain (arthralgia), or muscle aches (myalgia) (indicative of temporal arteritis)?"
  - "Have you experienced tearing or nasal congestion (as in cluster headache)?"
  - "Have you experienced altered mental status, fever, rash, or neck stiffness (meningitis)?"
  - "Have you fallen or had a head injury (possibly traumatic brain injury or intracranial hemorrhage)?"
  - "Have you experienced aura, numbness, tingling, weakness, or speech problem (characteristic of migraine or stroke)?"
  - "Have you noticed eye pain or redness, loss of vision, or change in the appearance of your eye (indicative of acute angle closure glaucoma)?"
- Frequency: "Is this pain an isolated or recurring event? How frequent are the episodes? Is this headache similar to past headaches? If so, what prompted you to seek medical care on this occasion?"
- Palliative factors: "Does anything make the pain better? If so, what?"
  - Medications (type, dose, frequency), strategies, positions, or alternative therapies (massage, chiropractor, acupuncture)
  - Success or failure of each strategy
- Provocative factors: "Does anything make the pain worse? If so, what?"
  - Foods
  - Position (upright, supine, or dependent)
  - Light (photophobia)
  - Noise (phonophobia)
- **Past medical history (PMH)/past surgical history (PSH):** Hypertension, cancer, polymyalgia rheumatica, systemic lupus erythematosus, glaucoma, migraine, concussion, brain surgery, ventricular shunt
- **Medications (MEDS):** Anticoagulants (adherence, international normalized ratio [INR] monitoring, most recent INR level), migraine medications (adherence)
- **Social history (SH):** Smoking, use of alcohol (EtOH), use of street drugs (specifically cocaine or other sympathomimetic agents), occupation, interference with daily activities
- **Family history (FH):** Brain cancer, cerebral aneurysm, sudden death, migraine

APPROACH TO SEIZURE: HISTORY

- Seizures are broadly classified as primary and secondary seizures, depending on whether the seizure itself is a problem in isolation or a result of some inciting event. It is important to consider this distinction in order to document the history appropriately.

Primary Seizure
- Seizure disorder or epilepsy
- Seizure recurrence (usually triggered by nonadherence to an antiseizure medication regimen, sleep deprivation, drug interactions, intercurrent illness or infection, or psychologic stress)

Secondary Seizure (Age-Based Approach)
* **Pediatric:** Fever, infection, inborn errors of metabolism, congenital adrenal hyperplasia
* **Adult:** Use of street drugs (cocaine or other sympathomimetic agents), prescription medications (selective serotonin reuptake inhibitors [SSRIs], neuroleptic agents, lithium), drug withdrawal (alcohol, benzodiazepines), infection (meningitis, encephalitis), hypotension, hypoxia (respiratory illness, shortness of breath), hypoglycemia (diabetes), metabolic derangement (vomiting, diarrhea, dehydration, renal dysfunction, liver disease), and pregnancy (eclampsia)

DD$_X$: VITAMINS C
* **V**ascular: Intracranial hemorrhage
* **I**nfectious: Meningitis, encephalitis
* **T**raumatic: Head injury, post–brain injury seizure
* **M**etabolic: Hypocalcemia, hypoglycemia, hyponatremia, hypoxia
* **I**diopathic/**i**atrogenic: Nonadherence with antiseizure medication regimen, drug interactions
* **N**eoplastic: Brain tumor
* **S**ubstance abuse and **p**sychiatric: Drug withdrawal, sympathomimetic agents, serotonin syndrome, neuroleptic malignant syndrome, pseudoseizure

DD$_X$: Other
* Epilepsy, eclampsia (pregnancy)

History
* Use **ChLORIDE FPP** to delineate the presenting concern, and ask the patient questions as follows:
  * **C**haracter: If bystanders were present, use their collateral history to determine the appearance of the seizure.
  * **O**nset: "When did the seizure begin? Did you experience an aura before the seizure?"
  * **D**uration: "How long did the seizure last?" Inquire about duration of ictal and postictal phases.
  * **E**vents associated:
    * "Did you experience features suggestive of generalized tonic-clonic seizure: incontinence, tongue or cheek biting, injury, myalgias?"
    * "Did you experience loss of consciousness, motor activity, or postictal symptoms?"
  * **F**requency: "Have you had any similar past episodes?"
    * If the patient has epilepsy, establish frequency of seizure, typical quality and recovery.
    * Establish whether there has been any recent change in pattern.
  * **P**rovocative factors: "Does anything make these seizures worse? If so, what?"
    * Explore alternative causes: vasovagal syncope (light-headedness, nausea, diaphoresis, visual changes); cardiac syncope (palpitation, chest pain, shortness of breath); pregnancy; infectious entity (fever, rash, nuchal rigidity, cough, abdominal pain, vomiting, diarrhea)
    * Consider potential age-based causes, and ask questions to differentiate between these.
    * If the patient has epilepsy, ask about common triggers for recurrence.
* **PMH/PSH:** Epilepsy, seizure disorder, traumatic brain injury, cancer
* **MEDS:** Antiseizure medications (check adherence and plasma levels), SSRIs, neuroleptics, lithium, new medications (antibiotics; drug interactions)
* **SH:** Smoking, use of EtOH, use of street drugs, drug withdrawal

Pearl: Seizure versus Syncope
* **Syncope** is a sudden loss of consciousness as a result of transient hypotension, hypoxia, or cardiac dysrhythmia. Syncope is often preceded by a brief interruption in cerebral blood flow that leads to depressed mental status and transient neurologic

signs that mimic seizure, including myoclonic jerks, twitching, facial grimacing, or automatisms.

- The neurologic manifestations of seizure are typically more violent, rhythmic, of longer duration, and followed by a postictal phase of depressed mental status or confusion.

CRANIAL NERVES: EXAMINATION

- Table 5-4 lists the cranial nerves and their general function along with a mnemonic.

Cranial Nerve I: Olfactory Nerve
Sensory: Smell
- Smell is often not formally assessed unless impairment of function is strongly suspected.

Cranial Nerve II: Optic Nerve
Sensory: Vision
- Visual acuity (Snellen chart)
- Visual field testing (confrontation):
  - Stand an arm's length away from the patient.
  - Instruct the patient to cover one eye and stare at your nose.
  - Ask the patient, "How many fingers do you see me holding up in the background while you stare at my nose?"
  - Hold one to five digits up at a time in each of the four quadrants of vision in random order.
  - Repeat for the opposite eye.
- Afferent component of pupillary reflex (light detection):
  - Shine a light toward the patient's pupil from the lateral aspect of the patient's face.
  - Avoid holding the light directly in patient's field of view: fixation will result in pupillary constriction or dilation as a result of accommodation.
  - The normal finding is pupil constriction.

Table 5-4 Cranial Nerve Examination

Cranial Nerve	Naming Memory Tool			Function Memory Tool		
	Name of Nerve	**Initial**	**Mnemonic**	**Function**	**Initial**	**Mnemonic**
I	**O**lfactory	**O**	**O**n	**S**ensory	**S**	**S**ome
II	**O**ptic	**O**	**O**ld	**S**ensory	**S**	**S**ay
III	**O**culomotor	**O**	**O**lympus's	**M**otor	**M**	**M**arry
IV	**T**rochlear	**T**	**T**owering	**M**otor	**M**	**M**oney
V	**T**rigeminal	**T**	**T**ops	**B**oth	**B**	**B**ut
VI	**A**bducens	**A**	**A**	**M**otor	**M**	**M**y
VII	**F**acial	**F**	**F**inn	**B**oth	**B**	**B**rother
VIII	**A**uditory	**A**	**A**nd	**S**ensory	**S**	**S**ays it is
IX	**G**lossopharyngeal	**G**	**G**erman	**B**oth	**B**	**B**ad
X	**V**agus	**V**	**V**iewed	**B**oth	**B**	**B**usiness
XI	**S**pinal accessory	**S**	**S**ome	**M**otor	**M**	**M**arrying
XII	**H**ypoglossal	**H**	**H**awks	**M**otor	**M**	**M**oney

Adapted from Diepenbrock NH. *Quick Reference to Critical Care*. 3rd ed. Philadelphia: Lippincott Williams & Wilkins; 2008 [p. 23].

Cranial Nerve III: Oculomotor Nerve
Motor
- Efferent component of pupillary reflex (pupil constriction)
- All extraocular movements (except those controlled by cranial nerves IV and VI)
  - Instruct the patient, "Follow my finger (or light) with your eyes, but do not move your head."
  - Move an object through six cardinal directions of gaze (Figure 5-10).

Cranial Nerve IV: Trochlear Nerve
Motor
- Extraocular movement (superior oblique nerve)
  - Moves eye down and in (see Figure 5-10)

Cranial Nerve V: Trigeminal Nerve
Motor
- Muscles of mastication (masseter and temporalis nerves) (Figure 5-11)
  - Instruct the patient, "Clench your teeth."
  - Palpate the masseter and temporalis muscles bilaterally for presence and symmetry of contraction.

Sensory
- Afferent component of corneal reflex (corneal sensation)
- Facial sensation:
  - Three main branches (V1, V2, and V3; Figure 5-12) need to be tested independently for sensation of light touch and discrimination between sharpness and dullness (Figure 5-13).
  - Instruct the patient, "Tell me when you feel the cotton touching your face."
  - Ask the patient, "Does this feel sharp or dull?"
  - Compare sensation on the right side with that on the left side by lightly touching the forehead, cheek, and the lateral aspect of the chin.
  - Ask the patient, "Does this (right side) feel the same as this (left side)?"

Cranial Nerve VI: Abducens Nerve (see Figure 5-10)
Motor
- Extraocular movement (lateral rectus muscle)
  - Abducts eyes from midposition

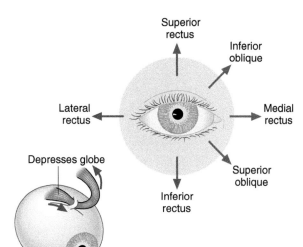

Figure 5-10 Extraocular movements with demonstration of superior oblique function. (From Hall T. *PACES for the MRCP with 250 Clinical Cases.* 2nd ed. Philadelphia: Elsevier; 2008 [p. 409, Figure 3.49].)

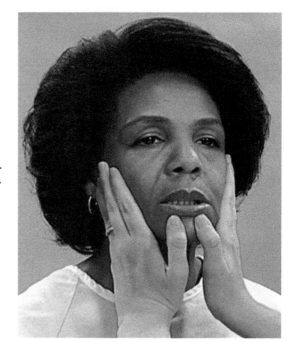

Figure 5-11 Technique for examination of the trigeminal nerve motor function. (From Seidel HM, Ball JW, Dains JE, et al. *Mosby's Guide to Physical Examination.* 6th ed. St. Louis: Mosby; 2006 [p. 777, Figure 22-12].)

Figure 5-12 Divisions of trigeminal nerve sensory branches: ophthalmic division (V1), maxillary division (V2), and mandibular division (V3). (From Swartz MH. *Textbook of Physical Diagnosis: History and Examination.* 6th ed. Philadelphia: Elsevier; 2010 [p. 656, Figure 22-10].)

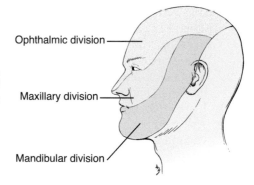

Ophthalmic division

Maxillary division

Mandibular division

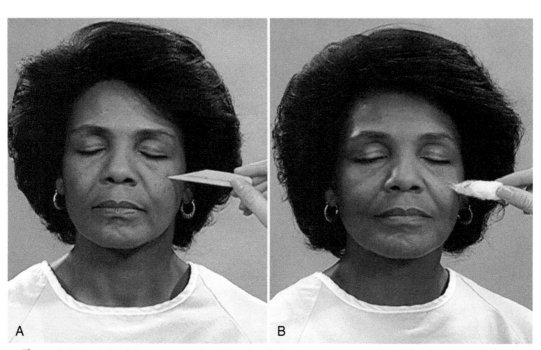

A   B

Figure 5-13 Techniques for sensory testing of the trigeminal nerve. **A,** Discrimination of sharpness versus dullness. **B,** Light touch. (From Seidel HM, Ball JW, Dains JE, et al. *Mosby's Guide to Physical Examination.* 6th ed. St. Louis: Mosby; 2006 [p. 778, Figure 22-13].)

Cranial Nerve VII: Facial Nerve (Figure 5-14)

Motor

- Efferent component of the corneal reflex (eyelid closure)
- Muscles of facial expression: assess for presence and symmetry of muscle function by instructing the patient as follows:
  - "Raise your eyebrows."
  - "Close your eyes as tight as you can" (attempt to open the eyelids to test muscle strength).
  - "Smile and show me your top teeth."
  - "Puff out your cheeks and do not let me push the air out."

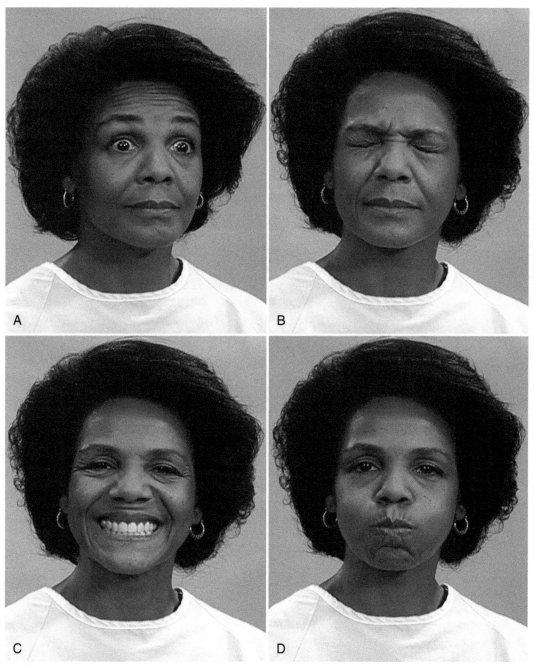

Figure 5-14 Facial nerve examination. Ask the patient to do the following: **A,** "Raise eyebrows." **B,** "Close your eyes as tight as you can, and do not let me open them." **C,** "Smile and show me your teeth." **D,** "Puff out your cheeks, and do not let me push the air out." (From Seidel HM, Ball JW, Dains JE, et al. *Mosby's Guide to Physical Examination.* 6th ed. St. Louis: Mosby; 2006 [p. 779, Figure 22-14, *A, C, E, F*].)

Sensory: Taste
- Anterior two thirds of tongue. Assess function by asking the patient, "Do your foods taste normal?"
  - Taste is often not formally assessed unless impairment of function is strongly suspected.
  - Formal evaluation of taste requires application of various tastes (sweet, salty, sour) to each specific taste region of the tongue.

Cranial Nerve VIII: Auditory (Vestibulocochlear) Nerve
Sensory: Hearing
- Assess for detection and symmetry of light finger rub in each ear.
  - Instruct the patient, "Lift your hand on the side where you hear a noise"; alternate sides randomly.
  - Ask the patient, "Do both sides sound the same?"

Weber Test (Lateralization) (Figure 5-15)
- Strike the tuning fork.
- Place the stem of the tuning fork firmly on the crown of the patient's head.
- Ask the patient, "Do you hear the sound on one side or the middle?"
- A normal response is equal sound in both ears (normal sensory and conductive hearing).
- An abnormal response is lateralization:
  - Ipsilateral conductive hearing loss
  - Contralateral sensorineural hearing loss

Rinne Test (Air Versus Bone Conduction) (see Figure 5-15)
- Strike the tuning fork.
- Place the stem of the tuning fork firmly on the patient's mastoid bone.
- Ask the patient, "Tell me when the buzzing stops."
- Hold the tuning fork 1 to 2 cm from the patient's ipsilateral ear canal.
- Ask the patient, "Do you hear it now?"
- In a normal response, air conduction is greater than bone conduction.
- In an abnormal response:
  - Air conduction is the same as bone conduction, or bone conduction is greater than air conduction (conductive hearing loss).

Cranial Nerve IX: Glossopharyngeal Nerve
Motor
- Pharyngeal muscles: Assess for symmetry and function.
  - Ask the patient, "Are you having any difficulty swallowing?"
  - Instruct the patient, "Say 'ahhh'": assess for presence and symmetry of palate rise.

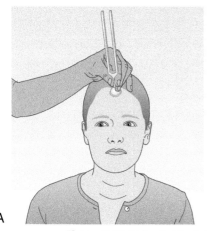
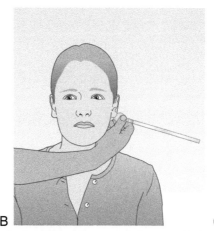
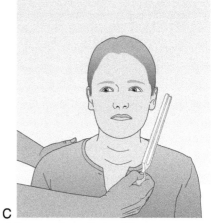

A   B   C

Figure 5-15 Weber test for lateralization **(A)** and Rinne test for bone conduction **(B)** versus air conduction **(C).** (From Hall T. *PACES for the MRCP with 250 Clinical Cases.* 2nd ed. Philadelphia: Elsevier; 2008 [p. 386, Figure 3.23].)

Sensory: Taste
- Posterior third of tongue
  - Taste is often not formally assessed unless impairment of function is strongly suspected.
  - Formal evaluation of taste requires application of a bitter-tasting substance to the posterior third of the tongue.
- Afferent component of the gag reflex (pharyngeal sensation)

Cranial Nerve X: Vagus Nerve
Motor
- Efferent component of the gag reflex (pharyngeal muscle contraction)

Sensory
- Pharyngeal sensation
- Visceral sensation

Cranial Nerve XI: Spinal Accessory Nerve (Figure 5-16)
Motor
- Trapezius and sternocleidomastoid muscles
  - Instruct the patient, "Shrug your shoulders."
  - Instruct the patient, "Turn your head right; turn your head left."
  - Test both muscles against resistance and assess for symmetry.

Cranial Nerve XII: Hypoglossal Nerve (Figure 5-17)
Motor
- Tongue musculature
  - Observe the tongue at rest for asymmetry, fasciculations, or atrophy.
  - Instruct the patient, "Stick your tongue out and straight down toward your chin": assess for symmetry or deviation.
  - Note speech articulation.

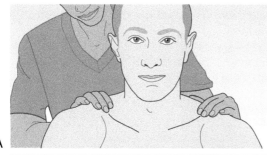

A

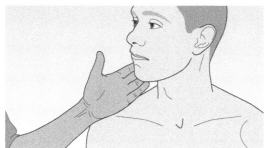

B

Figure 5-16 Spinal accessory nerve examination: trapezius contraction **(A)** and sternocleidomastoid contraction **(B).** (From Hall T. *PACES for the MRCP with 250 Clinical Cases.* 2nd ed. Philadelphia: Elsevier; 2008 [p. 387, Figure 3.24].)

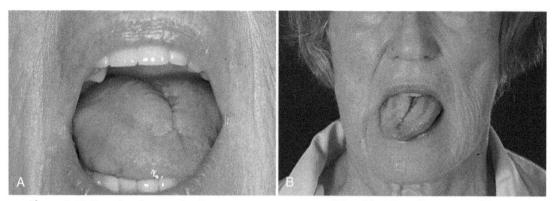

Figure 5-17 Hypoglossal nerve palsy. Note tongue asymmetry at rest **(A)** and deviation with protrusion **(B).** (From Hall T. *PACES for the MRCP with 250 Clinical Cases.* 2nd ed. Philadelphia: Elsevier; 2008 [p. 421, Figure 3.62].)

COORDINATION AND CEREBELLAR FUNCTION: EXAMINATION (Figure 5-18)

- Test of rapid alternating movements:
  - Instruct the patient to use one hand to slap the palm of the contralateral hand or ipsilateral thigh alternately with palm and dorsum of hand.
  - Have the patient repeat on opposite side.
- Finger tap:
  - Instruct the patient to repetitively tap the pad of the thumb with the tip of the index finger of the same hand.
  - Have the patient repeat on opposite side.
- Finger-nose test (Figure 5-18, *A*):
  - Stand an arm's length away from the patient (your arm should be fully extended for patient to reach you).
  - Have the patient touch his or her nose.
  - Instruct the patient to alternate rapidly between touching your fingertip and his or her own nose.
  - Have the patient repeat on opposite side.
- Heel-to-shin test (Figure 5-18, *B*):
  - Have patient run the heel of one foot carefully down the shin of the opposite leg.
  - Have the patient repeat on opposite side.
- Tandem gait test:
  - Instruct the patient to walk by placing one foot in front of the other with the heel of the leading foot touching the toe of the trailing foot.

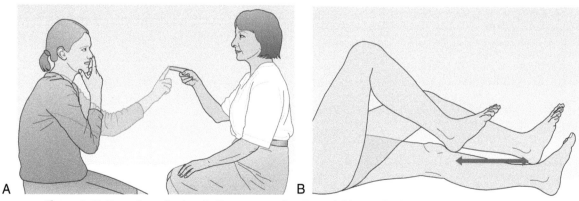

Figure 5-18 Tests of coordination. **A,** Finger-nose testing. **B,** Heel-shin coordination. (From Hall T. *PACES for the MRCP with 250 Clinical Cases.* 2nd ed. Philadelphia: Elsevier; 2008 [p. 392, Figure 3.28].)

- Romberg test:
  - Have patient stand comfortably with feet apart (shoulder width) and with hands resting at the sides.
  - Instruct the patient to close the eyes and maintain this position for 1 minute.
  - Observe for any instability.

SPINAL CORD FUNCTION: EXAMINATION

- If the cervical spine is the suspected area of abnormality, the examination must encompass the upper limbs, torso, perianal region, and lower limbs (Figure 5-19). In contrast, if the thoracic or lumbar spine is the suspected area of abnormality, examination of the perianal area and lower limbs is adequate.

Tone
- To evaluate muscular tone, have the patient relax the limb being examined. Under normal circumstances, the muscle maintains a slight amount of muscular tone and resistance to passive movement. In the early phase of spinal cord injury, the tone may be flaccid because the efferent signals to muscle are interrupted. Eventually, tone increases as a result of loss of inhibitory signals.
- Upper extremity:
  - Hold the patient's wrist and hand in your dominant hand.
  - Support the patient's elbow with your nondominant hand.
  - Gently flex and extend the patient's digits, wrist, and elbow.
  - Gently move the patient's shoulder through its range of motion.
- Lower extremity:
  - Hold the patient's foot and ankle with your dominant hand.
  - Support the patient's thigh with your nondominant hand.
  - Gently flex and extend at the ankle and knee.
- Assess for jerking or cog-wheeling, flaccidity, or resistance suggestive of increased tone.

Power
- Muscle strength or power must be described or graded in a standardized manner so that it is universally understood by various health care providers and compared over time (Table 5-5).
- The upper limb is supplied by the spinal nerves of C5 to T1, and the lower limb is supplied by the spinal nerves of L2 to S1. Each myotome must be evaluated and graded through a comparison of the right and left sides (Table 5-6).

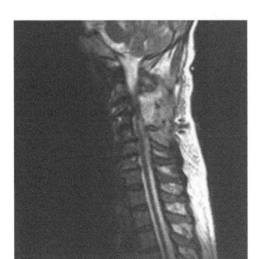

Figure 5-19 Cervical myelopathy. Compression of dural sac and spinal cord as a result of severe spinal degeneration. (Courtesy of Dr. Osama Loubani, Dalhousie University, Halifax, Nova Scotia.)

Table 5-5 Grading of Muscle Power

Grade	Description
0	No muscle contraction
1	Flicker or trace of contraction
2	Active movement when gravity is eliminated
3	Active movement against gravity
4	Active movement against gravity and some resistance
5	Active movement against resistance

Table 5-6 Examination of Myotomes

Upper Limb		Lower Limb	
C5	Elbow flexion	L2	Hip flexion
C6	Wrist extensors	L3	Knee extension
C7	Elbow extension	L4	Ankle dorsiflexion
C8	Finger flexion (DIP of middle digit)	L5	Long toe extensor
T1	Finger abduction	S1	Ankle plantar flexors

From American Spinal Injury Association. *Standard neurological classification of spinal cord injury,* www.asia-spinalinjury.org/publications/2006_Classif_worksheet.pdf; 2006. Accessed 16.09.10. DIP, Distal interphalangeal joint.

Deep Tendon Reflexes (Figure 5-20)
- Ensure appropriate draping while exposing the target tendons.
- Position patient in seated, semi-sitting, or supine position.
- Ensure that patient is relaxed.
- Strike tendon with appropriately weighted and sized reflex hammer:
  - Upper extremity: Biceps (C5 to C6), triceps (C6 to C7), and brachioradialis (C5 to C6) reflexes.
  - Lower extremity: Patellar (L2 to L4) and ankle (S1).
- Use reinforcement techniques if the patient is unable to voluntarily relax muscular tone; for example, ask the patient to firmly hook hands together and forcefully pull the arms against one another (Jendrassik maneuver).
- Assign a grade to each reflex (Table 5-7).

Plantar Response (L5 to S1) (Figure 5-21)
- Using a blunt object, apply firm constant pressure to the sole of the foot, starting at the heel.
- Drag the object toward the small toe, arching along the metatarsophalangeal joints of the digits toward the great toe.
- Observe for response of toes:
  - A normal response is downward flexion of the toes.
  - An abnormal response is dorsiflexion of the great toe, with or without abduction of remaining digits (Babinski's sign). Babinski's sign may be seen as a normal response in infants; in adults, it typically represents a pathologic process along the corticospinal tracts.

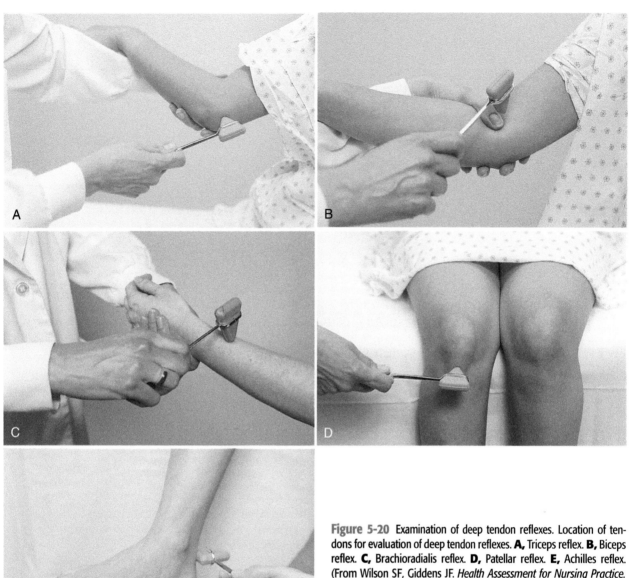

Figure 5-20 Examination of deep tendon reflexes. Location of tendons for evaluation of deep tendon reflexes. **A,** Triceps reflex. **B,** Biceps reflex. **C,** Brachioradialis reflex. **D,** Patellar reflex. **E,** Achilles reflex. (From Wilson SF, Giddens JF. *Health Assessment for Nursing Practice.* 4th ed. St. Louis: Mosby; 2009 [Figure 16-26].)

Table 5-7 Grading of Deep Tendon Reflexes

Grade	Description
0	Absent
1+	Trace or diminished
2+	Average
3+	Brisker than average
4+	Very brisk, hyperactive, with clonus

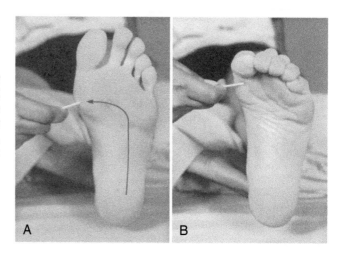

Figure 5-21 Plantar response examination. **A,** To elicit the plantar reflex, the examiner applies firm, constant pressure along the lateral surface of the sole, starting at the heel and moving along the ball of the foot, ending beneath the great toe. **B,** The normal response to plantar stimulation is flexion of all the toes. (From Barkauskas VH, Baumann LC, Darling-Fisher CS. *Health and Physical Assessment.* 3rd ed. St. Louis: Mosby; 2008 [p. 484, Figures 19-42, 19-43].)

Sensation
Light Touch and Pin-Pinch Testing
- Expose the patient's key dermatomal areas (outlined in Figure 5-22) while maintaining appropriate draping technique.
- Perform light touch test and pin-pinch test in all key dermatomal areas.
- Compare right and left sides.
- If abnormality at the sensory level is suspected, move the sensory stimulus from the insensate area to a sensate area to accurately delineate sensory level.

Proprioception
- Awareness of the position of one body part in relation to another
- Position sense

Finger (Figure 5-23, *A*)
- Isolate the patient's digit being tested from any contact with adjacent digits.
- Hold the digit firmly at the distal interphalangeal (DIP) joint (pressing inward from lateral aspects with the index finger and thumb of one hand).
- Use your other hand to gently move the patient's distal phalanx randomly to the up or down position.
- Ask patient periodically, "Is your finger up or down?"

Great Toe (Figure 5-23, *B*)
- Isolate the patient's great toe from contact with the adjacent toe.
- Hold the toe firmly at the interphalangeal (IP) joint (pressing inward from lateral aspects of IP joint with the index finger and thumb of one hand).
- Ask the patient to close his or her eyes.
- Use your other hand to gently move the patient's distal phalanx randomly to the up or down position.
- Ask patient periodically, "Is your toe up or down?"

Vibration
- Strike the tuning fork.
- Place the stem of the vibrating tuning fork firmly on the ball of the patient's great toe (Figure 5-24) or finger.
- Ask patient, "Do you feel the vibration?"
- Instruct the patient, "Tell me when the vibration stops."
- If patient unable to feel vibration on the ball of the great toe, move stimulus progressively to interphalangeal joint of great toe and ankle until patient can detect vibration.

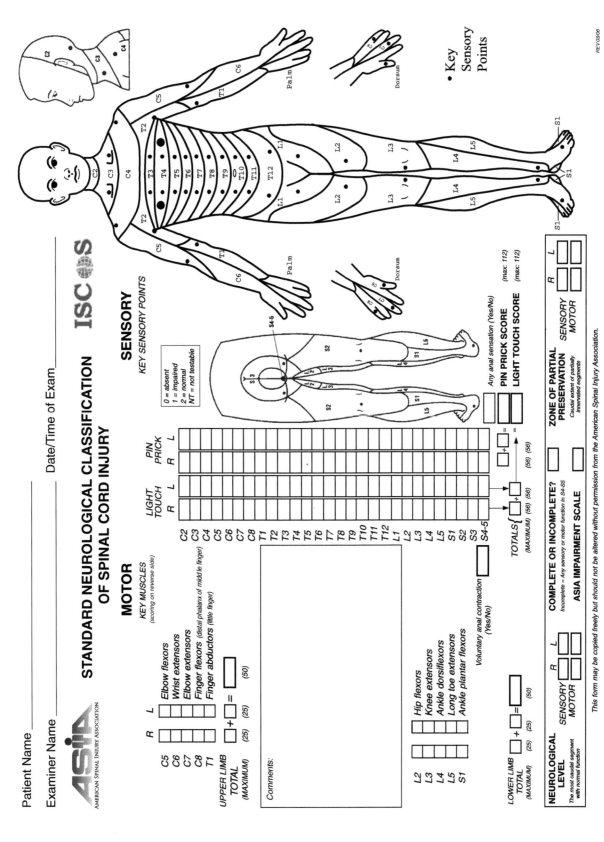

Figure 5-22 Dermatomal sensory examination. Key dermatomal areas to be tested are indicated by a *dot*. (From *American Spinal Injury Association*. *Standard Neurological Classification of Spinal cord injury*. www.asia-spinalinjury.org/publications/2006_Classif_worksheet.pdf., 2006. Accessed 06.09.10.)

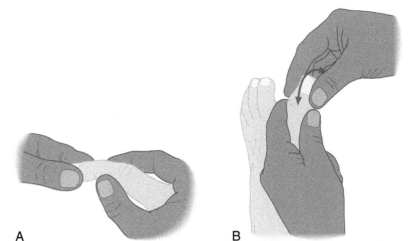

Figure 5-23 Examination of proprioception in a finger **(A)** and toe **(B).** (From Hall T. *PACES for the MRCP with 250 Clinical Cases.* 2nd ed. Philadelphia: Elsevier; 2008 [p. 397, Figure 3.31].)

A   B

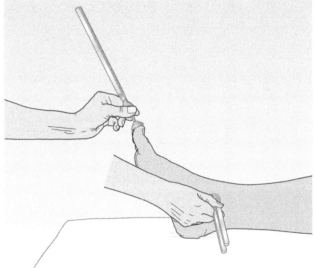

Figure 5-24 Examination of vibration sense. (From Hall T. *PACES for the MRCP with 250 Clinical Cases.* 2nd ed. Philadelphia: Elsevier; 2008 [p. 397, Figure 3.32].)

Digital Rectal Examination
- Using appropriate in-line spinal immobilization technique, roll the patient to one side.
- Assess anal tone by digital rectal examination (see Figure 3-5).
- Assess anal and perianal sensation with light touch and pin-pinch testing.
- Preservation of anal tone or sensation represents sacral sparing, which is indicative of an incomplete spinal cord injury with the potential for salvaging urinary and fecal continence.

Evidence: Digital Rectal Examination in Blunt Trauma
- In a 2005 retrospective study of patients who had sustained blunt trauma,[1] the sensitivity and specificity of decreased rectal tone on digital rectal examination were found to be 50% (95% confidence interval [CI] 37% to 63%) and 93% (95% CI 91% to 94%), respectively, for diagnosis of spinal cord injury. These results are further proof that normal tone on digital rectal examination is not adequate information to exclude spinal cord injury. A prospective study would offer a more accurate estimation.

DIFFERENTIATE UPPER MOTOR NEURON AND LOWER MOTOR NEURON DISEASE: EXAMINATION

Upper Motor Neuron Findings*
- Increased tone
- Increased deep tendon reflexes
- Weakness

Lower Motor Neuron Findings
- Decreased tone
- Decreased deep tendon reflexes
- Weakness
- Atrophy
- Fasciculations

MENINGISMUS: EXAMINATION

- Level of consciousness:
  - Assess with AVPU scale.
- Amoss's sign or Hoyne's sign:
  - Patient spontaneously assumes posture of flexed knees and hips, with the back in extreme lordosis, and neck extended.
- Nuchal rigidity:
  - Place patient supine.
  - Gently flex the neck forward.
  - Assess for rigidity.
- Brudzinski's sign (see Figure 5-25, *A*):
  - Position the patient supine.
  - Passively flex the patient's neck.
  - Assess for resulting flexion of the hips or knees.
- Kernig's sign (Figure 5-25, *B*):
  - Position the patient supine or sitting.
  - Flex the patient's hips to 90 degrees.
  - Extend the patient's knee.
  - Assess for resulting resistance or pain in back or thigh.
- Jolt accentuation:
  - Position the patient supine or sitting.
  - Ask the patient to turn his or her head rapidly and repeatedly from right to left.
  - Assess for worsening of headache.

---

*In the acute phase of illness, an upper motor neuron lesion may actually manifest with flaccid paralysis, decrease in tone, and decrease in or absence of deep tendon reflexes.

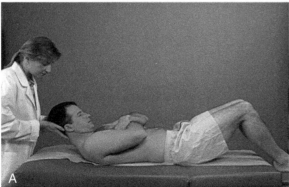
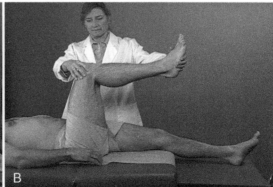

Figure 5-25 Examination for meningismus. **A,** Brudzinski's sign. **B,** Kernig's sign. (From Seidel HM, Ball JW, Dains JE, et al. *Mosby's Guide to Physical Examination.* 6th ed. St. Louis: Mosby; 2006 [p. 792, Figure 22-29].)

Evidence: Physical Examination for Meningitis

- The physical examination has some clinical utility in the evaluation for meningitis, although the accuracy of each specific test is limited by a paucity of contemporary and prospective studies. The absence of all three findings of fever, neck stiffness, and altered mental status can essentially preclude the diagnosis of meningitis.
- Tests for meningeal irritation—including nuchal rigidity, Kernig's sign, and Brudzinski's sign—have low sensitivity, and absence of these findings does not exclude the diagnosis of meningitis.
- Although not widely recognized or used, jolt accentuation is a useful diagnostic test with sensitivity of 97% and specificity of 60%. A negative result of a jolt accentuation test essentially excludes the diagnosis of meningitis, while a positive result mandates a lumbar puncture.[2]

SEIZURE: HISTORY

> **INSTRUCTIONS TO CANDIDATE: A 27-year-old man with a history of epilepsy presents to the emergency department after a generalized tonic-clonic seizure. Obtain a focused history to determine possible causes.**

DD$_X$: VITAMINS C
- **V**ascular: Intracranial hemorrhage
- **I**nfectious: Meningitis, encephalitis
- **T**raumatic: Head injury, post–brain injury seizure
- **M**etabolic: Hypocalcemia, hypoglycemia, hyponatremia, hypoxia
- **I**diopathic/**i**atrogenic: Nonadherence to an antiseizure medication regimen, drug interactions
- **N**eoplastic: Brain tumor
- **S**ubstance abuse and **p**sychiatric: Sympathomimetic agents, serotonin syndrome, neuroleptic malignant syndrome, drug withdrawal (e.g., EtOH), pseudoseizure

DD$_X$: Other
- Epilepsy

History
- Ask the patient the following:
  - **Character:** "Did anyone witness the seizure? What did it look like?"
    - Focal versus general (loss of consciousness)
    - Tonic phase, clonic phase
    - Postictal phase
    - Similarity to past seizures
  - **Onset:** "Did you know you were going to have a seizure? Did you experience an aura? What were you doing at the time? Did you fall?"
  - **Duration:** "How long did the seizure last? Did you have more than one? If more than one, did you regain consciousness between seizures?"
  - **Events associated:**
    - Generalized tonic-clonic seizure: "Were you incontinent of urine? Did you bite your tongue or cheek? Do your muscles hurt?"
    - Neurologic symptoms: "Did you experience numbness, tingling, weakness, or difficulty speaking? Did anyone notice if you had a facial droop?"
    - "Did you suffer a head injury recently or in the past (traumatic brain injury)?"
    - Vasovagal syncope: "Did you have symptoms such as light-headedness, nausea, vomiting, or sweating before you lost consciousness?"
    - Cardiac syncope: "Did you experience palpitations, chest pain, shortness of breath, or fainting without warning?"
  - **Frequency:** "How often do you have seizures? When was your last seizure? Was anything different about this seizure in comparison with the other ones you have had? Why did you come to the emergency department for this one?"

- ▪ Provocative factors: "Do you know what might have caused this seizure?"
  - ◆ Sleep deprivation
  - ◆ Stress
  - ◆ Alcohol
  - ◆ Nonadherence to an antiseizure medication regimen
  - ◆ Infection or illness
  - ◆ Drug interaction
  - ◆ Street drug use
- **PMH/PSH:** Epilepsy (year of diagnosis, seizure control, medications used), malignancy
- **MEDS:** Antiseizure medication (type, dose, frequency, and adherence), antibiotics
- **SH:** Smoking, use of EtOH, use of street drugs (cocaine or other sympathomimetic agents), driving status
- **FH:** Brain cancer, epilepsy

TEMPORAL ARTERITIS: HISTORY AND PHYSICAL EXAMINATION

INSTRUCTIONS TO CANDIDATE: An 83-year-old man presents with progressive headache and vision loss in the right eye over 7 days. Obtain a focused history, and perform a focused physical examination.

DD$_X$: VITAMINS C
- **V**ascular: Migraine, subarachnoid hemorrhage, temporal arteritis
- **I**nfectious: Cerebral abscess, meningitis, sinusitis
- **T**raumatic: Head injury, concussion, intracranial hemorrhage (epidural hematoma, subdural hematoma, subarachnoid hemorrhage)
- **I**diopathic/iatrogenic: Post–lumbar puncture headache
- **N**eoplastic: Brain tumor
- **S**ubstance abuse and psychiatric: Carbon monoxide poisoning

DD$_X$: Other
- Tension headache, cluster headache, acute angle closure glaucoma, occipital neuralgia

History
- Ask the patient the following:
  - ▪ **Character:** "Describe your headache. Is the pain throbbing? Sharp? Achy? Tight? Is this the worst headache of your life?"
  - ▪ **Location:** "Where exactly does your head hurt: one side? Both sides? Neck? One or both eyes? Does one spot hurt more than any other?"
  - ▪ **Onset:** "When did the pain start? Did it start gradually or suddenly? Was the pain maximal at onset?"
  - ▪ **Radiation:** "Does the pain move anywhere (neck, one or both eyes, jaw)?"
  - ▪ **Intensity:** "How severe is the pain on a scale of 1 to 10, with 1 being mild pain and 10 being the worst? If the pain was not at its worst when the headache started, how long did it take to reach its maximum? How does the headache affect your activities of daily living?"
  - ▪ **Duration:** "How long has the pain been there? Is it getting better, getting worse, or staying the same?"
  - ▪ **Events associated:**
    - ◆ "Have you experienced nausea, vomiting, or fainting (possibly indicative of subarachnoid hemorrhage)?"
    - ◆ "Have you noticed any loss of vision, jaw pain with chewing (claudication), joint pain (arthralgia), or muscle aches (myalgia) (indicative of temporal arteritis)?
    - ◆ "Have you had watery eyes or nasal congestion (as in cluster headache)?"
    - ◆ "Have you been drowsy or confused? Have you had fever, rash (petechiae, purpura), or neck stiffness (indicative of meningitis)?"
    - ◆ "Have you had a fall or a head injury leading up to the headache (possibly traumatic brain injury or intracranial hemorrhage)?"

- ◆ "Did you experience an aura, numbness, tingling, weakness, or any difficulty speaking (characteristic of migraine or stroke)?"
- ◆ "Did you have eye pain or redness, loss of vision, or change in the appearance of your eye (indicative of acute angle closure glaucoma)?"
  - ▪ Frequency: "Have you ever had a headache like this before? How often do you get headaches like this? Is there anything different about this headache compared to the other ones you've had? Why did you come to the hospital/office for this one?"
  - ▪ Palliative factors: "Does anything make the headache better? If so, what?"
    - ◆ Analgesic medications (type, dose, frequency)
    - ◆ Alternative strategies (massage, chiropractor, alternative medicine)
    - ◆ Position (upright, supine, or dependent)
    - ◆ Quiet
    - ◆ Dark
  - ▪ Provocative factors: "Does anything make the headache worse? If so, what?"
    - ◆ Position (upright, supine, or dependent)
    - ◆ Light (photophobia)
    - ◆ Noise (phonophobia)
- **PMH/PSH:** Hypertension, cancer, polymyalgia rheumatic, systemic lupus erythematosus, glaucoma, stroke, atrial fibrillation, migraine, brain surgery, ventricular shunt
- **MEDS:** Anticoagulants (INR monitoring, recent INR level), migraine medications (adherence)
- **SH:** Smoking, use of EtOH, use of street drugs (cocaine or other sympathomimetic agents)
- **FH:** Brain cancer, cerebral aneurysm, sudden death, migraine

Physical Examination

- **Vital signs (Vitals):** Evaluate heart rate (HR), blood pressure (BP), respiratory rate (RR), and temperature.
  - ▪ Be alert for the combination of hypertension, bradycardia, and irregular respirations that accompany raised intracranial pressure (ICP) (Cushing's response)
- **General:** Assess the patient's general appearance, noting any apparent distress or exanthem.
- **Level of consciousness:** Assess with the AVPU scale or GCS.
- **Head, eyes, ears, nose, and throat (HEENT):**
  - ▪ Head: Assess for tender points on scalp, scalp laceration or hematoma, and tenderness at the temporal artery.
  - ▪ Eyes: Check for cloudy cornea, irregular pupil, injection, tearing, anisocoria, and intraocular pressure.
  - ▪ Ears: Determine whether tympanic membrane is intact, and check for otitis externa, hemotympanum, and otorrhea.
  - ▪ Nose: Assess for maxillary sinus tenderness and rhinorrhea.
- **Cranial nerve examination** as outlined on pp. 150-155.
- **Assess for meningismus** as outlined on p. 163, including Amoss's sign or Hoyne's sign, nuchal rigidity, Brudzinski's sign, Kernig's sign, and jolt accentuation.
- **Screening neurologic examination:**
  - ▪ Assess gait.
  - ▪ Assess motor function.
    - ◆ Pronator drift: Instruct the patient to hold both arms extended with palms up for 10 seconds. Observe for downward drift or even subtle pronation of forearm or curling of fingertips on one side.
    - ◆ Leg drift: Instruct the patient to lift each leg for 5 seconds. Observe for any downward drift on one side.
  - ▪ Evaluate sensation of touch in extremities.
  - ▪ Perform tests of coordination and cerebellar function as outlined on pp. 156-157.

FACIAL DROOP: HISTORY AND PHYSICAL EXAMINATION

INSTRUCTIONS TO CANDIDATE: A 29-year-old woman presents with unilateral facial droop. Obtain a focused history, and perform a focused physical examination in order to differentiate between upper and lower motor neuron disease.

DD$_X$: VITAMINS C
* Vascular: Stroke, intracranial hemorrhage
* Infectious: Acute otitis media, otitis externa, parotitis, herpes zoster oticus, Lyme disease
* Traumatic: Mandible fracture, blunt injury to face, laceration
* Idiopathic/iatrogenic: Bell palsy, post–facial surgery condition
* Neoplastic: Brain tumor, facial neuroma, acoustic neuroma, parotid tumor, cholesteatoma

History
* Ask the patient the following:
   * **Character:** "What changes in your appearance have you noticed?"
   * **Location:** "Which part of your face specifically looks different? Forehead? Eyes? Smile?"
   * **Onset:** "When did this problem start? Was it sudden or gradual?"
   * **Duration:** "How long has your face appeared this way? Is the problem getting better, getting worse, or staying the same?"
   * **Events associated:**
      * "Have you suffered a head or face injury?"
      * "Does your face hurt?"
      * "Have you recently had a cough, sore throat, runny nose, or sinus congestion?"
      * "Have you had fever? Pain in your ears? Ear discharge?"
      * "Do you have a rash?"
      * "Have you experienced any weight loss or loss of appetite (constitutional symptoms)?"
      * Neurologic symptoms: "Have you experienced numbness, tingling, weakness, difficulty speaking, hearing loss, or ringing in your ears (tinnitus)?"
   * **Frequency:** "Has this problem ever happened before?"
* **PMH/PSH:** Chickenpox, malignancy, atrial fibrillation, hypertension, dyslipidemia, diabetes
* **MEDS**
* **SH:** Smoking, use of EtOH, use of street drugs
* **FH:** Brain cancer

Physical Examination
* **Vitals:** Evaluate HR, BP, RR, and temperature.
* **General:** Assess the patient's general appearance, noting any obvious facial asymmetry or drooling. Pay attention to the patient's phonation and articulation of speech.
* **HEENT:**
   * **Head:** Check whether the parotid gland is tender or swollen. Check for facial injury or hematoma. Palpate the mandible for tenderness or deformity.
   * **Eyes:** Assess for ptosis, ability to close the eye, injection, tears, and dry eyes.
   * **Ears:** Assess for pain on manipulation of external ear, edematous external ear canal, qualities of the tympanic membrane (e.g., injected, dull, bulging), hemotympanum, and hearing.
* **Cranial nerve examination** as outlined on pp. 150-155. Test forehead and lower two thirds of facial musculature in isolation.
* **Screening neurologic examination:** Assess gait, motor function (pronator drift, leg drift), and sensation of touch in extremities.

Pearl: Distinguishing Upper and Lower Motor Neuron Disease in Facial Paralysis
* Pathologic processes of the facial nerve (lower motor neuron; Figure 5-26) result in paresis or paralysis of one entire side of the face. With disease of the upper motor neuron, function of voluntary muscles of the forehead is preserved, inasmuch as the forehead musculature has bilateral cortical innervations (Figure 5-27). In assessing patients with facial paralysis, you must test specifically for preservation of the forehead musculature on the affected side. Bell palsy is a lower motor neuron disorder, and the entire face, including the forehead, is thus involved.

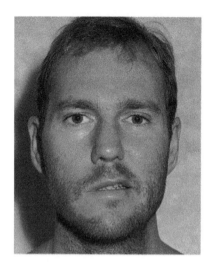

Figure 5-26 Right facial palsy. (From Swartz MH. *Textbook of Physical Diagnosis: History and Examination.* 6th ed. Philadelphia: Elsevier; 2010 [p. 666, Figure 21-17].)

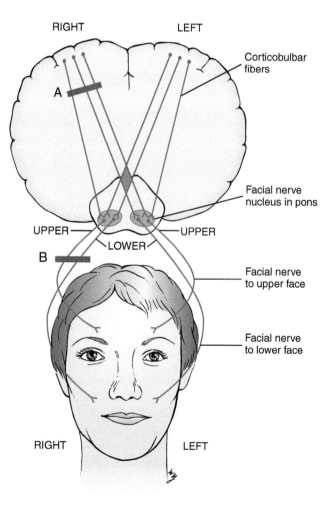

Figure 5-27 Types of facial weakness. Upper motor neuron lesion **(A)** produces a motor nerve palsy that causes weakness of the contralateral side of the lower face but spares the contralateral side of the forehead. Lower motor neuron lesion **(B)** produces a motor nerve palsy that causes total paralysis of the ipsilateral side of the face. (From Swartz MH. *Textbook of Physical Diagnosis: History and Examination.* 6th ed. Philadelphia: Elsevier; 2010 [p. 666, Figure 21-16].)

SAMPLE CHECKLISTS

Headache: History

> **INSTRUCTIONS TO CANDIDATE: A 23-year-old woman with a history of migraine presents to her family physician with increased frequency and severity of headaches. Obtain a focused history.**

Key Points	Satisfactorily Completed
Introduces self to patient	❏
Determines how the patient wishes to be addressed	❏
Washes hands	❏
Explains purpose of the encounter	❏
Completes history in a logical manner	❏
Asks about character of headache:	
• Elicits descriptors	❏
• Asks whether this is the worst headache of the patient's life	❏
• Asks whether the headache differs from previous headaches	❏
Asks about location of headache:	
• Specific location of maximal pain	❏
• Lateralization	❏
Asks about onset of headache:	
• Gradual versus sudden	❏
• Maximal at onset or time to maximal pain	❏
Asks whether headache radiates	❏
Asks about intensity of pain (pain scale)	❏
Asks about duration of pain:	
• Duration	❏
• Whether headache is getting better, getting worse, or staying the same	❏
Asks about events associated with headache:	
• Nausea, vomiting, or both	❏
• Trauma	❏
• Pregnancy	❏
• Neurologic symptoms (numbness, tingling, speech abnormalities)	❏
• Explores alternative diagnoses	❏
• Fever, rash, neck stiffness (meningitis)	❏
• Muscle strain, vise-like headache (tension headache)	❏
• Tearing, nasal congestion (cluster headache)	❏
Establishes frequency of headaches:	
• Frequency	❏
• Change in frequency or pattern	❏
Asks about palliative factors (medications, alternative treatments, position)	❏
Asks about provocative factors:	
• Light (photophobia)	❏
• Sound (phonophobia)	❏
• Migraine triggers	❏
Asks about past medical history	❏

Continued

Key Points	Satisfactorily Completed
Asks about medications:	
• Types of medications	❑
• Adherence to medication regimen	❑
Asks about allergies	❑
Asks about social history:	
• Smoking	❑
• Use of EtOH (red wine)	❑
• Use of street drugs	❑
• Interference with daily life or work	❑
Asks about family history	❑
Makes appropriate closing remarks	❑

Ataxia: Physical Examination

INSTRUCTIONS TO CANDIDATE: A 61-year-old man presents to the emergency department with unsteady gait. Perform a focused physical examination.

Key Points	Satisfactorily Completed
Introduces self to patient	❑
Determines how the patient wishes to be addressed	❑
Washes hands	❑
Explains the nature of the examination to the patient	❑
Examines the patient in a logical manner	❑
General:	
• Observes for tremor	❑
• Observes the patient ambulating	❑
• Characterizes the patient's gait	❑
• Comments on the quality of the patient's speech (e.g., phonation)	❑
Performs screening motor examination:	
• Pronator drift	❑
• Leg drift	❑
Performs screening sensory examination:	
• Ability to detect touch over four extremities	❑
Performs examination of coordination and cerebellar function:	
• Rapid alternating movements	❑
• Finger tap	❑
• Finger-nose test	❑
• Heel-shin test	❑
• Tandem gait	❑
• Romberg test	❑
Drapes the patient appropriately	❑
Makes appropriate closing remarks	❑

Meningitis: Physical Examination

INSTRUCTIONS TO CANDIDATE: A 17-year-old woman presents to the emergency department with fever, rash, and headache (Figure 5-28). Perform a focused physical examination.

Key Points	Satisfactorily Completed
Introduces self to patient	❏
Determines how the patient wishes to be addressed	❏
Washes hands	❏
Explains the nature of the examination to the patient	❏
Examines the patient in a logical manner	❏
Evaluates vital signs (HR, BP, RR, and temperature)	❏
General:	
• Notes overall general appearance or apparent distress	❏
• Evaluates skin, noting any exanthem (see Figure 5-28)	❏
• Evaluates position (Amoss's or Hoyne's sign)	❏
Establishes level of consciousness:	
• Makes correct AVPU scale determination	❏
Examines for meningismus:	
• Nuchal rigidity	❏
• Brudzinski's sign	❏
• Kernig's sign	❏
• Jolt accentuation	❏
Performs cranial nerve examination	❏
Performs screening neurologic examination	❏
Drapes the patient appropriately	❏
Makes appropriate closing remarks	❏

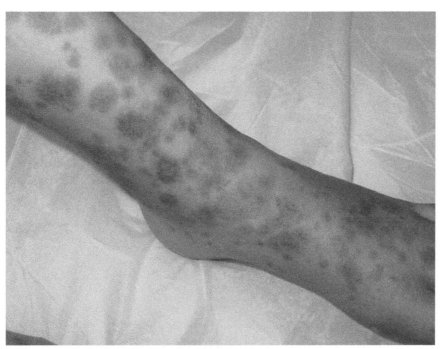

Figure 5-28 Purpuric lesions on the left lower extremity. (Courtesy of Dr. Peter Green, Dalhousie University, Halifax, Nova Scotia.)

ADVANCED SKILLS

APPROACH TO ALTERED LEVEL OF CONSCIOUSNESS: HISTORY

DD_X: VITAMINS C
- **V**ascular: Stroke (ischemic or hemorrhagic)
- **I**nfectious: Cerebral abscess, encephalitis, meningitis, sepsis
- **T**raumatic: Traumatic brain injury, intracranial hemorrhage, hypotension
- **M**etabolic: Hypoglycemia, hypoxia, electrolyte disturbance
- **I**diopathic/iatrogenic: Prescription medications
- **N**eoplastic: Brain tumor
- **S**ubstance abuse and psychiatric: Accidental toxic exposure, drug withdrawal, use of street drugs, malingering, mental illness
- **O**ther: Postictal state

Cause (Age-Based Approach)
- **Pediatric patient:** Trauma (fall, nonaccidental trauma), ingestion (prescription medications, toxins in the home), infection (fever, rash, cough, rhinorrhea, vomiting, diarrhea), metabolic derangement (vomiting, diarrhea, dehydration)
- **Adult patient:** Trauma (head injury), ingestion (prescription medications, street drugs, drug-drug interactions, drug withdrawal), infection (cough, vomiting, diarrhea, dysuria/frequency/urgency, fever, rash, anorexia), intracranial hemorrhage (use of anticoagulants, head injury, hypertension)
- **Geriatric patient:** Trauma (fall, nonaccidental trauma), medications (see "Pearl: Altered Mental Status in the Geriatric Patient" on p. 173), infection (fever, rash, cough, vomiting, diarrhea, cellulitis, urinary symptoms), metabolic derangement (vomiting, diarrhea, dehydration, cancer, liver disease, renal dysfunction, furosemide), intracranial hemorrhage (headache, hypertension, head injury, use of anticoagulants), malignancy (headache, neurologic symptoms, history of cancer that metastasizes to brain, smoking, constitutional symptoms [weight loss, anorexia]), change in environment

History
- Collateral information becomes very important in obtaining the history of a patient who is confused or has altered mentation. Attempt to obtain as much history as possible from the patient themselves. Additional valuable information can be obtained from family members, caretakers, medical records, or paramedics who attended to the patient.
- The patient's belongings should be searched for evidence of street or prescription drug use.
- Use the **ChLORIDE FPP** mnemonic to delineate the presenting concern, and ask the patient or caregiver the following questions:
  - **Character:** Determine quality of mental status change (confusion, combativeness, depressed level of consciousness).
  - **Onset:** "When was the change was noticed? Was the change sudden or gradual in onset?"
  - **Duration:** "How long did the confusion last? Was he or she confused the entire time? Was the confusion variable throughout the day? Did the level of confusion seem to be related to the time of day?"
  - **Events associated:**
    - "Did you have shortness of breath (respiratory cause)?"
    - "Did you have chest pain or palpitations (cardiac cause)?"
    - "Did you have fever, rash, nuchal rigidity, cough, abdominal pain, vomiting, or diarrhea (infectious cause)?"
    - "Did you have a seizure, headache, head injury, weakness, loss or change in sensation of your skin, or difficulty speaking (neurologic cause)?"
    - "Did you have vomiting or diarrhea (hypovolemia)?"

- Frequency: "Have you had any similar past episodes? What was the cause then?"
- Provocative factors: Consider potential age-stratified causes, and ask questions to differentiate between these.
- **PMH/PSH:**
  - **Pediatric patient:** Ask specifically about developmental disability, diabetes, inborn errors of metabolism, psychiatric illness, and sickle cell disease.
  - **Adult and geriatric patient:** Ask specifically about atrial fibrillation, cancer, diabetes, human immunodeficiency virus (HIV) infection, hypertension, liver disease, renal dysfunction, psychiatric illness, and stroke.
- **MEDS:** Anticoagulants, antihistamines, benzodiazepines, opioids, antibiotics, anticonvulsants, lithium

Pearls: Altered Mental Status in the Geriatric Patient
- The most common cause of confusion in elderly persons is medication side effects and polypharmacy.
- The medications that most commonly lead to confusion in elderly persons are antihistamines, benzodiazepines, and opioids.
- For elderly patients, it is essential to carefully review all medications for these common culprits and for drug-drug interactions.

APPROACH TO STROKE: HISTORY

DD$_X$: VITAMINS C
- **Vascular:** Ischemic stroke (thrombosis or embolism), hemorrhagic stroke, transient ischemic attack, arterial dissection, vasculitis
- **Traumatic:** Traumatic intracranial hemorrhage
- **Metabolic:** Todd's paralysis (postseizure), hypoglycemia

History
- Ask the patient the following:
  - **Character:**
    - If bystanders were present, use their collateral history to determine the appearance of the stroke.
    - Specifically inquire about facial droop, expressive or receptive aphasia, hemiparesis, upper limb or lower limb involvement, sensory abnormality, neglect, and depressed mental status.
  - **Onset:** "Specifically, when did this problem begin?" If time at onset is unknown, determine when the patient was last seen appearing normal.
  - **Duration:** "How long did symptoms last? Has there been any improvement? Specifically, which abnormalities have resolved and which ones remain?"
  - **Events associated:**
    - "Have you experienced headache, fainting, or vomiting (hemorrhagic stroke)?"
    - "Did you have a seizure?" Residual unilateral hemiparesis may persist after seizure (Todd's paralysis) and may mimic stroke.
    - "Have you been injured recently?"
  - **Frequency:** "Have you experienced any similar past episodes? If so, what was the diagnosis at the time, and were any investigations or treatments undertaken?"
- **PMH/PSH:** Risk factors (atrial fibrillation, diabetes, dyslipidemia, family history, hypertension, smoking); cancer
- **MEDS:**
  - If the patient is taking anticoagulants for atrial fibrillation or another reason, determine medication adherence, frequency of INR monitoring, and recent INR levels.
  - Determine whether the patient is taking new medications (recent antibiotics, drug interactions).
- **SH:** Smoking, use of EtOH, use of street drugs

APPROACH TO NEUROPATHIC PAIN: HISTORY

DD$_X$: VITAMINS C

- **V**ascular: Poststroke pain
- **I**nfectious: Epidural abscess, discitis, apical lung pneumonia, postherpetic neuralgia, HIV neuropathy
- **T**raumatic: Posttraumatic spinal cord injury, spinal fracture, dislocation, or ligamentous injury with spinal cord or nerve compression
- **M**etabolic: Diabetes, nutritional deficiency
- **I**diopathic/**i**atrogenic: Postsurgical pain, postradiation myelopathy
- **N**eoplastic: Primary brain or spinal cord tumor, metastatic cancer with spinal cord or nerve involvement or compression
- **S**ubstance abuse and psychiatric: Alcohol neuropathy, diethyltoluamide (DEET)

History

- Ask the patient the following:
  - **Character:** "Describe the pain. Is it sharp, burning, hot, or like an electric shock? Do you feel numbness or tingling? Does you skin hurt if you brush it lightly (allodynia)?"
  - **Location:** "Where is the pain the worst?"
  - **Onset:** "When did the pain first begin? Was the onset sudden or gradual? What were you doing when the pain started?"
  - **Radiation:** "Does the pain radiate to other places? Where does it radiate (dermatomal pattern, or peripheral nerve pattern)? Where do you feel the pain (sensory level)?"
  - **Intensity:** "How severe is the pain on a scale of 1 to 10, with 1 being mild pain and 10 being the worst pain you have ever had?"
  - **Duration:** "How long has the pain lasted? Has the pain been progressive or intermittent? Is there a time when the pain is worse?" Neuropathic pain is typically worse at the end of the day.
  - **Events associated:**
    - "Have you had weight loss, loss of appetite, or pain keeping you awake at night (symptoms suggestive of malignancy)?"
    - "Have you experienced incontinence of urine or stool, numbness in the anogenital area, muscular weakness, or loss of sensation (cauda equina syndrome)?"
    - "Have you recently had a rash or shingles (postherpetic neuralgia)?"
    - "Have you experienced fainting or light-headedness when moving from lying to sitting or sitting to standing position (orthostasis, autonomic neuropathy)?"
    - "Have you recently had an infection or used intravenous (IV) drugs (epidural abscess)?"
  - **Frequency:** "Is the pain constant or intermittent?"
  - **Palliative factors:** "Does anything relieve the pain?"
    - Medications (type, dose, frequency), strategies, positions, or alternative therapies (massage, chiropractor, acupuncture)
    - Success or failure of each strategy
  - **Provocative factors:** "Does anything make the pain worse?"
    - Position, movement, exertion
    - A single identifiable inciting event
- **PMH/PSH:** Alcoholism, cancer, degenerative disc disease, diabetes, HIV infection, herpes zoster (shingles); spinal surgery, other surgery
- **MEDS:** All medications (prescription and non-prescription) used to manage the pain
- **SH:** Smoking, use of EtOH, use of street drugs (specifically inquire about IV drug use); occupation; interference with daily activities

Pearl: Red Flags of Neuropathic Pain
- The following historical features should alert the clinician to the possibility of a life- or limb-threatening cause of neuropathic pain. These features may be indicative of malignancy, epidural abscess, or other causes of spinal cord compression, cauda equina syndrome, or advanced spinal nerve compression.
  - Progressive nature of pain
  - Muscular weakness
  - Numbness
  - Urinary or fecal incontinence
  - Urinary retention
  - Fever
  - IV drug use
  - Constitutional symptoms
  - History of cancer that metastasizes to bone

COMA: PHYSICAL EXAMINATION

- Establish level of consciousness: AVPU scale, Glasgow Coma Scale
- Evaluate vital signs (HR, BP, RR, oxygen saturation, blood glucose, temperature)

Cranial Nerves
- Cranial nerve II: Observe response to sudden visual threat (blink?).
- Cranial nerves II, III: Observe pupillary reflex.
- Cranial nerves III, IV, VI: Evaluate spontaneous eye movements.
- Cranial nerves V, VII: Assess corneal reflex.
- Cranial nerves IX, X: Assess gag reflex.

Vestibuloocular Reflexes (Bilaterally)
- Oculocephalic testing (Doll's Eyes):
  - Position the patient supine.
  - Hold the patient's eyes open, and rotate his or her head to the side.
  - In a normal reflex, eyes move in the opposite direction.
  - An abnormal reflex is absence of the doll's-eye movement (indicative of brainstem dysfunction).
- Caloric stimulation:
  - Position the patient supine.
  - Perform otoscopic examination to ensure integrity of the tympanic membrane.
  - Have an assistant hold the patient's eyes open.
  - Inject cold water into the ear canal, and observe for nystagmus.
  - Repeat with warm water.
  - A normal response is **COWS** ("**c**old **o**pposite, **w**arm **s**ame"), which refers to the rapid phase of horizontal nystagmus.
  - An abnormal response is the absence of nystagmus (indicative of brainstem dysfunction).

Ophthalmoscopic Examination
- Look for signs of raised ICP (papilledema, loss of venous pulsations):
  - Vitreous hemorrhage, subhyaloid retinal hemorrhage, signs of raised ICP, or a combination of these is suggestive of subarachnoid hemorrhage.
- Look for signs of basal skull fracture:
  - Hemotympanum, otorrhea (revealed by otoscopic examination)
  - Raccoon eyes, Battle's sign, rhinorrhea
- Assess sensory and motor responses to painful stimuli.
- Evaluate deep tendon reflexes.
- Evaluate plantar reflex.

SPINAL INJURY: HISTORY AND PHYSICAL EXAMINATION

> **INSTRUCTIONS TO CANDIDATE: A 25-year-old unrestrained male driver in a motor vehicle collision presents to the emergency department immobilized on a backboard and with a cervical collar; he is complaining of neck pain. Obtain a focused history, and perform a focused physical examination to determine need for cervical spine radiography and presence of spinal cord injury.**

DD$_X$: VITAMINS C
- **V**ascular: Vertebral artery dissection
- **T**raumatic: Cervical spine fracture, dislocation, or ligamentous injury; muscle strain
- **I**diopathic/**i**atrogenic: Pressure sores caused by spine board immobilization

History
- History of incident:
  - The patient's position in car (front seat versus back seat; driver versus passenger)
  - Whether the patient was restrained and the type of restraint used, if applicable (shoulder belt versus lap belt)
  - Description of collision, speed
  - Whether patient has been ambulatory since the collision
- Ask the patient the following:
  - **Character:** "What does your neck pain feel like? Sharp? Tight? Achy?"
  - **Location:** "Where exactly does your neck hurt? Midline? Laterally? Does one spot hurt more than any other?"
  - **Onset:** "When did the pain start: immediately? Or was it delayed? After you were immobilized?"
  - **Radiation:** "Does the pain move anywhere, such as to your head or limbs?"
  - **Intensity:** "How severe is the pain on a scale of 1 to 10, with 1 being mild pain and 10 being the worst?"
  - **Duration:** "How long has the pain been there? Is it getting better, getting worse, or staying the same?"
  - **Events associated:**
    - "Are you experiencing numbness, tingling, or muscle weakness (high-risk symptoms of spinal cord injury)?"
    - "Have you been drinking alcohol or using any drugs (intoxication)?" This limits utility of the clinical examination in diagnosing spine injury or spinal cord injury.
    - "Did you lose consciousness? Do you remember the event (amnesia)?"
  - **Palliative factors:** "Does anything make the neck pain better? If so, what?"
    - Analgesic medications administered by paramedics (type, dose, frequency)
  - **Provocative factors:** "Does anything make the neck pain worse? If so, what?"
    - Spine board
    - Collar
    - Movement of limbs
- **PMH/PSH:** Spinal surgery, degenerative disc disease, rheumatoid arthritis, osteoporosis, ankylosing spondylitis
- **MEDS:** Analgesics administered by paramedics, steroids, anticoagulants
- **SH:** Smoking, use of EtOH, use of street drugs

Physical Examination
- **Vitals:** Evaluate HR, BP, RR, and temperature.
- **General:** Assess the patient's general appearance, noting any apparent distress and spontaneous limb movement.

- **Spine:** Follow these procedures:
  - Have an assistant maintain manual in-line cervical spine immobilization.
  - Remove cervical collar.
  - With the help of four assistants, remove the patient from the spine board, using in-line manual immobilization technique.
  - When the patient is log-rolled onto his side, palpate the spine from the top of the cervical spine to the coccyx.
  - Note any areas of tenderness or deformity.
  - Reapply the cervical collar, and instruct the patient not to move.
- **Level of consciousness:** Determine GCS score by evaluating eye opening, verbal response, and motor response (p. 144).
- **Motor examination:**
  - Evaluate upper extremities (elbow flexion, elbow extension, wrist extension, finger flexion, finger abduction).
  - Evaluate lower extremities (hip flexion, knee extension, ankle dorsiflexion, ankle plantar flexion, long toe extension).
- **Sensory examination:**
  - Perform light touch test and pin-pinch testing in all key dermatomal areas (see Figure 5-22).
- **Digital rectal examination:**
  - If motor or sensory abnormality is detected, perform digital rectal examination for evidence of rectal sparing (see Figure 3-8).
  - Assess anal tone and sensation.
  - Maintain manual in-line spinal immobilization throughout.

Evidence: Cervical Spine Radiography in Blunt Trauma
- The Canadian C-Spine Rule[3] is a clinical decision tool used to determine whether a patient who has suffered blunt trauma requires evaluation with a cervical spine (c-spine) radiograph.
- The tool consists of three questions to make this determination:
  - Does the patient have any high-risk factor (age ≥65 years, dangerous mechanism, or paresthesias in extremities) that necessitates radiography?
  - Does the patient have any low-risk factor present (i.e., simple rear-end motor vehicle collision, sitting position in emergency department, being ambulatory at any time since injury, delayed onset of neck pain, or absence of midline cervical spine tenderness) that allows safe assessment of range of motion?
  - If a low-risk factor is present, is the patient able to actively rotate neck 45 degrees to the left and right?
- This tool has a sensitivity of 100% (95% CI 98% to 100%) and a specificity of 42.5% (95% CI 40% to 44%) in the clinical setting and therefore can be used to safely identify patients who do not require radiography.[3]

CAUDA EQUINA SYNDROME: HISTORY AND PHYSICAL EXAMINATION

INSTRUCTIONS TO CANDIDATE: A 76-year-old man with history of prostate cancer presents with back pain, weakness of lower limbs, and urinary incontinence. Obtain a focused history, and perform a focused physical examination.

DD$_X$: VITAMINS C
- **V**ascular: Spinal cord infarction, aortic dissection
- **I**nfectious: Epidural abscess, discitis
- **T**raumatic: Spinal fracture, dislocation, or ligamentous injury with spinal cord compression or cauda equina syndrome
- **N**eoplastic: Primary or metastatic neoplasm with erosion or compression of spinal cord or cauda equina, spinal cord tumor

History
- Ask the patient the following:
  - **Character:** "What does your back pain feel like: sharp? Achy? Burning? Shooting?"
  - **Location:** "Where exactly does your back hurt (midline, laterally)? Where along the length of spine does it hurt? Does one spot hurt more than any other?"
  - **Onset:** "When did the pain start? Was the onset sudden or gradual? Has the pain been getting progressively worse? Specifically, was there something that triggered the pain?"
  - **Radiation:** "Does the pain move anywhere (buttocks, limbs, perineum)?"
  - **Intensity:** "How severe is the pain on a scale of 1 to 10, with 1 being mild pain and 10 being the worst?"
  - **Duration:** "How long has the pain been there? Is it getting better, getting worse, or staying the same?"
  - **Events associated:**
    - "Have you experienced any injuries or falls (spinal fracture, dislocation, or ligamentous injury)?"
    - "Do you have numbness or tingling? If so, where, exactly?"
    - "Have you experienced incontinence of urine or stool, numbness in the anogenital area, muscular weakness, or loss of sensation (cauda equina syndrome or spinal cord compression)?"
    - "Have you had a fever or recent infection? Do you use IV drugs? Do you have any disease of your immune system? Do you take steroid medication (immunocompromise)?" Positive answers to these may be indications of epidural abscess or discitis.
    - "Have you had fever, chills, night sweats, weight loss, anorexia, or weakness (constitutional symptoms)?"
  - **Palliative factors:** "Does anything make the back pain better? If so, what?"
    - Analgesic medications (type, dose, frequency)
    - Position
  - **Provocative factors:** "Does anything make the back pain worse? If so, what?"
    - Position
    - Palpation
- **PMH/PSH:** Spinal surgery, degenerative disc disease, disc herniation, osteoporosis, malignancy, known metastases, hypertension, ankylosing spondylitis
- **MEDS:** Analgesics, steroids, chemotherapy
- **SH:** Smoking, use of EtOH, use of street drugs (ask specifically about IV drug use)

Physical Examination
- **Vitals:** Evaluate HR, BP, RR, and temperature.
- **General:** Assess the patient's general appearance, noting any apparent distress, spontaneous movement of limbs, or cachexia.
- **Spine examination:**
  - Test range of motion.
  - Palpate along the length of the spine, noting any areas of tenderness or deformity.
- **Tone:**
  - Evaluate tone of upper extremities.
  - Evaluate tone of lower extremities.
- **Motor examination:**
  - Evaluate upper extremities (elbow flexion, elbow extension, wrist extension, finger flexion, finger abduction).
  - Evaluate lower extremities (hip flexion, knee extension, ankle dorsiflexion, ankle plantar flexion, long toe extension).
- **Sensory examination:**
  - Perform light touch test and pin-pinch testing in all key dermatomal areas (see Figure 5-22).
- **Deep tendon reflexes:**
  - Evaluate patellar reflex.
  - Evaluate plantar reflex (check for Babinski's sign).

- **Digital rectal examination** (see Figure 3-8):
  - Evaluate anal tone.
  - Evaluate anal and perineal sensation.

HEAD INJURY: HISTORY AND PHYSICAL EXAMINATION

> **INSTRUCTIONS TO CANDIDATE: A 42-year-old man presents to the emergency department after being struck in the head with a baseball bat. Perform a focused physical examination to determine severity of injury and need for computed tomographic (CT) scan.**

DD$_X$: VITAMINS C
- Traumatic: Scalp contusion, scalp laceration, skull fracture, epidural hematoma, subdural hemorrhage, subarachnoid hemorrhage

Physical Examination
- **Vitals:** Evaluate HR, BP, RR, and temperature.
  - Be alert for the combination of hypertension, bradycardia, and irregular respirations that accompany raised ICP (Cushing's response).
- **General:** Assess the patient's general appearance, noting any apparent distress, vomiting, or obvious injury above the clavicles.
- **Level of consciousness:** Determine GCS score by evaluating eye opening, verbal response, and motor response (p. 144).
- **HEENT:**
  - **Head:** Assess for scalp contusion, scalp hematoma, laceration, and depressed skull fracture.
  - Eyes: Check whether the pupils are of equal size; check for "raccoon eyes"; perform funduscopic examination (for papilledema, retinal hemorrhage).
  - Ears: Check for hemotympanum, otorrhea, and Battle's sign.
  - Nose: Assess for rhinorrhea and epistaxis.
- **Cranial nerve examination** as outlined on pp. 150-155.
- **Screening neurologic examination:**
  - Assess gait.
  - Assess motor function (pronator drift, leg drift).
  - Evaluate sensation of touch in extremities.
  - Perform tests of coordination and cerebellar function as outlined on pp. 156-157.

Evidence: Computed Tomography in Minor Head Injury
- The Canadian CT Head Rule[4] is a clinical decision tool used to determine whether a patient who has suffered a minor head injury (GCS score of 13 to 15 and loss of consciousness, definite amnesia, or witnessed disorientation) requires a CT scan of the brain.
- The tool recommends a CT scan for any patient who has suffered a minor head injury and has any of the following *high-risk features:*
  - Is the patient's GCS score <15 at 2 hours after injury?
  - Is an open or depressed skull fracture suspected?
  - Does the patient show one or more signs of basal skull fracture (i.e., hemotympanum, cerebrospinal fluid otorrhea or rhinorrhea, Battle's sign, raccoon eyes)?
  - Has the patient had two or more episodes of vomiting?
  - Is the patient ≥65 years old?
  - Does the patient have a *medium-risk feature?*
    - Amnesia ≥30 minutes before impact
    - Dangerous mechanism: Pedestrian struck by vehicle, occupant ejected from motor vehicle, or person falling from elevation of more than 3 feet or 5 stairs.

- The high-risk factors have a sensitivity of 100% (95% CI 92% to 100%) for predicting the need for neurosurgical intervention. The moderate-risk factors have a sensitivity of 98.4% (95% CI 96% to 99%) for predicting clinically important brain injury.
- This tool can be used to safely identify patients who do not need CT brain for minor head injury.[4]

SAMPLE CHECKLIST

Stroke: History

> **INSTRUCTIONS TO CANDIDATE:** A 76-year-old woman with a history of atrial fibrillation presents to the emergency department with concerns that she may have suffered a "slight" stroke. Obtain a focused history.

Key Points	Satisfactorily Completed
Introduces self to patient	❑
Determines how the patient wishes to be addressed	❑
Washes hands	❑
Explains purpose of the encounter	❑
Completes history in a logical manner	❑
Asks for a specific description of the incident:	
• Which side of the body was affected	❑
• Presence of muscle weakness	❑
• Presence of sensory abnormality	❑
• Presence of expressive aphasia	❑
• Presence of receptive aphasia	❑
• Presence of depressed mental status	❑
Asks about onset of stroke:	
• Specific time at onset	❑
• If time at onset is unknown, last time the patient was seen appearing normal	❑
Asks about symptoms:	
• Duration of symptoms	❑
• Complete or partial resolution of symptoms	❑
• Remaining deficits	❑
Asks about events associated with the event:	
• Headache	❑
• Syncope	❑
• Vomiting	❑
• Palpitations	❑
Asks about frequency of symptoms:	
• Whether the patient has had previous similar episodes	❑
• Whether the patient has undergone investigations or treatments for similar episodes	❑
Asks about past medical history:	
• Atrial fibrillation	❑
• Diabetes	❑
• Hypertension	❑
• Dyslipidemia	❑
Asks about medications:	
• Anticoagulants (dose, route, frequency)	❑
• Inquires about INR testing and recent results	❑
• New medications (e.g., antibiotics)	❑
Asks about allergies	❑

Key Points	Satisfactorily Completed
Asks about social history:	
• Smoking	❑
• Use of EtOH	❑
• Use of street drugs	❑
• Living situation and social supports	❑
Asks about family history	❑
Makes appropriate closing remarks	❑

REFERENCES

1. Guldner GT, Brzenski AB. The sensitivity and specificity of the digital rectal examination for detecting spinal cord injury in adult patients with blunt trauma. *Am J Emerg Med.* 2006;24: 113-117.

2. Attia J, Hatala R, Cook DJ, et al. The rational clinical exam: does this adult patient have meningitis? *JAMA.* 1999;281:175-181.

3. Stiell IG, Wells GA, Vandemheen KL, et al. The Canadian C-Spine Rule for radiography in alert and stable trauma patients. *JAMA.* 2001;286:1841-1848.

4. Stiell IG, Wells GA, Vandemheen KL, et al. The Canadian CT Head Rule for patients with minor head injury. *Lancet.* 2001;357:1391-1396.

CHAPTER 6

Musculoskeletal System

ESSENTIAL SKILLS

APPROACH TO MUSCULOSKELETAL PAIN: HISTORY

- **ID:** Age, sex
- Ask the patient the following:
  - **C**haracter: "What is the pain like? Sharp? Dull?"
  - **L**ocation: "From where does the pain originate? From which joint(s) or region(s)?"
  - **O**nset: "When did the pain start? How did it come on (sudden versus gradual)?"
  - **R**adiation: "Does the pain move anywhere?"
  - **I**ntensity: "How severe is the pain on a scale of 1 to 10, with 1 being mild pain and 10 being the worst? How does it affect your activities of daily living (dressing,

getting to bathroom, taking care of yourself, cooking, cleaning, shopping, getting around)? Is the pain getting better, getting worse, or staying the same?"
- **Duration:** "How long have you had the pain (acute versus chronic)?"
- **Events associated:**
  - "Have you had any falls?" This is especially important for an elderly patient.
  - "Do you have morning stiffness? Swelling? Redness?"
  - "Have you experienced joint clicking or locking?"
  - "Do you have muscle pain (cramps)? Wasting?"
  - "Is your movement limited? Do you have weakness?"
  - "Is any numbness or tingling associated with the pain?"
  - "Have you had fever or chills?"
  - "Have you been injured recently? What was the mechanism of injury?"
  - "Do you participate in occupational activities or sports? Do you perform repetitive movements (e.g., typing)?"
- **Frequency:** "Have you ever had this pain before? How often does the pain come (intermittent versus constant)?"
- **Palliative factors:** "Does anything make the pain better? If so, what?"
  - Rest
  - Activity
  - Analgesic medications
  - Application of heat or cold
- **Provocative factors:** "Does anything make the pain worse? If so, what?"
  - Rest
  - Activity (particular movements)
- **Past medical history (PMH)/past surgical history (PSH):** Arthritis, gout, pseudogout, osteoporosis, connective tissue disease, past injuries, previous surgical procedures, other medical problems
- **Medications (MEDS):** Nonsteroidal anti-inflammatory drugs (NSAIDs), acetaminophen, narcotics, acetylsalicylic acid (ASA), steroids, or immunosuppressants, alternative therapies (e.g., glucosamine)
- **Allergies**
- **Social history (SH):** Smoking, use of EtOH, use of street drugs, sexual history, use of mobility aids (e.g., wheelchair, walker, cane), and occupation
- **Family history (FH):** Arthritis, osteoporosis, or connective tissue disease

APPROACH TO MUSCULOSKELETAL PAIN: EXAMINATION

Inspection
- Begin inspecting the patient's gait, posture, and movements from the time you enter the room.
- When you examine a joint, it is always important to examine the contralateral joint for comparison. As you inspect, note any asymmetry, and use the SEADS mnemonic:
  - **S**welling
  - **E**rythema, **e**cchymosis
  - **A**trophy
  - **D**eformity
  - **S**kin changes

Palpation
- It is important to examine above and below the joint in question because pain and other symptoms may be referred. This is especially important in trauma, when further injuries might be overlooked in the presence of an "obvious" fracture. It is equally important in patients with neurologic conditions that alter pain perception or in those who cannot communicate their symptoms accurately (e.g., very young children, patients with dementia, or patients with altered level of consciousness).

- When you palpate, examine the contralateral joint for comparison. Note any asymmetry, and use the TEST CA mnemonic:
  - Tenderness
  - Effusion
  - Swelling
  - Temperature
  - Crepitus
  - Atrophy

Range of Motion

- **Active range of motion (ROM):** While you immobilize the joint proximal to the joint being examined, instruct the patient to move the joint being examined (Figure 6-1). ROM should be symmetric (compare left with right). If there appears to be limitation in active ROM, test the passive ROM also.
- **Passive ROM:** The examiner performs these maneuvers; the patient's efforts are not needed. Move the joint in question through the same range of movement as in active ROM. Passive and active ROM should be nearly equal (passive ROM often exceeds active ROM slightly).

Grading Power (Oxford Scale)

- 5: Normal (active movement against resistance)
- 4: Active movement against gravity and some resistance
- 3: Active movement against gravity
- 2: Active movement when gravity eliminated
- 1: Flicker or trace of contraction
- 0: No muscle contraction

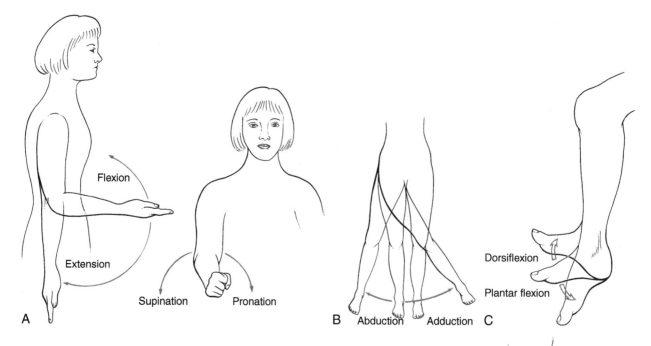

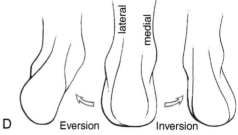

Figure 6-1 Skeletal muscle movements. **A,** Muscle movements of the elbow. **B,** Muscle movements of the hip joint. **C** and **D,** Muscle movements of the ankle joint. (From Swartz M. *Textbook of Physical Diagnosis: History and Examination.* 6th ed. Philadelphia: Elsevier; 2010 [pp. 592, Figure 20-8; p. 595, Figure 20-14, *B*; p. 597, Figure 20-18].)

Neurovascular Assessment
- It is important to perform a neurovascular assessment of injured extremities.
- Check distal pulses and capillary refill. Assess the skin color (cyanosis, erythema, pallor) and temperature by using the dorsum of your hand, and compare them with those of the contralateral limb.
- Test sensation, and map areas of decreased sensation.
- **Compartment syndrome** is a limb-threatening emergency resulting from increased pressure in an anatomic compartment that compromises associated nerves and circulation. It is characterized by pain disproportionate to the injury or clinical findings, paresthesias, and increased pain on passive stretch of involved muscles.

Special Tests
- These are specific to the joint being examined (e.g., Tinel's sign and occiput-to-wall distance).

CERVICAL SPINE: EXAMINATION

Patient Positioning
- Cooperative patients with *acute* injuries to the cervical spine should be examined in the supine position with the head and neck immobilized. Examination should be limited to light palpation of the cervical spine and soft tissues of the neck until injury of the spine is clinically or radiographically excluded.
- Patients without acute injury should be examined while sitting, with the neck, upper back, and shoulders exposed.

Inspection
- Inspect the neck in a resting position, noting its normal lordotic curve (Figure 6-2). Observe any resting rotation or lateral flexion.

Palpation
- Palpate the cervical spine for tenderness, spasm, or mass; start at the base of the skull and palpate down to the spinous prominence (C7). Palpate the trapezius, sternocleidomastoid muscle, and paraspinal muscles.

Range of Motion
- Begin the evaluation by inspecting the patient's active ROM. Instruct the patient to put his or her chin to the chest (flexion), look up at the ceiling (extension), turn the head from side to side (rotation), and touch ear to shoulder (lateral flexion).
- To measure ROM specifically, use the central axis of the torso and a line through the vertex of the skull as a reference. Normal ranges are as follows:
  - Flexion: 45 degrees
  - Extension: 50 degrees
  - Rotation: 70 degrees
  - Lateral flexion: 45 degrees
- If the active ROM is limited, test the passive ROM by placing your hands on either side of the patient's head to guide the neck through the same motions (flexion, extension, rotation, and lateral bending).

Grading Power
- Repeat the motions elicited for ROM, using an opposing force. Grade the muscle power according to the Oxford scale.

Special Tests
- With the patient standing with his or her back against a wall, measure the **occiput-to-wall distance.** The inability to touch the occiput against the wall is abnormal. This measurement may be used to follow the progression of ankylosing spondylitis and

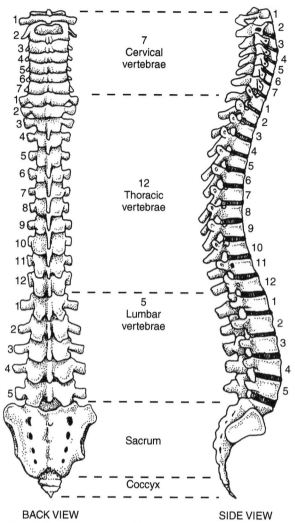

7
Cervical
vertebrae

12
Thoracic
vertebrae

5
Lumbar
vertebrae

Sacrum

Coccyx

BACK VIEW   SIDE VIEW

Figure 6-2 Vertebral column. (From Marx JA, Hockberger RS, Walls RM, eds. *Rosen's Emergency Medicine: Concepts and Clinical Practice.* 5th ed. St. Louis: Mosby; 2002 [p. 330, Figure 36-1, *A*].)

can also be used as part of the assessment for osteoporosis and associated chronic spinal fractures.

- Ask the patient to simultaneously rotate and laterally flex the neck toward the affected side. Reproduction of radicular symptoms **(Spurling's sign)** is suggestive of cervical root impingement.
- The **compression test** is less specific than Spurling's sign for identifying cervical root impingement. Perform this test with the patient sitting. Exert an axial load by applying downward pressure on the patient's head. Reproduction or exacerbation of radicular pain is suggestive of cervical nerve root impingement.
- **Lhermitte's sign** is nonspecific, but its presence should prompt thorough neurologic evaluation. It is associated with conditions such as vitamin B_{12} deficiency, multiple sclerosis, and cervical disc disease (nerve impingement) and refers to the presence of electric-like shocks that radiate down the back in response to forward flexion of the neck.

Neurologic Correlates
- A patient with spinal injury, spinal cord injury, or nerve root symptoms should have a complete neurologic examination, including assessment of sensory, motor, and reflexes in all limbs.

- Deficits associated with specific nerve roots (Figure 6-3):
  - C4: Abnormal sensation in the necklace distribution; weakness in elevation of scapulae
  - C5: Abnormal sensation in the anterolateral shoulder; deltoid and biceps weakness and diminished biceps reflex
  - C6: Abnormal sensation in the lateral hand (thumb) and forearm; biceps and wrist extensor weakness and diminished biceps reflex
  - C7: Abnormal sensation in the index and middle fingers and in the dorsal arm; triceps and digit extensor weakness and diminished triceps reflex
  - C8: Abnormal sensation in the small finger and medial arm; hypothenar and hand flexor weakness

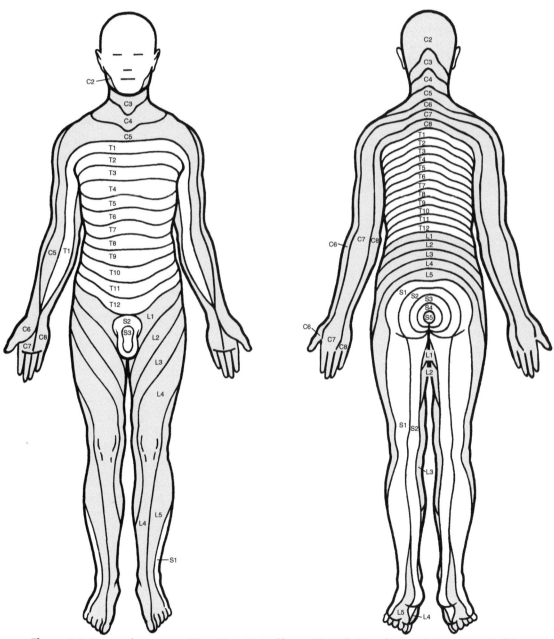

Figure 6-3 Sensory dermatomes. (From Marx JA, Hockberger RS, Walls RM, eds. *Rosen's Emergency Medicine: Concepts and Clinical Practice.* 5th ed. St. Louis: Mosby; 2002 [p. 347, Figure 36-22].)

Pearl
- **Torticollis** is painful lateral deviation of the neck in association with contralateral sternocleidomastoid muscle tenderness or spasm.

THORACIC SPINE: EXAMINATION

Patient Positioning
- Cooperative patients with *acute* injuries to the thoracic spine should be examined only in the supine position. With the help of two or more assistants, log rolling the patient allows palpation of the thoracolumbar spine and soft tissues and minimizes further spinal injury.
- Patients without acute traumatic injuries are best examined standing, wearing an examining gown that opens in the back (to expose the thoracic spinal area).

Inspection
- Inspect the thoracic spine in a resting position, noting the normal slight upper thoracic kyphosis and thoracolumbar lordosis (see Figure 6-2).
- The posterior ribs, shoulder height, scapulae, and iliac crests should be symmetric in upright and flexed positions. Asymmetry may be suggestive of scoliosis (Figure 6-4).

Palpation
- Palpate each spinous process. This may be facilitated by having the patient lean forward, resting his or her elbows on a bed or chair back. Begin palpating at the level of C7 to T1, which is typically prominent and easily identified. The L4 process sits on the line joining the iliac crests posteriorly (Figure 6-5). Note any tenderness or step deformities that may be indicative of spondylolisthesis.
- Palpate the paraspinal muscles for bulk, tenderness, mass, or spasm.
- Place your hands over the scapulae, and ask the patient to bend forward. Note the position of your hands; their height should be symmetric. This technique may reveal subtle scoliosis.

Percussion
- Percuss each vertebra with the hypothenar aspect of your closed fist. Deep pain in response to percussion is nonspecific but may be indicative of degenerative disease, malignancy, or infection.

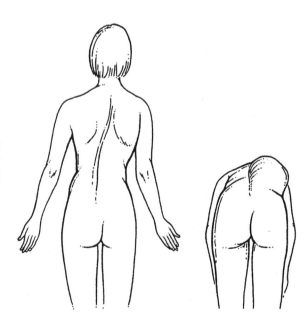

Figure 6-4 Inspecting for scoliosis. (From Swartz M. *Textbook of Physical Diagnosis: History and Examination.* 3rd ed. Philadelphia: Saunders; 1998 [p. 634, Figure 22-28].)

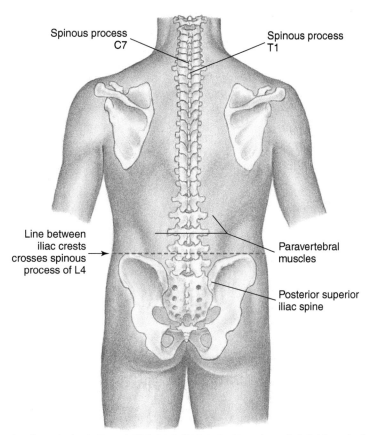

Spinous process
C7

Spinous process
T1

Line between
iliac crests
crosses spinous
process of L4

Paravertebral
muscles

Posterior superior
iliac spine

Figure 6-5 Landmarks on the back. (From Seidel HM, Ball JW, Dains JE, et al. *Mosby's Guide to Physical Examination.* 6th ed. St. Louis: Mosby; 2006 [p. 710, Figure 21-19].)

Range of Motion

- Inspect the patient's active ROM. With the patient standing, instruct him or her to touch his or her toes (forward flexion). With the patient in flexion, palpate the spinous processes, noting the normal increased interspinous distance. **Finger-to-floor distance** can be used to measure the extent of flexion. The normal range varies considerably, but this measurement can be used to monitor disease progression in ankylosing spondylitis.
- Using your hands to fix the pelvis, ask the patient to bend backward (extension), bend laterally (lateral flexion), and to rotate from side to side. There is little extension in the thoracic spine itself because of the angulation of the spinous processes. Normal ranges are as follows:
  - Extension: 30 degrees
  - Lateral flexion: 35 degrees
  - Rotation: 30 degrees
- Observe for the normal reversal from thoracolumbar lordosis to kyphosis in flexion. Failure to reverse may be an indication of degenerative disease.

Pearl

- Thoracic disc herniation typically occurs in the mid-lower thoracic spine and manifests with radicular pain down the back or along the ribs. A central disc herniation may manifest with weakness, spasticity below the level of the lesion, or bowel or bladder dysfunction.

LUMBAR SPINE AND SACROILIAC JOINTS: EXAMINATION

Patient Positioning

- Cooperative patients with *acute* injuries to the lumbar spine should be examined only in the supine position. With the help of two or more assistants, log rolling the patient allows palpation of the thoracolumbar spine and soft tissues and minimizes further spinal injury.
- Patients without acute traumatic injuries are best examined standing, wearing an examining gown that opens in the back (to expose the lumbosacral spinal area).

Inspection

- Inspect the lumbosacral spine in a resting position, noting the normal lumbar lordotic curve. Note any asymmetry of the iliac crests.

Palpation

- Palpate each spinous process. The L4 process sits on the line joining the iliac crests posteriorly (see Figure 6-5). Note any tenderness or step deformities that may be indicative of spondylolisthesis. Palpate for tenderness over the posterior superior iliac spine and sacroiliac joints.
- Palpate the paraspinal muscles for bulk, tenderness, mass, or spasm.

Percussion

- Percuss each vertebra with the hypothenar aspect of your closed fist. Deep pain in response to percussion is nonspecific but may be an indication of degenerative disease, malignancy, or infection.

Range of Motion

- Inspect the patient's active ROM. With the patient standing, instruct him or her to touch his or her toes (forward flexion). With the patient in flexion, palpate the spinous processes, noting the normal increased interspinous distance. **Finger-to-floor distance** can be used to measure the extent of flexion. The normal range varies considerably, but this measurement is useful in monitoring disease progression in ankylosing spondylitis.
- Using your hands to fix the pelvis, ask the patient to bend backward (extension), bend laterally (lateral flexion), and rotate from side to side. Normal ranges are as follows:
  - Extension: 30 degrees
  - Lateral flexion: 35 degrees
  - Rotation: 30 degrees
- Observe for the normal reversal from thoracolumbar lordosis to kyphosis in flexion. Failure to reverse may be an indication of degenerative disease.

Special Tests

- **Sacroiliac joint pain** can be reproduced by placing the patient in a supine position with the contralateral hip and knee flexed and the ipsilateral hip hyperextended over the edge of the bed. This maneuver reproduces pain in sacroiliitis.
- Radicular pain from L5 or S1 roots can be reproduced by several techniques that stretch the sciatic nerve roots:
  - **Straight leg raising** is usually performed with the patient supine and legs extended. The symptomatic leg is passively raised off the bed (knee extended). A positive test result is worsened pain in the affected leg at hip flexion of <60 to 70 degrees.
  - The **bowstring sign** is elicited by passively raising the patient's symptomatic leg off the bed with the knee in slight flexion until just below the threshold for radicular pain. The bowstring sign is pain that is then elicited through firm compression of the popliteal fossa (pain radiates from the knee to the back).

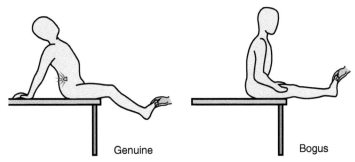

Genuine Bogus

Figure 6-6 Reassessing positive straight leg raising in the seated position. (Adapted from Munro JF, Campbell IW, eds. *Macleod's Clinical Examination.* 10th ed. Edinburgh: Churchill Livingstone; 2000 [p. 271, Figure 8-13, *B* and *C*].)

- **Lasègue's sign** is elicited by passively raising the patient's symptomatic leg off the bed with the knee in slight flexion until just below the threshold for radicular pain. Lasègue's sign is worsening of pain with passive dorsiflexion of the ankle.
- Tests for radicular pain may also be performed with the patient in a sitting position and may unveil inconsistencies (Figure 6-6).
- **Crossed-over** or bilateral leg pain in response to these maneuvers may be suggestive of a central disc herniation or cauda equina involvement.
- **Schober's test** is initiated with the patient in a standing position. Identify the **dimples of Venus** (sacroiliac joints), and make a mark on the skin at the midline. Using a measuring tape, make a second mark 10 cm above. Ask the patient to bend forward. Remeasure the distance between the two marks (Figure 6-7). It normally measures at least 15 cm. Reduced expansion of the interspinous distance may be suggestive of ankylosing spondylitis.

Evidence

- In general, physical examination techniques to assess back pain are not reliable[1] (Table 6-1). Most studies of the usefulness of clinical examination for diagnosis of lumbar radiculopathy have been performed in surgical settings with populations in which this condition is highly prevalent. Assessments of muscle weakness (ankle dorsiflexion, extension of great toe), muscle wasting, impaired reflexes, and sensory deficits were each noted to have poor sensitivity but higher specificity for diagnosing radiculopathy (results could not be pooled because of heterogeneity). Straight leg raising was found to be relatively sensitive (92%; 95% confidence interval [CI] 87% to 95%) with poorer specificity (28%; 95% CI 18% to 40%). The crossed-over straight leg raise is less sensitive (28%; 95% CI 22% to 35%) and more specific (90%; 95% CI 85% to 94%).[2]

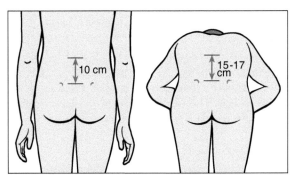

Figure 6-7 Schober's test. (Adapted from Munro JF, Campbell IW, eds. *Macleod's Clinical Examination.* 10th ed. Edinburgh: Churchill Livingstone; 2000 [p. 269, Figure 8-10].)

Table 6-1	Usefulness of Clinical Examination in the Diagnosis of Lumbar Radiculopathy	
Clinical Feature	**+LR (95% CI)**	**−LR (95% CI)**
Straight leg raising	1.3 (1.1–1.4)	0.30 (0.24–0.39)
Crossed-over straight leg raising	2.1 (1.6–2.8)	0.86 (0.83–0.89)

From van der Windt DA, Simons E, Riphagen II, et al. Physical examination for lumbar radiculopathy due to disc herniation in patients with low-back pain, *Cochrane Database Syst Rev.* 2010;2:CD007431.

CI, Confidence interval; −LR, negative likelihood ratio; +LR, positive likelihood ratio.

Pearls

- Herniated lumbar discs most commonly occur at the levels of L4 to L5 and L5 to S1. Lateral disc herniation at these levels may produce neurologic findings in the distribution of L5 and S1 nerve roots, respectively.
- Signs of **cauda equina syndrome** include diminished saddle sensation, reduced rectal tone, and urinary retention. Patients with back pain and bowel or bladder symptoms should be examined for sensation in the saddle distribution and rectal tone. Postvoid residual urine should be quantified as well.
- New onset of atraumatic back pain or tenderness, particularly in patients aged <18 or >60 years, should raise suspicion of serious illness, such as malignancy, pancreatitis, ruptured abdominal aortic aneurysm, or aortic dissection. A thorough physical examination for thoracic or abdominal causes of referred back pain must be performed.

SHOULDER: EXAMINATION

Patient Positioning

- The patient should be draped in a manner to allow full exposure of the shoulder and comparison with the other side. An examining gown tied under the arms will leave the shoulders exposed while covering the chest and breasts.

Inspection

- Inspect for SEADS.

Palpation

- While you palpate the shoulder, be alert for TEST CA, and note any asymmetry.
- Palpate the sternoclavicular joint, following the clavicle laterally to the acromioclavicular joint (Figure 6-8). Palpate the acromion, spine, and body of the scapula. The coracoclavicular joint is situated just medial and inferior to the acromioclavicular joint. The greater tubercle of the humerus and humeral head are palpated laterally beneath the deltoid muscle. The glenohumeral joint is typically not palpable beneath the overlying musculature.
- Palpate the supraspinatus, infraspinatus, deltoid, and biceps areas for tenderness. The tendon of the long head of the biceps is palpable in the groove medial to the greater tuberosity (Figure 6-9). The subacromial bursa lies deep to the deltoid and just lateral to the acromion. The supraspinatus tendon wraps anteriorly over the glenohumeral joint, inserting on the greater tuberosity.

Range of Motion

- Movement of the shoulder combines motions of the scapula and glenohumeral joint.
- Inspect the patient's active ROM in the affected shoulder, and compare it with that of the contralateral shoulder. Instruct him or her to raise the arms forward (flexion)

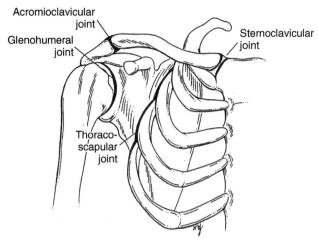

Figure 6-8 Bony anatomy of the shoulder. (From Swartz M. *Textbook of Physical Diagnosis: History and Examination.* 6th ed. Philadelphia: Elsevier; 2010 [p. 591, Figure 20-5].)

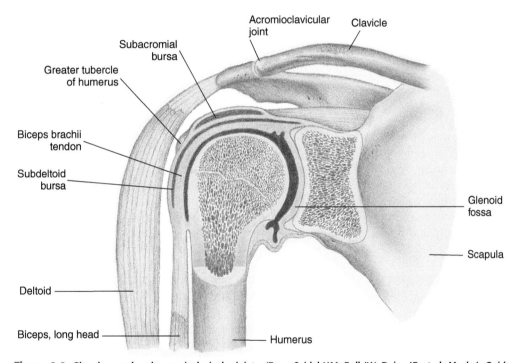

Figure 6-9 Glenohumeral and acromioclavicular joints. (From Seidel HM, Ball JW, Dains JE, et al. *Mosby's Guide to Physical Examination.* 6th ed. St. Louis: Mosby; 2006 [p. 696, Figure 21-6].)

and straight over the head and extend them backward (extension). Ask him or her to lift the arms laterally overhead (abduction) and swing them across the chest (adduction). Assess internal and external rotation with the elbows flexed; instruct the patient to put his or her hands behind the head (external rotation) and behind the back (internal rotation). Normal ranges are as follows:

- Forward flexion: 180 degrees
- Extension: 45 degrees
- Abduction: 180 degrees
- Adduction: 45 degrees
- Internal and external rotation: 90 degrees

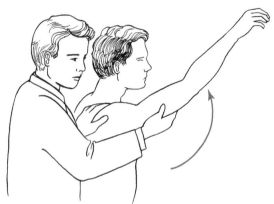

Figure 6-10 The Neer impingement test. (Adapted from Marx JA, Hockberger RS, Walls RM, eds. *Rosen's Emergency Medicine: Concepts and Clinical Practice.* 5th ed. St. Louis: Mosby; 2002 [p. 601, Figure 46-39].)

- If the active ROM is limited, test the passive ROM by guiding the shoulder through the same motions (flexion, extension, abduction, adduction, internal and external rotation).

Grading Power
- Repeat the motions elicited for ROM, using an opposing force. Grade the muscle power according to the Oxford scale.
- Reduced strength, particularly for abduction and external rotation, is common with acute and chronic injuries of the rotator cuff.

Special Tests
- The **drop test** is performed by asking the patient to actively abduct the shoulder 90 degrees. Inability to maintain this position is a positive result and is suggestive of a significant rotator cuff tear.
- The **Neer impingement test** is performed on the patient's right shoulder by fixing the scapula (with your left hand) and flexing the glenohumeral joint (with your right hand) as you stand behind the patient (Figure 6-10). Note that the forearm is pronated. This action impinges on the subacromial bursa between the greater tuberosity and the acromion (see Figure 6-9). The presence of pain with this maneuver is a positive result and may be an indication of subacromial bursitis.

Evidence
- The Neer test for impingement has a sensitivity of 79% (95% CI 75% to 82%) and a specificity of 53% (95% CI 48% to 58%), limiting its use as a diagnostic tool.[3] The drop test has a positive likelihood ratio (+LR) in the range of 2.9 to 5.0 and a less impressive negative likelihood ratio (−LR) in the range of 0.74 to 0.92.[3]

Pearl
- A patient with shoulder pain should have an examination of the neck to rule out referred pain. Elicit Spurling's sign, and perform the cervical compression test to detect cervical root impingement or radiculopathy as a source of shoulder pain.

ELBOW: EXAMINATION

Patient Positioning
- Expose both arms (for comparison purposes) from shoulder to fingers.

Inspection
- Inspect the elbow in its resting position for SEADS. The normal carrying angle is 5 to 20 degrees (Figure 6-11).

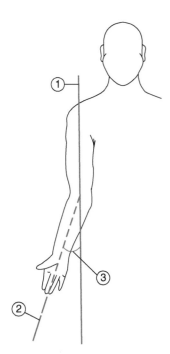

Figure 6-11 Carrying angle *(3)* is formed by the intersection of lines drawn parallel to the long axis of the humerus *(1)* and ulna *(2)*. (From Marx JA, Hockberger RS, Walls RM, eds. *Rosen's Emergency Medicine: Concepts and Clinical Practice.* 5th ed. St. Louis: Mosby; 2002 [p. 558, Figure 45-5].)

Palpation

- While you palpate the elbow, be alert for TEST CA, and note any asymmetry.
- Palpate the olecranon, the medial and lateral condyles of the humerus, and the radial head (Figure 6-12). Palpate the forearm and humerus, including the wrist and shoulder joints.
  - An elbow effusion is best palpated in the anatomic triangle formed by the radial head, lateral condyle, and olecranon.
- Palpate the ulnar nerve (between the olecranon and medial epicondyle), the olecranon bursa (normally not palpable), the common extensor insertion at the lateral epicondyle, and the common flexor insertion at the medial epicondyle.

Range of Motion

- Begin by inspecting the patient's active ROM in the affected elbow, and compare it with that in the contralateral elbow. Instruct the patient to bend his or her elbow (flexion) and straighten the elbow (extension). Pronation and supination are assessed

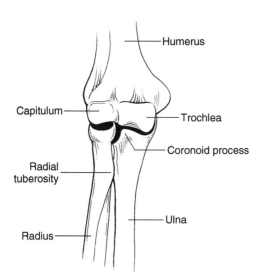

Figure 6-12 Bony anatomy of the elbow. (From Swartz M. *Textbook of Physical Diagnosis: History and Examination.* 6th ed. Philadelphia: Elsevier; 2010 [p. 592, Figure 20-8].)

with the elbow flexed to 90 degrees and the thumb pointing straight up (neutral position). Normal ranges are as follows:

- Flexion: 150 degrees
- Extension: 0 degrees (mild *symmetric* hyperextension is within normal limits)
- Supination: 90 degrees
- Pronation: 90 degrees

- If the active ROM is limited, test the passive ROM by guiding the elbow through the same motions (flexion, extension, supination, and pronation).

Grading Power

- Repeat the motions elicited for ROM, using an opposing force. Grade the muscle power according to the Oxford scale.

Special Tests

- By using forced wrist extension, evaluate for **tennis elbow.** Tenderness over the common extensor insertion at the lateral epicondyle is suggestive of lateral epicondylitis, or tennis elbow.
- By using forced wrist flexion, evaluate for **golfer's elbow.** Tenderness over the common flexor insertion at the medial epicondyle is suggestive of medial epicondylitis, or golfer's elbow.

Pearls

- In the setting of injury, an abnormal or asymmetric carrying angle may be indicative of a supracondylar fracture.
- Olecranon bursitis, otherwise known as **student's elbow,** is suggested by the presence of point tenderness, swelling, and fluctuance over the olecranon.

WRIST: EXAMINATION

Patient Positioning

- Expose both arms (for comparison purposes) from elbows to fingertips.

Inspection

- Inspect the dorsal and volar surfaces of the wrist for SEADS.

Palpation

- While you palpate the wrist, be alert for TEST CA, and note any asymmetry.
- Palpate the patient's wrist, using both your hands with thumbs positioned dorsally and index fingers against the volar surface. The wrist joint includes the distal radius and ulna and the carpal bones (Figure 6-13). Identify landmarks, including the radial and ulnar styloid processes and the distal radioulnar articulation.
- The **anatomic snuffbox** is bordered by the abductor pollicis longus/extensor pollicis brevis and extensor pollicis longus muscles. The scaphoid is palpable within the snuffbox (Figure 6-14). The scaphoid tubercle is palpated at the base of the thenar eminence with the wrist in extension.
- **Lister's tubercle** is a bony prominence on the dorsum of the wrist (dorsal tubercle of the radius). The scapholunate joint is just distal to Lister's tubercle and is a common site of ligamentous injury.
- The pisiform is palpated at the base of the hypothenar muscles.
- Palpate the extensor and flexor tendons as they cross the wrist joint (Figure 6-15).
- Palpate the forearm. Palpate the radial and ulnar pulses.

Range of Motion

- Begin by inspecting the patient's active ROM in the affected wrist, and compare it with that of the contralateral wrist, beginning with the wrist in a neutral position, fingers extended.

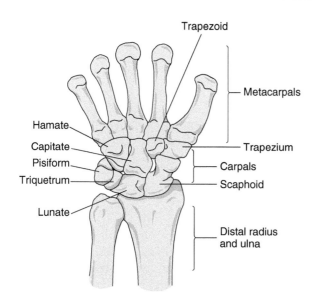

Trapezoid

Metacarpals

Hamate

Capitate

Pisiform

Triquetrum

Lunate

Trapezium

Carpals

Scaphoid

Distal radius
and ulna

Figure 6-13 Bony anatomy of the wrist. (From Marx JA, Hockberger RS, Walls RM, eds. *Rosen's Emergency Medicine: Concepts and Clinical Practice.* 5th ed. St. Louis: Mosby; 2002 [p. 535, Figure 44-1].)

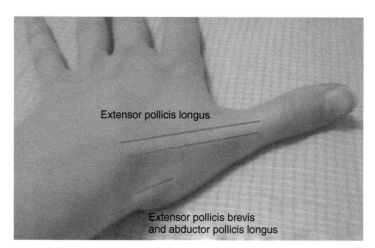

Extensor pollicis longus

Extensor pollicis brevis
and abductor pollicis longus

Figure 6-14 Anatomic snuffbox.

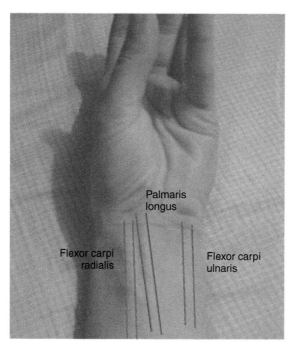

Palmaris
longus

Flexor carpi
radialis

Flexor carpi
ulnaris

Figure 6-15 Flexor tendons of wrist.

- Instruct the patient to bend the wrist up and down (flexion and extension) and from side to side (radial and ulnar deviation). Normal ranges are as follows:
  - Flexion: 90 degrees
  - Extension: 70 degrees
  - Ulnar deviation: 50 degrees
  - Radial deviation: 20 degrees
- If the active ROM is limited, test the passive ROM by guiding the wrist through the same motions (flexion, extension, ulnar and radial deviation).

Grading Power

- Repeat the motions elicited for ROM, using an opposing force. Grade the muscle power according to the Oxford scale.

Special Tests

- **Phalen's test:** Ask the patient to hold both wrists in full flexion with the dorsal surfaces pressed together (the opposite of prayer hands) for approximately 60 seconds. Numbness or paresthesias in the distribution of the median nerve are suggestive of carpal tunnel syndrome.
- **Tinel's sign:** Percuss the volar aspect of the wrist over the median nerve. Numbness or paresthesias in the distribution of the median nerve are suggestive of carpal tunnel syndrome.
- **Finkelstein's test:** Instruct the patient to place his or her thumb in the palm of the closed fist. Ask the patient to deviate the wrist in the ulnar direction. This test stretches the extensor pollicis brevis and abductor pollicis longus and produces pain in patients with de Quervain tenosynovitis.

Evidence

- Table 6-2 describes the usefulness of two clinical examination techniques performed to evaluate carpal tunnel syndrome.

HAND: EXAMINATION

Patient Positioning

- Expose both arms (for comparison purposes) from elbows to fingertips.

Inspection

- Inspect the dorsal and volar surfaces of the hand for SEADS (Figure 6-16).
- Note specifically any pattern of joint inflammation or thickening and any contractures.
- Note any asymmetry or atrophy of the intrinsic muscles of the hand, including the thenar eminence, hypothenar muscles, and interossei.

Palpation

- While you palpate the hand, be alert for TEST CA, and note any asymmetry.
- Palpate the individual bones of the hands, including the carpals, metacarpals, and phalanges.

Table 6-2	Usefulness of Clinical Examination in the Diagnosis of Carpal Tunnel Syndrome	
Clinical Feature	**+LR (95% CI)**	**−LR (95% CI)**
Phalen's test	1.3 (1.1–1.6)	0.7 (0.6–0.9)
Tinel's sign	1.4 (1.0–1.9)	0.8 (0.7–1.0)

Modified from D'Arcy CA, McGee S. The rational clinical examination: does this patient have carpal tunnel syndrome? *JAMA.* 2000;283:3110-3117.
CI, Confidence interval; −LR, negative likelihood ratio; +LR, positive likelihood ratio.

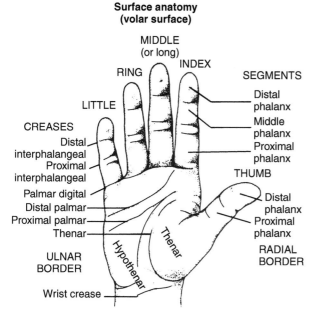

**Surface anatomy
(volar surface)**

MIDDLE
(or long)

RING   INDEX

LITTLE

SEGMENTS

Distal
phalanx

Middle
phalanx

Proximal
phalanx

THUMB

CREASES

Distal
interphalangeal

Proximal
interphalangeal

Palmar digital

Distal palmar

Proximal palmar

Thenar

Thenar

Hypothenar

Distal
phalanx

Proximal
phalanx

RADIAL
BORDER

ULNAR
BORDER

Wrist crease

Figure 6-16 Surface anatomy of the hand. (From Marx JA, Hockberger RS, Walls RM, eds. *Rosen's Emergency Medicine: Concepts and Clinical Practice.* 5th ed. St. Louis: Mosby; 2002 [p. 494, Figure 43-1].)

- Palpate the metacarpophalangeal (MCP) joints in slight flexion. Place your thumb on either side of the patient's extensor tendon dorsally, with your index fingers supporting the palmar aspect of the joint.
- Using the index finger and thumb of both your hands, palpate each interphalangeal joint, compressing each joint from lateral and anteroposterior directions. Check the stability of each joint in all directions (dorsal, volar, radial, and ulnar).

Range of Motion
- Begin by inspecting the patient's active ROM in the affected hand, and compare it with that in the contralateral hand.
- Instruct the patient to bend the fingers forward at the knuckles (MCP joints) and then stretch them back (flexion and extension). Have the patient make a fist (finger flexion), stretch the fingers apart (abduction), and touch them together again (adduction). Normal ranges are as follows:
  - MCP joint: 90 degrees flexion, 30 degrees extension
  - Proximal interphalangeal (PIP) joint: 120 degrees flexion, 0 degrees extension
  - DIP joint: 70 degrees flexion, 0 degrees extension
- If the active ROM is limited or if asymmetry is present, test the passive ROM by gently guiding the hand joints through the same planes of movement.

Grading Power
- Repeat the motions elicited for ROM, using an opposing force. Grade the muscle power according to the Oxford scale.
  - Lumbrical muscles: flexion of the MCP joint with interphalangeal joints in extension
  - Flexor digitorum superficialis: flexion of the PIP joint with immobilization of the MCP joint
  - Flexor digitorum profundus: flexion of the distal interphalangeal (DIP) joint with immobilization of the PIP joint
  - Dorsal interossei (digit abduction) and volar interossei (digit adduction)
  - Thenar eminence: opposition of thumb and small finger (the hypothenar muscles also play a role), elevation of the thumb from the palm against resistance
  - Adductor pollicis: gripping a sheet of paper between the thumb and index metacarpal

Pearls

- Symmetric involvement of the MCP and PIP joints is suggestive of rheumatoid arthritis. Digits tend to swell in a fusiform manner.
- Degenerative osteoarthritis affects the PIP and DIP joints but rarely affects the MCP joints. **Heberden nodes** occur at the DIP joints, and **Bouchard nodes** occur at the PIP joints.
- Atrophy of the intrinsic hand muscles may occur as a result of systemic disease (e.g., extrahepatic sign of liver disease) or joint disease and disuse or may be secondary to specific nerve dysfunction (e.g., advanced carpal tunnel syndrome is characterized by atrophy of the thenar eminence supplied by the median nerve).

HIP: EXAMINATION

Patient Positioning

- For inspection, the patient should be standing.
- For palpation, the patient should be supine.

Inspection

- Inspect the hips anteriorly and posteriorly with the patient in a standing position, noting any SEADS.
- Observe the stance, posture, and gait.
- Note any asymmetry in the height of the iliac crests or the gluteal folds (see Figure 6-5).

Palpation

- While you palpate the hip and pelvis, be alert for TEST CA, and note any asymmetry.
- Palpate the anterior superior iliac spine (ASIS), femurs, and greater trochanters (Figure 6-17). Exerting pressure on both sides of the pelvis simultaneously, test its stability.

Range of Motion

- Begin by inspecting the patient's active ROM in the affected hip, and compare it with that in the contralateral hip. Place the patient in a supine position, and instruct him or her to lift the straightened leg from the examining table (hip flexion). Have the patient lower the leg and swing it outward (abduction) and then medially (adduction). Instruct the patient to flex the knee and rotate it outward, placing the lateral aspect of the foot on the contralateral knee (external rotation), and then rotate it inward (internal rotation). Have the patient stand and extend the leg backward without arching the back (extension). Normal ranges are as follows:
  - Flexion: 90 to 120 degrees
  - Extension: Up to 30 degrees

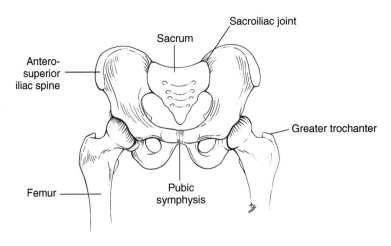

Figure 6-17 Bony anatomy of the hip and pelvis. (Adapted from Swartz M. *Textbook of Physical Diagnosis: History and Examination.* 6th ed. Philadelphia: Elsevier; 2010 [p. 595, Figure 20-13].)

- Abduction: Up to 45 degrees
- Adduction: Up to 30 degrees
- External rotation: 45 degrees
- Internal rotation: 40 degrees
- If the active ROM is limited, test the passive ROM by guiding the hip through the same motions (flexion, extension, abduction, adduction, external and internal rotation).

Grading Power
- Repeat flexion, extension, abduction, and adduction, using an opposing force. Grade the muscle power according to the Oxford scale.

Special Tests
- Perform the **Trendelenburg test** to detect weak hip abductors. Stand behind the patient, and ask him or her to stand on one leg and then on the other. Note any change in the level of the iliac crests or gluteal folds during this maneuver. If the iliac crest drops toward the non–weight-bearing side, it is indicative of weakness of the hip abductors in the weight-bearing limb.
- Measure **true leg length** from the ASIS to the medial malleolus (measuring tape crosses the knee medially). Discrepancy within 1 cm is acceptable.
- Consider performing **auscultatory percussion** in patients with acute onset of hip pain. While auscultating with the bell of the stethoscope over the pubic symphysis, percuss the patella. Compare the auscultated percussion notes in the right and left hips. A diminished percussion note in the painful hip may be indicative of a fracture.

Evidence
- Although many orthopedic evaluations rely heavily on the use of imaging, auscultatory percussion can be a useful in predicting the likelihood of occult hip fracture (+LR 6.7; 95% CI 3.0 to 15.1; and −LR 0.05; 95% CI 0.03 to 0.09).[4]

KNEE: EXAMINATION

Patient Positioning
- Expose both knees (for comparison purposes) from groin to ankles.

Inspection
- Inspect the knee in flexed and extended positions for SEADS.
- Effusions are best observed through inspection of the suprapatellar region. The anteromedial depression may be obliterated if the effusion is large.
- Observe the stance, posture, and gait.
- **Genu varum** (bow-legged deformity) is considered to be present when there is >2.5 cm of space between the knees with the medial malleoli together.
- **Genu valgum** (knock-knees) is considered to be present when there is >2.5 cm of space between the medial malleoli when the knees are together.

Palpation
- While you palpate the knee, be alert for TEST CA, and note any asymmetry.
- Palpate the patella, tibial tuberosity, tibial condyles, and femoral epicondyles (Figure 6-18).
- The normal knee is cooler than its surrounding tissue. Palpate for temperature with the dorsum of your hand, using the midthigh and shin for comparison. To determine symmetry, compare with the contralateral knee.
- Examining for effusions:
  - Immobilize the patella with the thumb and index finger (suprapatellar). Use the free hand to "milk" the medial aspect of the knee (upward strokes). If a downward stroke is used on the lateral aspect of the knee, fluid is displaced and may be visible as a bulge medially, known as the **bulge sign.**

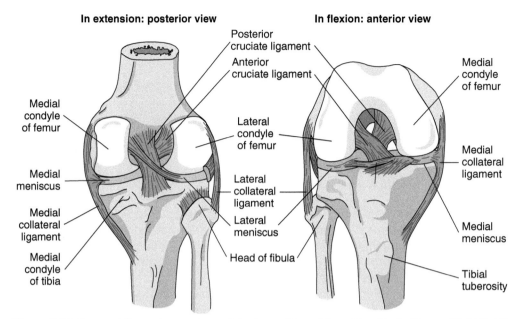

In extension: posterior view   **In flexion: anterior view**

Figure 6-18 Bony and ligamentous anatomy of the knee. (Adapted from Marx JA, Hockberger RS, Walls RM, eds. *Rosen's Emergency Medicine: Concepts and Clinical Practice.* 5th ed. St. Louis: Mosby; 2002 [p. 675, Figure 50-1].)

- ▪ A large effusion can be assessed by immobilizing the knee and **balloting** the patella against the femur while maintaining suprapatellar compression with the immobilizing hand.
- • The quadriceps angle **(Q angle)** is measured with the knee extended. The angle is formed by intersecting lines drawn from the tibial tubercle to the ASIS and from the center of the patella to the ASIS. A normal Q angle is <10 to 15 degrees. An increased Q angle predisposes to dislocation of the patella.

Range of Motion
- • Begin by inspecting the patient's active ROM in the affected knee, and compare it with that in the contralateral knee. Instruct the patient to bend his or her knee (flexion) and straighten it (extension). Normal ranges are as follows:
  - ▪ Flexion: ≤130 degrees
  - ▪ Extension: 0 degrees (mild *symmetric* hyperextension is within normal limits)
- • If the active ROM is limited, test the passive ROM by guiding the knee through the same motions (flexion, extension).

Grading Power
- • Repeat the motions elicited for ROM, using an opposing force. Grade the muscle power according to the Oxford scale.

Special Tests
- • Ligaments, a fibrocartilaginous capsule, and the surrounding muscles stabilize the knee. Test the stability of the knee by using the following maneuvers with the patient in the supine position. These tests should be performed on both knees, to assess symmetry.
  - ▪ The **anterior drawer test** is performed with the knee flexed to 90 degrees and anchored on the examining table (the examiner sits on it). Place your fingers in the patient's popliteal fossa and your thumbs over the joint line anteriorly, and pull the tibia forward. A positive finding is a palpable step that develops with anterior force, indicative of a tear in the anterior cruciate ligament (ACL).
  - ▪ The **posterior drawer test** is performed in the same position as the anterior drawer test. Apply a backward force on the tibia. A positive finding is displacement of

the tibia of >5 mm posteriorly, indicative of a tear in the posterior cruciate ligament (PCL).

- **Lachman's test** is more sensitive than the anterior drawer test for detecting ACL injury, but the PCL must be intact. The patient's knee is flexed at 15 degrees. Your left hand stabilizes the patient's thigh, and your right hand grasps the tibia and pulls it anteriorly. Anterior displacement of the tibia of >5 mm (in comparison with contralateral knee) is an indication of injury to the ACL.
- The **collateral ligament stress test** is performed in two positions: knee extended and knee flexed to 30 degrees. Using one of your arms to support the patient's leg, rest your other hand on the knee to apply a varus or valgus stress. Medial joint line opening (in comparison with the normal knee) during valgus stress is indicative of injury to the medial collateral ligament, whereas lateral joint line opening on varus stress is indicative of lateral collateral ligament damage. Instability with the knee fully extended is indicative of a complete injury, whereas instability at 30 degrees may be indicative of more limited injury.
- **McMurray's test** is performed with the patient supine. Place your left hand on the patient's knee, ensuring that you are able to feel the joint line. Using your right hand to grasp the patient's foot, flex and extend the knee while simultaneously internally and externally rotating it. External rotation tests the medial meniscus, and internal rotation tests the lateral meniscus. Pain or palpable clicking in the joint line constitutes a positive test result.

Evidence

- Table 6-3 describes tests that are useful in the clinical examination for diagnosing knee injuries. In the studies from which these data were extracted, the clinical examinations were performed by orthopedic surgeons. Less experienced examiners would presumably not perform as well experts. Also, most of these tests are noted to be less accurate in patients with hemarthrosis (acute injury).[5]

Pearls

- Swelling over the patella itself is more often caused by prepatellar bursitis than by effusion.
- Unilateral swelling and erythema in a knee is almost always caused by a pathologic process.

Table 6-3	Usefulness of the Clinical Examination in the Diagnosis of Ligamentous or Meniscal Knee Injury	
Clinical Feature*	**+LR (95% CI)**	**−LR (95% CI)**
Anterior drawer test	3.8 (0.7–22)	0.3 (0.05–1.5)
Lachman's test	**25 (2.7–651)**	**0.1 (0.0–0.4)**
Overall examination for ACL injury	**25 (2.1–306)**	**0.04 (0.01–0.5)**
Overall examination for PCL injury	**21 (2.1–205)**	**0.05 (0.01–0.5)**
McMurray's test	1.3 (0.9–1.7)	0.8 (0.6–1.1)
Joint line tenderness (for meniscal injury)	0.9 (0.8–1.0)	1.1 (1.0–1.3)
Overall examination for meniscal injury	2.7 (1.4–5.1)	0.4 (0.2–0.7)

From Solomon DH, Simel DL, Bates DW, et al. The rational clinical examination: does this patient have a torn meniscus or ligament of the knee? Value of the physical examination. *JAMA*. 2001;286:1610-1620.

*In the studies from which the data were extracted, the clinical examinations were performed by orthopedic surgeons.

ACL, Anterior cruciate ligament; CI, confidence interval; −LR, negative likelihood ratio; +LR, positive likelihood ratio; PCL, posterior cruciate ligament.

Boldface represents findings associated with positive likelihood ratios ≥5 or with negative likelihood ratios ≤0.2. These are said to be moderate- to high-impact items.

KNEE PAIN: HISTORY

> **INSTRUCTIONS TO CANDIDATE: A 62-year-old man complains of "terrible" knee pain. Obtain a detailed history, exploring possible causes.**

DD$_X$: VITAMINS C
- **V**ascular: Vasculitis
- **I**nfectious: Septic arthritis
- **T**raumatic: Hemarthrosis
- **A**utoimmune/allergic: Rheumatoid arthritis, systemic lupus erythematosus, scleroderma, ankylosing spondylitis, reactive arthritis, rheumatic fever, and sarcoidosis
- **M**etabolic: Gout, pseudogout, apatite-related arthropathy
- **I**diopathic/iatrogenic: Osteoarthritis
- **N**eoplastic: Metastasis, primary tumor of bone or cartilage, and paraneoplastic syndrome

History
- Ask the patient the following:
  - **Character:** "What does the pain feel like? Do you have any stiffness?"
  - **Location:** "Where is the pain (in which knee and in what part of the knee)? Do you have pain in any other joints (distal versus proximal, monoarticular versus polyarticular)?"
  - **Onset:** "How did the pain start (sudden versus gradual)? Does it begin in the morning, during the day, or in the evening? Does it take >30 minutes after waking for the joints to 'loosen up' (morning stiffness)?"
  - **Radiation:** "Does the pain move anywhere? Down your leg or up your leg?"
  - **Intensity:** "How severe is the pain on a scale of 1 to 10, with 1 being mild pain and 10 being the worst pain? How does it affect your activities of daily living?"
  - **Duration:** "How long does the pain last (constant versus intermittent, acute versus chronic)?"
  - **Events associated:**
    - "Have you noticed redness, swelling, or deformity?"
    - "Do you have limitation of movement or weakness?"
    - "Have you sustained trauma (recent or past)? Are you taking anticoagulants? Do you have a bleeding disorder (hemarthrosis)?"
    - "Are you having diarrhea or stomatitis?"
    - "Have you noticed skin changes such as rashes, nodules, psoriasis, tophi, or shiny skin?"
    - "Have you had conjunctivitis, oral ulcers, a sexually transmitted disease, or enthesopathy (reactive arthritis)?"
    - "Do you have Raynaud phenomenon?"
    - "Have you had constitutional symptoms (fever, chills, night sweats, weight loss, anorexia, or asthenia)?"
    - "Have your medications changed recently?"
  - **Frequency:** "Has this ever happened to you before? How often does it happen?"
  - **Palliative factors:** "Does anything make the pain better? If so, what?"
    - Activity versus rest (activity exacerbates osteoarthritis, whereas rest worsens inflammatory arthritides)
    - Antiinflammatory medications
  - **Provocative factors:** "Does anything make the pain worse? If so, what?"
    - Activity versus rest
    - Weight bearing (osteoarthritis)
    - Stair climbing (patellofemoral arthritis)
- **PMH/PSH:** Arthritis, inflammatory bowel disease, bleeding diathesis, lung disease, renal disease, psoriasis, sexually transmitted disease, human immunodeficiency

Clinical Feature	+LR (95% CI)	−LR (95% CI)
Age >80	3.5 (1.8–7)	0.86 (0.73–1.0)
Diabetes	2.7 (1–6.9)	0.93 (0.83–1.0)
Rheumatoid arthritis	2.5 (2–3.1)	0.45 (0.32–0.72)
Recent joint surgery	**6.9 (3.8–12)**	0.78 (0.64–0.94)
Hip or knee prosthesis	3.1 (2–4.9)	0.73 (0.57–0.93)
Skin infection	2.8 (1.7–4.5)	0.76 (0.60–0.96)
Skin infection in the presence of prosthesis	**15.0 (8.1–28)**	0.77 (0.64–0.93)
HIV infection	1.7 (1–2.8)	0.47 (0.25–0.9)

Table 6-4 Usefulness of Risk Factors in the Diagnosis of Septic Arthritis in Adults

From Margaretten ME, Kohlwes J, Moore D, et al. Does this adult patient have septic arthritis? *JAMA.* 2007;297:1478-1488.

CI, Confidence interval; HIV, human immunodeficiency virus; −LR, negative likelihood ratio; +LR, positive likelihood ratio.

Boldface represents findings associated with positive likelihood ratios ≥5 or with negative likelihood ratios ≤0.2. These are said to be moderate- to high-impact items.

(HIV) infection, or connective tissue disease; trauma, previous joint surgery, or arthroscopy
- **MEDS:** NSAIDs, ASA, steroids, warfarin, or allopurinol
- **SH:** Smoking, use of EtOH, use of street drugs, intravenous drug use, recent travel, multiple sexual partners, and unprotected sex
- **FH:** Arthritis, connective tissue disease, or inflammatory bowel disease

Evidence (Table 6-4)
- Few investigators have evaluated the use of clinical examination techniques to diagnose septic arthritis. Fever provides less useful information than intuition would suggest (sensitivity 57%; 95% CI 52% to 62%). Joint pain (sensitivity 85%; 95% CI 78% to 90%) and joint swelling (sensitivity 78%; 95% CI 71% to 85%) appear to be more common symptoms.[6]

CARPAL TUNNEL SYNDROME: PHYSICAL EXAMINATION

INSTRUCTIONS TO CANDIDATE: A 33-year-old administrative assistant complains of tingling and pain in her right hand that wakes her up from sleep at night. Perform a focused physical examination.

DD$_X$: VITAMINS C (Carpal Tunnel Syndrome)
- Traumatic: Chronic repetitive use syndrome
- Autoimmune/allergic: Rheumatoid arthritis
- Metabolic: Diabetes mellitus, hypothyroidism, acromegaly, gout, and obesity
- Idiopathic
- Congenital/genetic: Congenitally narrowed carpal tunnel

DD$_X$: Other
- Pregnancy

Patient Positioning
- Expose both arms (for comparison purposes) from elbows to fingertips.

Inspection
- Inspect the dorsal and volar surfaces of the hand for SEADS.
- Note any asymmetry or atrophy of the intrinsic muscles of the hand, including the thenar eminence, hypothenar muscles, and interossei.
  - Thenar atrophy is observed as a concavity of the eminence best noted when inspected tangentially.

Palpation
- While you palpate the hand, be alert for TEST CA, and note any asymmetry.
- Palpate the individual bones of the hands, including the carpals, metacarpals, and phalanges. Palpate the MCP and interphalangeal joints.

Range of Motion
- Begin by inspecting the patient's active ROM in the affected hand, and compare it with that in the contralateral hand.
- Instruct the patient to bend the fingers forward at the knuckles (MCP joints) and then stretch them back (flexion and extension); to make a fist (finger flexion); and to stretch the fingers apart (abduction) and touch them together again (adduction).
- Ask the patient to oppose the thumb and small finger (opposition), point the thumb up as if hitchhiking (extension), and point it across the palm (flexion). Also ask the patient to abduct and adduct the thumb.
- If the active ROM is limited or if asymmetry is present, test the passive ROM by gently guiding the wrist through the same planes of movement.

Grading Power
- The **thumb abduction test** helps the examiner detect weakness of the abductor pollicis brevis muscle, which is innervated solely by the median nerve. Ask the patient to raise his or her thumb perpendicular to the palm against resistance. Weakness is characteristic of median nerve neuropathy or carpal tunnel syndrome.
- Repeat the motions elicited for ROM, using an opposing force. Grade the muscle power according to the Oxford scale.

Special Tests
- Test two-point discrimination and vibration sense (low-frequency tuning fork). Decreased pain sensation in the distribution of the median nerve, specifically along the palmar aspect of the index finger in comparison with the ipsilateral small finger, is suggestive of carpal tunnel syndrome (hypalgesia). By mapping sensation, you may delineate any nerve root involvement.
- Test the brachioradialis (C5 to C6), biceps (C5 to C6), and triceps (C7) reflexes to delineate any nerve root involvement.
- In **Phalen's test** the patient holds both wrists in full flexion with the dorsal surfaces pressed together (the opposite of prayer hands) for approximately 60 seconds. Numbness or paresthesias in the distribution of the median nerve are suggestive of carpal tunnel syndrome.
- To test for **Tinel's sign,** percuss the volar aspect of the wrist over the median nerve. Numbness or paresthesias in the distribution of the median nerve are suggestive of carpal tunnel syndrome.
- For the **flick test,** ask the patient what maneuver he or she performs when experiencing symptoms. If the patient demonstrates a flicking motion of the hands, the flick test is said to be positive.

Evidence
- Table 6-5 lists data on the usefulness of common clinical examination techniques for carpal tunnel syndrome.[7] The flick test may not have the clinical utility suggested by earlier studies; a 2004 study revealed that its sensitivity was only 37%.[8]

Table 6-5	Usefulness of Clinical Examination in the Diagnosis of Carpal Tunnel Syndrome		
Clinical Feature	**+LR (95% CI)**	**−LR (95% CI)**	
Thenar atrophy	1.6 (0.9–2.8)	1.0 (0.9–1.0)	
Thumb abduction test	1.8 (1.4–2.3)	0.5 (0.4–0.7)	
Hypalgesia	3.1 (2.0–5.1)	0.7 (0.5–1.1)	
Two-point discrimination	1.3 (0.6–2.7)	1.0 (0.9–1.1)	
Abnormal vibration sense	1.6 (0.8–3.0)	0.8 (0.4–1.3)	
Phalen's test	1.3 (1.1–1.6)	0.7 (0.6–0.9)	
Tinel's sign	1.4 (1.0–1.9)	0.8 (0.7–1.0)	

Modified from D'Arcy CA, McGee S. The rational clinical examination: does this patient have carpal tunnel syndrome? *JAMA.* 2000;283:3110-3117.
CI, Confidence interval; −LR, negative likelihood ratio; +LR, positive likelihood ratio.

Pearls
- **Carpal tunnel syndrome** is a compression neuropathy whereby the median nerve (C5 to T1) is compressed within the carpal tunnel.
- It is often considered to be an overuse syndrome that results from gross or repetitive microtrauma, such as typing with improper (nonergonomic) wrist position.
- Common systemic causes decrease the volume of the carpal tunnel by increasing the size of the tendons from tissue infiltration or myxomatous enlargement. These causes include pregnancy, diabetes, hypothyroidism, acromegaly, gout, and obesity. Rheumatoid arthritis is a common inflammatory cause of carpal tunnel syndrome.

ANKYLOSING SPONDYLITIS: PHYSICAL EXAMINATION

> **INSTRUCTIONS TO CANDIDATE: A 29-year-old man with a known diagnosis of ankylosing spondylitis presents to your office for a recheck. Perform an appropriate physical examination.**

Inspection
- Inspect the back. Note any spinal deformity such as loss of lumbar lordosis and pronounced thoracic kyphosis. Look at the patient's gait, stance, and posture.
- Inspect for peripheral joint involvement (hips, shoulders, and knees).

Palpation
- **Sacroiliac joint pain** can be reproduced (to confirm the diagnosis of sacroiliitis) by placing the patient in a supine position with the contralateral hip and knee flexed and the ipsilateral hip hyperextended over the edge of the bed. This maneuver reproduces pain in sacroiliitis.
- **Enthesitis** is tenderness over tendinous insertions, found commonly at the chest wall, Achilles tendon, plantar fascia near the heel, tibial tuberosity, patella, and iliac crests.

Tests Requiring Active and Passive Range of Motion
- In ankylosing spondylitis, the spine shows a progressively more limited ROM.
- **FABERE** maneuvers at the hip joint (**f**lexion, **ab**duction, **e**xternal **r**otation, and **e**xtension) stress the sacroiliac joint and elicit pain.
- Lumbar spine: Flexion is the most affected movement, although extension, axial rotation, and lateral bending are also affected.

- **Schober's test** is initiated with the patient in a standing position. Identify the **dimples of Venus** (sacroiliac joints), and use a pen to make a mark on the skin at the midline. Using a measuring tape, make a second mark 10 cm above. Ask the patient to bend forward. Remeasure the distance between the two marks (see Figure 6-6). This distance is normally at least 15 cm. Reduced expansion is suggestive of ankylosing spondylitis.
- Cervical spine: ROM is decreased with lateral flexion, forward flexion, hyperextension, and rotation. Depending on the patient's position of function, a stoop forward may develop. With the patient standing with his or her back against a wall, measure the **occiput-to-wall distance.** The inability to touch the occiput against the wall is abnormal. This finding may be used to monitor disease progression.
- Chest expansion: The chest normally expands 5 cm from expiration to maximal inspiration. This should be measured at the fourth intercostal space in men and immediately below the breasts in women.

Extraarticular Manifestations

- Ocular: The most common extraarticular manifestation of ankylosing spondylitis is acute anterior uveitis or iridocyclitis. It is accompanied by photophobia and increased lacrimation.
- Cardiovascular system: Aortic regurgitation (see pp. 34-36 and checklist on p. 41) is the most common cardiac manifestation. Atrioventricular conduction abnormalities, ascending aortitis, and pericarditis can also occur but may be undetectable clinically.
- Respiratory system: Progressive fibrosis of the upper lobes rarely occurs and is usually a late finding. It usually manifests with cough and, in rare cases, with hemoptysis.

SAMPLE CHECKLISTS

Cervical Spine: Examination

INSTRUCTIONS TO CANDIDATE: Perform an examination of the cervical spine. Describe your actions.

Key Points	Satisfactorily Completed
Introduces self to the patient	❑
Determines how the patient wishes to be addressed	❑
Washes hands	❑
Explains nature of the examination to the patient	❑
Examines the patient in a logical manner	❑
Inspects:	
• Posterior	❑
• Lateral	❑
• Curvature: Note normal lordotic curvature with patient supine or with occiput to wall	❑
Notes any SEADS:	
• **S**welling	❑
• **E**rythema, **e**cchymosis	❑
• **A**trophy	❑
• **D**eformity	❑
• **S**kin changes	❑
Palpates the spine:	
• Patient positioning: sitting	❑
• Cervical spinous processes	❑
• Sternocleidomastoid muscle, trapezius muscles	❑
• Paraspinal muscles	❑
Notes any TEST CA:	
• **T**enderness	❑
• **E**ffusion	❑
• **S**welling	❑
• **T**emperature	❑
• **C**repitus	❑
• **A**trophy	❑
Tests active ROM:	
• Flexion	❑
• Extension	❑
• Rotation	❑
• Lateral flexion	❑
Tests passive ROM:	
• Flexion	❑
• Extension	❑
• Rotation	❑
• Lateral flexion	❑
Tests power:	
• Flexion	❑
• Extension	❑
• Rotation	❑
• Lateral flexion	❑
Measures occiput-to-wall distance	❑
Drapes the patient appropriately	❑
Makes appropriate closing remarks	❑

Lumbar Spine: Examination

INSTRUCTIONS TO CANDIDATE: Perform an examination of the lumbar spine. Describe your actions.

Key Points	Satisfactorily Completed
Introduces self to the patient	❏
Determines how the patient wishes to be addressed	❏
Washes hands	❏
Explains nature of the examination to the patient	❏
Examines the patient in a logical manner	❏
Inspects:	
• Gait	❏
• Normal lordotic curve	❏
• Any kyphosis or scoliosis	❏
Notes any SEADS:	
• **S**welling	❏
• **E**rythema, **e**cchymosis	❏
• **A**trophy	❏
• **D**eformity	❏
• **S**kin changes	❏
Palpates:	
• Patient positioning: sitting or standing	❏
• Lumbar spinous processes	❏
• Paraspinal muscles	❏
Notes any TEST CA:	
• **T**enderness	❏
• **E**ffusion	❏
• **S**welling	❏
• **T**emperature	❏
• **C**repitus	❏
• **A**trophy	❏
Tests ROM:	
• Finger-to-floor distance	❏
• Schober's test	❏
• Extension	❏
• Lateral flexion	❏
• Rotation	❏
Performs special tests:	
• Straight leg raising (sitting and standing)	❏
• Bowstring sign	❏
• Lasègue's sign	❏
Drapes the patient appropriately	❏
Makes appropriate closing remarks	❏

Shoulder: Examination

INSTRUCTIONS TO CANDIDATE: Perform an examination of the right shoulder. Describe your actions.

Key Points	Satisfactorily Completed
Introduces self to the patient	❏
Determines how the patient wishes to be addressed	❏
Washes hands	❏
Explains nature of the examination to the patient	❏
Examines the patient in a logical manner	❏
Inspects:	
• Anterior	❏
• Posterior	❏
• Comparison with contralateral shoulder (asymmetry)	❏
Notes any SEADS:	
• **S**welling	❏
• **E**rythema, **e**cchymosis	❏
• **A**trophy	❏
• **D**eformity	❏
• **S**kin changes	❏
Performs palpation:	
• Sternoclavicular joint	❏
• Acromioclavicular joint	❏
• Coracoclavicular joint	❏
• Greater tuberosity of humerus	❏
• Scapula	❏
• Supraspinatus, infraspinatus, deltoid, and biceps tendons	❏
Notes any TEST CA:	
• **T**enderness	❏
• **E**ffusion	❏
• **S**welling	❏
• **T**emperature	❏
• **C**repitus	❏
• **A**trophy	❏
Tests active ROM:	
• Flexion	❏
• Extension	❏
• Abduction	❏
• Adduction	❏
• Internal rotation	❏
• External rotation	❏
Tests passive ROM:	
• Flexion	❏
• Extension	❏
• Abduction	❏
• Adduction	❏
• Internal rotation	❏
• External rotation	❏

Continued

Key Points	Satisfactorily Completed
Tests power:	
• Flexion	❏
• Extension	❏
• Abduction	❏
• Adduction	❏
• Internal rotation	❏
• External rotation	❏
Performs special tests:	
• Impingement test	❏
• Drop test	❏
Bonus:	
• Recognizes neck as source of referred pain (Spurling's sign, compression test)	❏
Drapes the patient appropriately	❏
Makes appropriate closing remarks	❏

Elbow: Examination

INSTRUCTIONS TO CANDIDATE: Perform an examination of the left elbow. Describe your actions.

Key Points	Satisfactorily Completed
Introduces self to the patient	❏
Determines how the patient wishes to be addressed	❏
Washes hands	❏
Explains nature of the examination to the patient	❏
Examines the patient in a logical manner	❏
Inspects:	
• Carrying angle	❏
• Comparison with contralateral elbow for symmetry	❏
Notes any SEADS:	
• **S**welling	❏
• **E**rythema, **e**cchymosis	❏
• **A**trophy	❏
• **D**eformity	❏
• **S**kin changes	❏
Palpates:	
• Olecranon	❏
• Medial and lateral humeral condyles	❏
• Radial head	❏
• Medial epicondyle	❏
• Lateral epicondyle	❏
• Effusion (anatomic triangle formed by radial head, lateral condyle, and olecranon)	❏
Notes any TEST CA:	
• **T**enderness	❏
• **E**ffusion	❏
• **S**welling	❏
• **T**emperature	❏
• **C**repitus	❏
• **A**trophy	❏

Key Points	Satisfactorily Completed
Tests active ROM:	
• Flexion	❑
• Extension	❑
• Supination	❑
• Pronation	❑
Tests passive ROM:	
• Flexion	❑
• Extension	❑
• Supination	❑
• Pronation	❑
Tests power:	
• Flexion	❑
• Extension	❑
• Supination	❑
• Pronation	❑
Performs special tests:	
• Forced wrist extension (tennis elbow, lateral epicondyle tenderness)	❑
• Forced wrist flexion (golfer's elbow, medial epicondyle tenderness)	❑
Drapes the patient appropriately	❑
Makes appropriate closing remarks	❑

Hand and Wrist: Examination

INSTRUCTIONS TO CANDIDATE: Perform an examination of the right hand and wrist. Describe your actions.

Key Points	Satisfactorily Completed
Introduces self to the patient	❑
Determines how the patient wishes to be addressed	❑
Washes hands	❑
Explains nature of the examination to the patient	❑
Examines the patient in a logical manner	❑
Inspects:	
• Volar aspect	❑
• Dorsal aspect	❑
• Thenar eminence	❑
• Comparison with contralateral wrist and hand for symmetry	❑
Notes any SEADS:	
• **S**welling	❑
• **E**rythema, **e**cchymosis	❑
• **A**trophy	❑
• **D**eformity (e.g., swan neck deformity)	❑
• **S**kin changes	❑
Palpates:	
• Radioulnar groove	❑
• Radiocarpal groove	❑

Continued

Key Points	Satisfactorily Completed
• MCP joints	❏
• PIP joints	❏
• DIP joints	❏
• Interphalangeal joints (thumbs)	❏
Notes any TEST CA:	
• **T**enderness	❏
• **E**ffusion	❏
• **S**welling	❏
• **T**emperature	❏
• **C**repitus	❏
• **A**trophy	❏
Tests active ROM:	
• Flexion and extension of wrist	❏
• Ulnar and radial deviation of wrist	❏
• Flexion and extension of MCP joints	❏
• Flexion and extension of PIP and DIP joints (flexor digitorum superficialis/profundus)	❏
• Abduction and adduction of fingers	❏
• Opposition (finger to thumb)	❏
• Abduction and adduction of thumb	❏
Tests passive ROM:	
• Flexion and extension of wrist	❏
• Ulnar and radial deviation of wrist	❏
• Flexion and extension of MCP joints	❏
• Flexion and extension of PIP and DIP joints (flexor digitorum superficialis/profundus)	❏
• Abduction and adduction of fingers	❏
• Abduction and adduction of thumb	❏
Tests power:	
• Flexion and extension of wrist	❏
• Ulnar and radial deviation of wrist	❏
• Flexion and extension of MCP joints	❏
• Flexion and extension of PIP and DIP joints (flexor digitorum superficialis/profundus)	❏
• Abduction of fingers	❏
• Adduction of fingers (ability to grip piece of paper between fingers against resistance)	❏
• Opposition (finger to thumb)	❏
• Abduction of thumb	❏
• Adduction of thumb (ability to grip piece of paper between thumb and index metacarpal)	❏
Performs special tests:	
• Tinel's sign	❏
• Phalen's test	❏
Drapes the patient appropriately	❏
Makes appropriate closing remarks	❏

Back and Right Leg Pain: History

> **INSTRUCTIONS TO CANDIDATE: A 53-year-old man visits his family doctor complaining of back and right leg pain. Obtain a focused history.**

Key Points	Satisfactorily Completed
Introduces self to the patient	❏
Determines how the patient wishes to be addressed	❏
Washes hands	❏
Establishes the purpose of the encounter	❏
Establishes the presenting concern in the patient's own words	❏
History of back pain:	
• Characterizes the pain	❏
• Establishes the location of pain	❏
• Ascertains whether and to where pain radiates	❏
• Establishes the onset and pattern of the pain	❏
• Asks about history of injury or trauma	❏
• Asks about the patient's activities at time of pain onset	❏
• Establishes the duration of this particular episode of pain	❏
• Asks about the severity of the pain on a scale of 1 to 10	❏
• Asks about previous episodes of similar pain	❏
• Asks about the frequency with which the pain occurs	❏
• Asks about palliative factors (e.g., NSAIDs, rest, position)	❏
• Asks about provocative factors (e.g., movement)	❏
Inquires about associated symptoms:	
• Fever	❏
• Dyspnea	❏
• Diaphoresis	❏
• Nausea or vomiting, or both	❏
• Syncope	❏
• Unexplained weight loss	❏
Asks about relevant social history:	
• Smoking	❏
• Use of EtOH	❏
• Use of intravenous drugs	❏
• Physical activity	❏
Asks about past medical and surgical history:	
• Malignancy	❏
• HIV infection	❏
• Immunocompromise	❏
• Osteoporosis	❏
• Spinal fracture	❏
• Spinal surgery	❏
Asks about medications:	
• Prescription drugs (including steroids, other immunosuppressants)	❏
• Over-the-counter drugs	❏
Asks about allergies	❏
Makes appropriate closing remarks	❏

Radiculopathy: Physical Examination

> **INSTRUCTIONS TO CANDIDATE: Examine a patient with a suspected protrusion of the right L4–L5 or L5–S1 disc, which would be causing root compression.**

Key Points	Satisfactorily Completed
Introduces self to the patient	❏
Determines how the patient wishes to be addressed	❏
Washes hands	❏
Explains nature of the examination to the patient	❏
Examines the patient in a logical manner	❏
Inspects:	
• Gait	❏
• Normal lordotic curvature (loss is a sign of spasm)	❏
• Presence of any kyphosis or scoliosis	❏
• Any fasciculations in the lower limb	❏
Notes any SEADS:	
• **S**welling	❏
• **E**rythema, **e**cchymosis	❏
• **A**trophy (lower limbs, especially right leg)	❏
• **D**eformity	❏
• **S**kin changes	❏
Palpates:	
• Patient positioning: sitting or standing	❏
• Lumbar spinous processes	❏
• Sacroiliac joints	❏
• Paraspinal muscles	❏
Notes any TEST CA:	
• **T**enderness	❏
• **E**ffusion	❏
• **S**welling	❏
• **T**emperature	❏
• **C**repitus	❏
• **A**trophy	❏
Tests ROM:	
• Finger-to-floor distance	❏
• Schober's test	❏
• Extension	❏
• Lateral flexion	❏
• Rotation	❏
Tests power:	
• Plantar flexion (walking on toes): S1	❏
• Dorsiflexion (walking on heels): L4	❏
• Flexion of great toe	❏
• Extension of great toe: L5	❏
• Knee flexion	❏
Tests muscle tone in lower extremities:	
• Notes any clonus	❏
Performs special tests:	
• Straight leg raising	❏
• Bowstring sign	❏
• Lasègue's sign	❏

Key Points	Satisfactorily Completed
Assesses deep tendon reflexes:	
• Knee (comparison with contralateral knee): L4	❏
• Ankle (comparison with contralateral ankle): S1	❏
• Plantar (comparison with contralateral foot)	❏
Assesses sensation:	
• L4 dermatome: medial malleolus	❏
• L5 dermatome: web space between first and second toes	❏
• S1 dermatome: lateral aspect of foot	❏
• Perineum (saddle region)	❏
Performs rectal examination for tone	❏
Drapes the patient appropriately	❏
Makes appropriate closing remarks	❏

Hand (Rheumatoid Arthritis): Physical Examination

INSTRUCTIONS TO CANDIDATE: Perform a focused physical examination of the hand in a patient with a history of rheumatoid arthritis. Describe your actions and expected findings (Figures 6-19 and 6-20).

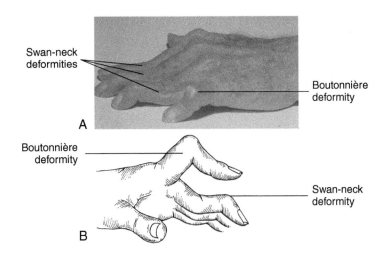

Figure 6-19 Swan-neck and boutonnière deformities in rheumatoid arthritis. (From Wilson SF, Giddens JF. *Health Assessment for Nursing Practice.* 2nd ed. St. Louis: Mosby; 2001 [p. 658, Figure 24-31].)

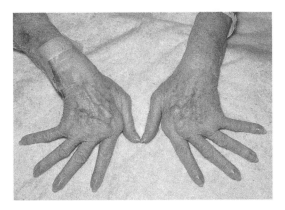

Figure 6-20 Ulnar deviation of the digits in rheumatoid arthritis. (From Swartz M. *Textbook of Physical Diagnosis: History and Examination.* 6th ed. Philadelphia: Elsevier; 2010 [p. 625, Figure 20-57].)

Key Points	Satisfactorily Completed
Introduces self to the patient	❑
Determines how the patient wishes to be addressed	❑
Washes hands	❑
Explains nature of the examination to the patient	❑
Examines the patient in a logical manner	❑
Inspects:	
• Comparison with contralateral hand for symmetry	❑
Notes any SEADS:	
• **S**welling (fusiform)	❑
• **E**rythema, **e**cchymosis	❑
• **A**trophy	❑
• **D**eformity	❑
• **S**kin changes (rheumatoid nodules)	❑
Identifies ulnar drift of digits	❑
Identifies subluxations	❑
Identifies "typical" rheumatoid deformities:	
• Swan-neck deformity	❑
• Boutonnière deformity	❑
Palpates:	
• Nodules	❑
• Tendons	❑
• MCP joints	❑
• PIP joints	❑
• DIP joints	❑
• Interphalangeal joints (thumbs)	❑
Notes any TEST CA:	
• **T**enderness	❑
• **E**ffusion	❑
• **S**welling	❑
• **T**emperature	❑
• **C**repitus	❑
• **A**trophy	❑
Tests active ROM:	
• Flexion and extension of MCP joints	❑
• Flexion and extension of PIP and DIP joints (flexor digitorum superficialis/profundus)	❑
• Abduction and adduction of fingers	❑
• Opposition (finger to thumb)	❑
• Abduction and adduction of thumb	❑
Tests passive ROM:	
• Flexion and extension of MCP joints	❑
• Flexion and extension of PIP and DIP joints	❑
• Abduction and adduction of fingers	❑
• Abduction and adduction of thumb	❑
Tests power:	
• Grip strength	❑
• Flexion and extension of MCP joints	❑
• Flexion and extension of PIP and DIP joints (flexor digitorum superficialis/profundus)	❑
• Abduction and adduction of fingers	❑
• Opposition (finger to thumb)	❑
• Abduction and adduction of thumb	❑
Drapes the patient appropriately	❑
Makes appropriate closing remarks	❑

Knee Injury: Physical Examination

> **INSTRUCTIONS TO CANDIDATE: An 18-year-old basketball player is brought to the emergency department by his friends. He injured his left knee and is unable to walk. Perform a focused physical examination of the knee, and describe your actions.**

Key Points	Satisfactorily Completed
Introduces self to the patient	❏
Determines how the patient wishes to be addressed	❏
Washes hands	❏
Explains nature of the examination to the patient	❏
Examines the patient in a logical manner	❏
Inspects:	
• Comparison with contralateral knee for symmetry	❏
• Patient's position of comfort	❏
Notes any SEADS:	
• **S**welling (suprapatellar convexity versus concavity)	❏
• **E**rythema, **e**cchymosis	❏
• **A**trophy	❏
• **D**eformity (e.g., genu valgum, genu varum)	❏
• **S**kin changes	❏
Palpates:	
• Patella	❏
• Tibial tuberosity	❏
• Tibial condyles	❏
• Femoral epicondyles	❏
• Balloting of the patella	❏
• Presence of bulge sign	❏
Notes any TEST CA:	
• **T**enderness	❏
• **E**ffusion: patellar tap, bulge sign	❏
• **S**welling	❏
• **T**emperature	❏
• **C**repitus: throughout the ROM	❏
• **A**trophy	❏
Tests active ROM:	
• Flexion	❏
• Extension	❏
Tests passive ROM:	
• Flexion	❏
• Extension	❏
Tests power:	
• Flexion	❏
• Extension	❏
Tests stability:	
• Collateral ligament stress test	❏
• Anterior drawer test or Lachman's test	❏
• Posterior drawer test	❏
Performs McMurray's test	❏
Determines Q angle	❏
Drapes the patient appropriately	❏
Makes appropriate closing remarks	❏

Ankle Injury: Physical Examination

> **INSTRUCTIONS TO CANDIDATE:** A 48-year-old woman presents to a walk-in clinic after twisting her right ankle. Perform a focused physical examination of her right ankle and foot, and describe your actions. Evaluate according to the components of the Ottawa Ankle and Foot rules.[9]

Key Points	Satisfactorily Completed
Introduces self to the patient	❏
Determines how the patient wishes to be addressed	❏
Washes hands	❏
Explains nature of the examination to the patient	❏
Examines the patient in a logical manner	❏
Inspects:	
• Inspection while patient bears weight and while patient sits	❏
• Comparison with contralateral ankle and foot for asymmetry	❏
Notes any SEADS:	
• **S**welling	❏
• **E**rythema, **e**cchymosis	❏
• **A**trophy	❏
• **D**eformity (e.g., pes planus, pes cavus)	❏
• **S**kin changes	❏
Palpates:	
• Medial malleolus	❏
• Lateral malleolus	❏
• Talus (anterior)	❏
• Calcaneus	❏
• Achilles tendon	❏
• Navicular bone	❏
• Metatarsals	❏
• MTP joints	❏
• Toes	❏
Notes any TEST CA:	
• **T**enderness	❏
• **E**ffusion	❏
• **S**welling	❏
• **T**emperature	❏
• **C**repitus	❏
• **A**trophy	❏
Tests active ROM:	
• Dorsiflexion	❏
• Plantar flexion	❏
• Inversion	❏
• Eversion	❏
• Flexion of great toe	❏
• Extension of great toe	❏
Tests passive ROM:	
• Dorsiflexion	❏
• Plantar flexion	❏
• Inversion	❏
• Eversion	❏

Key Points	Satisfactorily Completed
• Abduction and adduction of ankle	❏
• Flexion of great toe	❏
• Extension of great toe	❏
Tests stability:	
• Anterior drawer test	❏
• Inversion stress test	❏
• External rotation test	❏
Evaluates according to components of the Ottawa Ankle Rule:	
• Bone tenderness along the distal 6 cm of the posterior edge of the tibia or tip of the medial malleolus	❏
• Bone tenderness along the distal 6 cm of the posterior edge of the fibula or tip of the lateral malleolus	❏
• Inability to bear weight both immediately and in the emergency department for four steps	❏
Evaluates according to components of the Ottawa Foot Rule:	
• Bone tenderness at the base of the fifth metatarsal	❏
• Bone tenderness at the navicular bone	❏
• Inability to bear weight both immediately and in the emergency department for four steps	❏
Drapes the patient appropriately	❏
Makes appropriate closing remarks	❏

REFERENCES

1. May S, Littlewood C, Bishop A. Reliability of procedures used in the physical examination of non-specific low back pain: a systematic review. *Aust J Physiother.* 2006;52(2):91-102.
2. van der Windt DA, Simons E, Riphagen II, et al. Physical examination for lumbar radiculopathy due to disc herniation in patients with low-back pain. *Cochrane Database Syst Rev.* 2010;2:CD007431.
3. Hegedus EJ, Goode A, Campbell S, et al. Physical examination tests of the shoulder: a systematic review with meta-analysis of individual tests. *Br J Sports Med.* 2008;42(2):80-92; discussion, *Br J Sports Med.* 2008;42(2):92.
4. Tiru M, Goh SH, Low BY. Use of percussion as a screening tool in the diagnosis of occult hip fractures. *Singapore Med J.* 2002;43:467-469.
5. Solomon DH, Simel DL, Bates DW, et al. The rational clinical examination: does this patient have a torn meniscus or ligament of the knee? Value of the physical examination. *JAMA.* 2001;286:1610-1620.
6. Margaretten ME, Kohlwes J, Moore D, et al. Does this adult patient have septic arthritis? *JAMA.* 2007;297:1478-1488.
7. D'Arcy CA, McGee S. The rational clinical examination: does this patient have carpal tunnel syndrome? *JAMA.* 2000;283:3110-3117.
8. Hansen PA, Micklesen P, Robinson LR. Clinical utility of the flick maneuver in diagnosing carpal tunnel syndrome. *Am J Phys Med Rehabil.* 2004;83:363-367.
9. Stiell IG, Greenberg GH, McKnight RD, et al. Decision rules for the use of radiography in acute ankle injuries. *JAMA.* 1993;269:1127-1132.

CHAPTER 7

Dermatology

Peter Green, MD, FRCPC

ANATOMY

- The skin functions primarily as a barrier. It protects the internal environment against physical trauma, ultraviolet damage, and potentially infectious agents. Secondary functions include temperature regulation, sensation, vitamin D synthesis, body odor, and aesthetic appearance.
- Skin consists of the following elements (Figure 7-1): epidermis, dermis, appendageal structures, and subcutaneous fat.
  - The epidermis is an avascular structure composed of keratinocytes, cells that are constantly undergoing differentiation and migration to produce a dead layer of cells termed the *stratum corneum.*
  - The dermis is a vascular structure that also contains nerves and cutaneous appendages, such as eccrine and apocrine sweat glands, hair follicles, and sebaceous glands. The dermis is anchored to the epidermis by interlocking rete pegs (epidermal origin) to dermal papillae. The basement membrane zone is the interface between these two structures, and through a series of interactions, it effectively cements the two surfaces together. The dermis houses blood vessels (responsible for the erythema seen in many skin conditions) and nerves that provide sensation of touch, temperature, and pain.

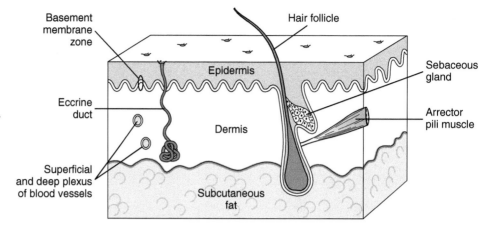

Figure 7-1 Anatomy of the skin.

- The underlying layer of fat provides insulation and functions also to cushion underlying structures (e.g., bone) against blunt trauma.

GLOSSARY OF SIGNS AND SYMPTOMS

Nonpalpable Primary Skin Lesions (Figure 7-2)
- A **macule** is a circumscribed nonpalpable area of skin discoloration with a diameter of ≤0.5 cm.
- A **patch** is a circumscribed nonpalpable area of skin discoloration with a diameter of >0.5 cm.

Palpable Primary Skin Lesions (Figure 7-3)
- A **papule** is a solid elevated lesion with a diameter of ≤0.5 cm.
- A **plaque** is an elevated lesion with a diameter of >0.5 cm but without significant depth.
- A **nodule** is a solid lesion in the skin with a diameter of >0.5 cm with considerable depth as measured by palpation.
- A **wheal** is an elevated white papule or plaque secondary to dermal edema that resolves within hours, leaving no cutaneous abnormality.

Fluid-Filled Primary Skin Lesions (Figure 7-4)
- A **vesicle** is a circumscribed fluid-filled lesion with a diameter of ≤0.5 cm.
- A **bulla** is a circumscribed fluid-filled lesion with a diameter of >0.5 cm.
- A **pustule** is a circumscribed lesion filled with pus.

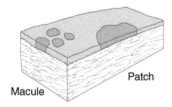

Figure 7-2 Nonpalpable primary skin lesions. (From Swartz M. *Textbook of Physical Diagnosis: History and Examination.* 6th ed. Philadelphia: Elsevier; 2010 [p. 150].

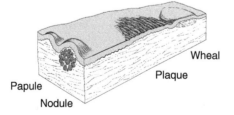

Figure 7-3 Palpable primary skin lesions. (Adapted from Swartz M. *Textbook of Physical Diagnosis: History and Examination.* 6th ed. Philadelphia: Elsevier; 2010 [p. 151].)

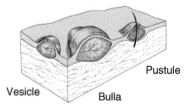

Figure 7-4 Fluid-filled primary skin lesions. (From Swartz M. *Textbook of Physical Diagnosis: History and Examination* 6th ed. Philadelphia: Elsevier; 2010 [p. 151].)

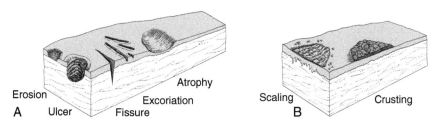

Figure 7-5 Secondary skin lesions below the skin plane **(A)** and above the skin plane **(B)**. **(A,** Adapted from Swartz M. *Textbook of Physical Diagnosis: History and Examination.* 6th ed. Philadelphia: Elsevier; 2010 [Figure 8-21]. **B,** From Swartz M. *Textbook of Physical Diagnosis: History and Examination.* 6th ed. Philadelphia: Elseiver; 2010 [Figure 8-22].)

Secondary Skin Lesions

- An **erosion** represents focal, partial-thickness loss of epidermis (Figure 7-5, *A*).
- An **ulcer** represents focal, complete-thickness loss of epidermis (see Figure 7-5, *A*).
- A **fissure** is a linear crack or cleavage in the skin (see Figure 7-5, *A*).
- An **excoriation** is a superficial loss of epidermis, often linear, created by scratching (see Figure 7-5, *A*).
- **Atrophy** in dermatology is loss of size as a result of thinning of part of the epidermis or dermis (see Figure 7-5, *A*).
- A **scale** is an abnormal accumulation or shedding of flakes of skin (representing stratum corneum) (see Figure 7-5, *B*).
- A **crust** is a dried deposit of serum, blood, or pus on the skin (see Figure 7-5, *B*).
- **Purpura** (a generic term) is any area of extravasation of blood into skin.
- **Petechiae** are palpable or nonpalpable extravasations of blood into skin involving an area of <0.5 cm.
- **Ecchymosis** is extravasation of blood into skin involving an area >2 cm.
- A **scar** is an area of induration or depression in the skin secondary to healing. It may be normal, hypertrophic (raised above the skin), or keloidal (spreading beyond original wound) in nature.

Arrangement

- Groups of lesions can be described according to certain patterns: grouped, linear, serpiginous, arcuate, nummular, annular, and reticular.
- Individual lesions may also be described as nummular or annular, such as a nummular plaque of eczema.

ESSENTIAL SKILLS

APPROACH TO DERMATOLOGIC EXAMINATION

- A complete dermatologic examination includes inspection of the following:
  - All hair-bearing and non–hair-bearing cutaneous surfaces
  - Hair
  - Mucous membranes
  - Nails
- In describing a cutaneous eruption (avoid the term "rash"), you should attempt to identify a primary lesion (e.g., papules in lichen planus, patches in vitiligo).

- Secondary changes may dominate the manifestation of the primary eruption, and a diligent search for primary lesions is key in these circumstances.
- It is helpful to document the color of the lesion, sharpness, surface contour, shape, and texture.
- Arrangement and distribution should be documented when describing a skin eruption.
- As in other areas of clinical examination, when you do not recognize something in the skin, use the **VITAMINS C** approach; it will enable you to expand your list of possibilities in the differential diagnosis and ensure that you do not forget relevant historical questions.
- By using the correct terminology to describe primary skin lesions and secondary changes, you communicate more effectively with colleagues, which ultimately benefits your patients.

ACNE: HISTORY AND FINDINGS

> **INSTRUCTIONS TO CANDIDATE: A 23-year-old woman presents with a history of facial acne unresponsive to over-the-counter (OTC) products. Obtain an appropriate history for facial acne in this setting, and identify the morphologic features of these facial lesions.**

DD$_X$: VITAMINS C
- **Vascular:** Rosacea (Figures 7-6 and 7-7)
- **Infectious:** Bacterial folliculitis
- **Traumatic:** Acne excoriée (Figure 7-8)
- **Metabolic:** Steroid acne (from either oral or topical steroids; Figure 7-9)
- **Idiopathic/iatrogenic:** Perioral dermatitis (iatrogenic steroid use; Figure 7-10)
- **Congenital/genetic:** Adenoma sebaceum in tuberous sclerosis
- **Other:** Acne vulgaris (Figure 7-11)

Assessment
- Consider the following:
  - **Character:** What is the nature of the acneiform eruption? Are primary lesions of acne vulgaris present (i.e., comedones [open and closed], papules, pustules, and nodules)? Is the acne predominantly noninflammatory (comedonal), inflammatory (papules, pustules, nodules), or mixed? (Rosacea and perioral dermatitis lack comedones, which is helpful in differentiating them from acne vulgaris.) Is scarring present (may occur with acne vulgaris), and is it linear or rectangular (in the absence of visible primary acne lesions, is suggestive of acne excoriée, implying excessive external manipulation of minimal acne)? Are lesions the same size and shape (monomorphic, more often seen in perioral dermatitis and steroid acne), or are their structures different? Are associated telangiectasias ("broken blood vessels") present? Is erythema (suggestive of rosacea), which can be fixed or transient, present on the nose and cheeks?
  - **Location:** Where do the lesions predominate: in areas rich in sebaceous glands, such as cheeks, forehead, upper chest, and back? Or is the distribution perioral, sparing cheeks, and forehead (perioral dermatitis)? Are papules and pustules predominantly on nose, cheeks forehead, and chin with significant background erythema and telangiectases (rosacea)? Are there unilateral papules and pustules (suggestive of bacterial folliculitis)?
  - **Onset:** Has the acne progressed gradually, or has the onset been acute over days? Sudden onset is suggestive of bacterial folliculitis.

- Intensity: Must be measured by the physician's assessment and the patient's perception of severity:
    - Are the lesions inflammatory (papules and pustules) versus noninflammatory (comedones)?
    - What is the extent of cutaneous involvement?
    - Is scarring present?
    - Are nodules present?
    - What is the psychologic impact on the patient?
- Duration: How long has the acne been present in its current state?
- Events associated:
    - Polycystic ovarian syndrome (PCOS): Are menses irregular? Is hirsutism, acanthosis nigricans, or insulin resistance present?
    - Rosacea: Does transient erythema (flushing) occur with alcohol, hot beverages, spicy foods, social stressors, or weather?
    - Acne excoriée or acne vulgaris with secondary excoriations: Does the patient manipulate (squeeze, pick, excoriate) the acne?
    - Adenoma sebaceum in tuberous sclerosis: Does the patient have a history of seizures, white patches (ash leaf macules), digital fibromas, tooth pits, or cutaneous collagenomas?
    - Has the patient used a topical moisturizer? Excessive, chronic application contributes to perioral dermatitis.
- Frequency: Is the acne of recent onset or a recurrent issue?
- Palliative factors: What treatments, if any, have worked?
    - Benzoyl peroxide (OTC or prescription), topical antibiotics or retinoids
    - Tetracyclines
    - Isotretinoin
- Provocative factors: Have topical treatments caused excess skin irritation? Has the acne worsened with the menstrual cycle? Does the patient apply excessive makeup to cover the acne? Does the patient manipulate the pimples (squeezing, popping), which may cause more inflammation or scarring? Does the patient believe that stress or diet causes the acne?
- **PMH:** PCOS, irregular menses
- **MEDS (including OTC medications):** Previous use of isotretinoin, recent use of oral steroids, use of oral contraceptive pill, use of antidepressants (may be suggestive of acne excoriée or a relative contraindication for isotretinoin)
- **Social history (SH):** Smoking, use of alcohol (EtOH), occupation, sexual activity (pregnancy is contraindicated during use of isotretinoin or tetracyclines)
- **FH:** Severe or scarring acne, rosacea

ECZEMA: HISTORY AND FINDINGS

INSTRUCTIONS TO CANDIDATE: An 8-year-old boy presents with a flare of his lifelong eczema. Obtain an appropriate history, focusing on factors responsible for this flare. Describe active skin findings and their distribution.

DD$_X$: VITAMINS C
- **Vascular:** Flare with intense heat and humidity, especially summer weather or intense exercise; cutaneous vasodilation exacerbates erythema and pruritus
- **Infectious:** Atopic dermatitis with secondary *Staphylococcus aureus* infection (Figure 7-12, C), eczema herpeticum (widespread herpes simplex 1) (Figure 7-12, B)
- **Autoimmune/allergic:** Atopic dermatitis with episodic flare (Figure 7-12), secondary allergic contact dermatitis to preservative or medicated ingredient in natural remedy
- **Idiopathic/iatrogenic:** Drug reaction

Assessment

- Consider the following:
  - **Character:** Is the dermatitis predominantly dry and scaly with chronically thickened skin? Are the lesions oozing and crusting (suggestive of secondary bacterial infection with *S. aureus*)? Are small, deep, intensely itchy vesicles present within the eczema (vesicular nature is suggestive of more acute flare of chronic atopic dermatitis or allergic contact dermatitis)? Is pruritus a prominent feature? Are painful, umbilicated vesicles present in a generalized or widespread distribution (eczema herpeticum)?
  - **Location:** Is the dermatitis predominantly on flexor surfaces (antecubital and popliteal fossae are the most common areas of eczema)? Are new areas flaring?
  - **Onset:** Has this flare developed quickly or been progressive?
  - **Radiation:** Is the eczema localized, or is there generalized involvement? Has the eczema spread beyond its usual areas of involvement?
  - **Intensity:** To what degree has the eczema affected the child's life? Is the itch bad enough to interfere with normal daily activities or interrupt sleep? Has the itch been severe enough to trigger excoriations or secondary infection?
  - **Duration:** How long has this particular flare lasted?
  - **Events associated:**
    - Has the child had fever or chills (suggestive of serious secondary infection or widespread involvement)?
  - **Frequency:** How often does the eczema flare and under what circumstances?
  - **Palliative factors:** How has the child's eczema been managed? How often are topical moisturizers or medicated ointment applied? (It is important to determine adherence to prescribed therapies.) How much of the medication has been used? (Make sure to look at the jar or tube to see how much is gone.) Does the patient prefer creams (slightly less effective but cosmetically more elegant) or ointments (consistency of petroleum jelly)?
  - **Provocative factors:** Is the child exposed to dust, pets, or wool? Is his skin excessively dry, which leads to further itch? Is he experiencing stress (which may be conducive to flares but is not the primary cause of eczema)? Has he started using any new topical products with potential allergens (fragrance, formaldehyde releasers, lanolin, preservatives)? Does his medicated cream "burn" the skin on contact (usually because of preservatives and not an allergic response but often a reason why patients stop therapy)?
- **PMH:** Hospital admission for eczema or use of oral antibiotics to manage secondary infection; asthma, rhinitis
- **MEDS:** Current prescription for topical therapy, recent oral antibiotics, or corticosteroids
- **Allergies:** Known medication allergies or documented allergies by skin testing; urticarial reactions to foods (egg, milk, peanut)
- **FH:** Atopic dermatitis, asthma

PAPULOSQUAMOUS ERUPTION: HISTORY AND FINDINGS

> **INSTRUCTIONS TO CANDIDATE:** A 23-year-old man presents with acute onset of multiple scaly, droplike plaques on the trunk after a sore throat. Obtain an appropriate history for a patient presenting with a new-onset papulosquamous eruption. Accurately describe the primary skin findings and their distribution.

DD$_X$: VITAMINS C

- **Infectious:** Secondary syphilis (Figure 7-13), tinea corporis, pityriasis versicolor (Figure 7-14), and pityriasis rosea (presumed viral) (Figure 7-15)
- **Autoimmune/allergic:** Guttate psoriasis, (Figure 7-16), allergic contact dermatitis
- **Idiopathic/iatrogenic:** Drug reaction
- **Neoplastic:** Cutaneous T-cell lymphoma (usually large plaques, chronic)

Assessment

- Consider the following:
  - **Character:** Are the plaques beefy red with thicker, adherent silvery scale (psoriatic plaques)? Are the plaques droplike (i.e., 1 to 2 cm, as in guttate psoriasis)? Is the eruption symmetric or asymmetric (tinea corporis)? Are the plaques pink with a collar of fine scale, and is there a larger herald patch that preceded the smaller plaques (pityriasis rosea)? Are copper-colored (yellowish) or "ham"-colored (reddish brown) scaly plaques on the palms or soles? Is lymphadenopathy present? Does the patient have oral ulceration (secondary syphilis)? Are subtle scaly plaques present with associated hypopigmentation (pityriasis versicolor)?
  - **Location:** Is the scalp concurrently involved with erythema and scale, often along the hair line (scalp psoriasis)? Are trunk and proximal extremities involved (guttate psoriasis and pityriasis versicolor)? Are scaly plaques involving the trunk and extremities, as well as the palms and soles, present (secondary syphilis)? Are the upper back and chest predominantly involved (pityriasis versicolor)? Are concurrent nail changes present (plaque psoriasis, tinea corporis)?
  - **Onset:** Was the onset acute (guttate psoriasis, pityriasis rosea, secondary syphilis), or has the condition been chronic (tinea corporis, pityriasis versicolor)?
  - **Radiation:** Is a "Christmas tree" pattern of scaly plaques on the trunk (pityriasis rosea)?
  - **Intensity:** What is the extent of eruption, and what is the intensity of pruritus?
    - Guttate psoriasis: Itch varies
    - Syphilis: Itch is usually minimal
    - Pityriasis rosea: Itch varies, is mild to marked
    - Pityriasis versicolor: Itch is asymptomatic to minimal
  - **Duration:** Has this condition lasted weeks or months? Guttate psoriasis and pityriasis rosea last approximately 6 to 8 weeks, even without treatment. Secondary syphilis lasts approximately 4 to 12 weeks.
  - **Events associated:**
    - Recent "strep throat" (which precedes guttate psoriasis)
    - Viral pharyngitis (which may precede pityriasis rosea)
    - Tinea unguium in toenails or fingernails, as a source of tinea corporis; exposure to an animal with "mangy" fur or potential to transfer fungal infection (e.g., cattle, cat, or dog)
    - Previous genital ulceration; fever, flulike symptoms, myalgia, stiff neck, and lymphadenopathy (secondary syphilis)
  - **Frequency:** Has the patient had a previous similar episode (guttate psoriasis)? Note: Pityriasis rosea rarely recurs.
  - **Palliative factors:** Has the patient tried any treatment to date?
  - **Provocative factors:** Does anything make the condition worse? Exercise or showering often makes any red lesion more pronounced as a result of increased vasodilation, and the lesion thus may be transiently more pruritic.
- **PMH:** Psoriasis (guttate flares may occur in isolation or with associated chronic plaque psoriasis), human immunodeficiency virus (HIV carries increased risk for syphilis)
- **MEDS:** Oral antibiotic for pharyngitis, often falsely implicated as reason for allergic reaction in guttate psoriasis
- **SH:** Risk factors for secondary syphilis such as infection with HIV and high-risk sexual practices (e.g., multiple partners, unprotected sex)

Pearls

- Secondary syphilis is a papulosquamous eruption that can vary considerably in clinical appearance with macules, papules, and plaques. Identification of risk factors; involvement of palms and soles; and the presence of lymphadenopathy, oral ulcers, and systemic symptoms are helpful in establishing the diagnosis.
- Pityriasis lichenoides, small-plaque parapsoriasis, and pityriasis rubra pilaris are more unusual papulosquamous eruptions in the differential diagnosis and are not described here.

ADVANCED SKILLS

HIVES: HISTORY

> **INSTRUCTIONS TO CANDIDATE:** A 34-year-old male nurse presents with a 1-week history of raised, markedly pruritic wheals in the skin (Figure 7-17). This has occurred daily and leaves no residual skin changes. Obtain an appropriate history for a patient presenting with hives.

DD$_X$: VITAMINS C
- **V**ascular: Urticarial vasculitis (hives that last longer than 24 hours and leave purpura)
- **I**nfectious: Erythema multiforme after *Mycoplasma* or herpes simplex infection (edematous target lesions with or without oral or mucosal involvement)
- **T**raumatic: Physical urticaria (pressure, vibration, cold, solar, and aquagenic)
- **A**utoimmune/**a**llergic: Acute urticaria, angioedema (hereditary or acquired), type 1 allergic reaction, and serum sickness or serum sickness–like reaction
- **I**diopathic/**i**atrogenic: Urticarial drug reaction

Assessment
- Consider the following:
  - **Character:** Are the plaques migratory (moving to different parts of skin)? Do they disappear, leaving no residual skin changes? Are they edematous and intensely pruritic? Are they large plaques or smaller papules (urticaria)? Does marked subcutaneous or more extensive swelling involve mucosal surfaces (angioedema)? Is residual purpura present (suggestive of urticarial vasculitis)?
  - **Location:** Are the wheals confined to skin? Is the airway involved (angioedema or type 1 allergic reaction)?
  - **Onset:** Has this problem been acute or chronic (6 weeks for urticaria)?
  - **Radiation:** Are the lesions regional or generalized?
  - **Intensity:** How severe is the itch (urticaria is markedly pruritic)?
  - **Duration:** Do individual lesions last <24 hours (indicative of urticaria or angioedema)? Do they last longer (indicative of urticarial vasculitis)?
  - **Events associated:**
    - Is the patient's throat swelling, or does it feel tight (angioedema, type 1 allergic reaction)?
    - Is there marked swelling, especially of the lips (angioedema)?
    - Does the patient have joint pain (serum sickness or serum sickness–like reaction)?
  - **Frequency:** Has the patient had repeated episodes of angioedema (hereditary or acquired angioedema)? How often do the hives occur?
  - **Palliative factors:** Has the patient tried anything for the hives, such as over-the-counter (OTC) antihistamines?
  - **Provocative factors:** Is the patient aware of physical triggers for the hives (e.g., pressure, vibration, cold, sweating, water)? Any food triggers (e.g., egg, seafood, strawberries)? Any exposure to latex products (possible type 1 latex allergy)? Has the patient had recent infectious symptoms?
- **Past medical history (PMH):** Any previous episodes of anaphylaxis; lupus (urticarial vasculitis); hepatitis; thyroid disease (rarely implicated in urticaria); lymphoma (acquired angioedema)
- **Medication (MEDS):** Any new medications; recent ingestion of nonsteroidal anti-inflammatory drugs (NSAIDs; trigger for urticaria); oral antibiotics (trigger for serum sickness–like reaction); angiotensin-converting enzyme inhibitor (trigger for angioedema); or radiocontrast dye
- **Allergies:** Known medication allergies or allergies documented by prick testing; check whether the patient carries an EpiPen
- **Family history (FH):** Hereditary angioedema (rare)

ERYTHEMA NODOSUM: HISTORY

INSTRUCTIONS TO CANDIDATE: A 35-year-old woman presents with a 1-week history of painful nodules, swelling, and "bruising" localized to the shins with no ulceration (Figure 7-18). Obtain an appropriate history to delineate the underlying cause and possible triggers for this eruption.

DD$_X$: VITAMINS C
- **V**ascular: Vasculitis (e.g., polyarteritis nodosa, thrombophlebitis)
- **I**nfectious: Cellulitis, deep fungal infection, tuberculosis
- **T**rauma
- **I**diopathic/iatrogenic: Idiopathic panniculitis
- **A**utoimmune/allergic: Systemic lupus erythematosus–associated panniculitis
- **M**etabolic: Pancreatic panniculitis
- **N**eoplastic: Lymphoma
- Co**n**genital/genetic: α_1-Antitrypsin deficiency panniculitis

Assessment
- Consider the following:
    - **Character:** Does the patient have discrete nodules that are red and tender? Are they palpable? Is associated bruising present? Is ulceration present? (Erythema nodosum does not ulcerate. Ulceration is more associated with vasculitis.) Is significant diffuse or circumferential unilateral erythema present (cellulitis)? Is a localized painful nodule with adjacent venous varicosities present (superficial thrombophlebitis)? Is surrounding purpura (palpable or nonpalpable) or livedo reticularis (netlike bluish discoloration) present (suggestive of vasculitis?)
    - **Location:** Are the nodules on the shins only? Are extensor surfaces of upper extremities involved (sometimes with erythema nodosum)?
    - **Onset:** Are the nodules of recent onset?
    - **Radiation:** Are both legs involved symmetrically, or are the nodules unilateral (less likely erythema nodosum, may be cellulitis)?
    - **Intensity:** How painful are the nodules? Do they interfere with walking?
    - **Duration:** How long have the nodules been present?
    - **Events associated:**
        - Did the patient have a sore throat before the nodules appeared? (Streptococcal pharyngitis may be a trigger for erythema nodosum.)
        - Does the patient have arthralgias? (These may accompany erythema nodosum.)
        - Does the patient feel systemically unwell? (This may be indicative of cellulitis, lymphoma, pancreatic disease, lupus, or vasculitis.)
        - Does the patient have a history of pulmonary symptoms of sarcoidosis? (Erythema nodosum associated with mild pulmonary sarcoid is Löfgren syndrome, which is most often asymptomatic.)
        - Has the patient traveled to areas with endemic tuberculosis, histoplasmosis, or coccidioidomycosis? (These are infectious triggers for erythema nodosum.)
        - Has the patient had fever or chills? (These may be indicative of infectious causes; low-grade fever may be seen with erythema nodosum.)
    - **Frequency:** Has the patient had previous similar episodes? (Erythema nodosum may be recurrent.)
    - **Palliative factors:** Does elevating the legs reduce discomfort (erythema nodosum)?
    - **Provocative factors:** Does anything make the discomfort worse? If so, what?
- **PMH:** Inflammatory bowel disease (IBD; associated with erythema nodosum), sarcoidosis, systemic lupus erythematosus (lupus panniculitis), pancreatic disease (pancreatic panniculitis), and pregnancy (trigger for erythema nodosum)
- **MEDS:** Recent ingestion of oral contraceptive pill or sulfa drug (trigger for erythema nodosum)

Pearls
- Erythema nodosum is the most common cause of panniculitis (inflammation of subcutaneous fat). Nodules in erythema nodosum last approximately 2 to 4 weeks; postinflammatory change lasts longer. If only bruising is present at the site of previous nodules, it may represent resolving erythema nodosum.
- A deep elliptical biopsy may be necessary to determine the exact cause.

LEG BLISTERS: HISTORY AND FINDINGS

> **INSTRUCTIONS TO CANDIDATE: A 28-year-old man presents with extensive linear blisters on the lower extremities that are weeping and crusting. He returned from a camping trip approximately 5 days ago. Obtain a focused history for this blistering eruption and, using accurate terminology, describe the skin findings.**

DD$_X$: VITAMINS C
- **V**ascular: Vasculitis (extensive accompanying purpura would be visible)
- **I**nfectious: Bacterial infection (bullous erysipelas or cellulitis), viral infection (herpes simplex, herpes zoster; Figures 7-19 and 7-20)
- **T**raumatic: Burn
- **A**utoimmune/allergic: Autoimmune blistering disorders (bullous pemphigoid, pemphigus vulgaris; Figure 7-21), bullous arthropod bites, acute allergic contact dermatitis (poison ivy, oak, or sumac; Figure 7-22)

Assessment
- Consider the following:
  - **C**haracter: Are the primary lesions vesicles (<0.5 to 1.0 cm) or bullae (>0.5 to 1.0 cm)? Are they grouped into small, grapelike clusters (herpes simplex) or along a dermatome (herpes zoster)? Are they arranged in a linear manner (allergic contact dermatitis)? Do the blisters rupture easily (pemphigus), or are they more tense (bullous pemphigoid)?
  - **L**ocation: Are the blisters more generalized (pemphigus, bullous pemphigoid) or localized? Are they unilateral? (Bilateral distribution would preclude cellulitis.) Do they involve the lip, lumbar spine, or other isolated area of skin (herpes simplex)? Are they limited to the lower extremity (allergic contact dermatitis to poison ivy, bullous erysipelas, cellulitis)?
  - **O**nset: Was the onset gradual or acute?
  - **R**adiation: Are the blisters linear or dermatomal?
  - **I**ntensity: What is the extent of cutaneous surface involved? (More extensive blisters are not likely to be herpes simplex [exception: eczema herpeticum; i.e., generalized herpes simplex infection].)
  - **D**uration: Do blisters rupture quickly (located more superficially) or remain tense (located deeper)?
  - **E**vents associated:
    - Are blisters present on the mucosal membranes (pemphigus, rarely bullous pemphigoid)?
    - Is associated itch present (allergic contact dermatitis, early phase of bullous pemphigoid)?
    - Has the patient had fever, chills, nausea, vomiting, and painful limb (bullous erysipelas, cellulitis, secondary bacterial infection of primary blistering process)?
    - Did the patient have preceding pain or burning sensation (herpes zoster)?
  - **F**requency: Has localized blistering recurred in the same area (herpes simplex)?
  - **P**alliative factors: Has topical therapy or systemic antihistamines resulted in any improvement in symptoms?
  - **P**rovocative factors: Has the patient been exposed recently to shrubbery or wooded areas (poison ivy, oak, or sumac)? Any new recent contacts (e.g., topical

moisturizer, itch creams with "-caine" suffix, or topical antibiotics as cause for allergic contact dermatitis)? Recent burn or trauma?

Physical Examination

- **Vital signs (Vitals):** Evaluate heart rate (HR), blood pressure (BP), and temperature. Fever is associated with bacterial infection but not with primary blistering disorders unless significant secondary infection is present.
- **General:** Evaluate patient's appearance. The patient may look well but is uncomfortable because of itch, or the patient may look unwell because of extensive blistering or infection.
- **Skin:** Examine all hair-bearing and non–hair-bearing cutaneous surfaces, hair, mucous membranes, and nails.

Pearls

- In a healthy individual, localized linear, unilateral bullae or vesicles on the lower extremity are probably caused by allergic contact dermatitis (e.g., poison ivy, oak, or sumac).
- On the lower extremity, a pattern of circumferential or extensive painful erythema with associated bullae and systemic symptoms is compatible with bullous erysipelas (sharply circumscribed erythema) or cellulitis (poorly circumscribed erythema).
- Herpes zoster is unusual on a lower extremity.
- Autoimmune blistering disorders such as pemphigoid or pemphigus are rare in young people and would not be localized exclusively to the lower extremity. They are mentioned here for the differential diagnosis of blistering diseases in general.

ANKLE ULCER: HISTORY AND FINDINGS

INSTRUCTIONS TO CANDIDATE: A 62-year-old man presents with a persistent ankle ulcer. Elicit historical risk factors for leg ulceration, and describe the relevant clinical features of this lesion.

DD$_X$: VITAMINS C

- **V**ascular: Venous stasis ulcer (Figure 7-23), arterial ulcer, and vasculitis
- **I**nfectious: Cellulitis
- **T**raumatic: Traumatic ulcer
- **A**utoimmune/**a**llergic: Vasculitis related to connective tissue disease
- **M**etabolic: Diabetic ulceration (Figure 7-24), necrobiosis lipoidica
- **I**diopathic/**i**atrogenic: Pressure ulcer, pyoderma gangrenosum
- **N**eoplastic: Squamous cell carcinoma, basal cell carcinoma, and lymphoma
- **S**ubstance abuse and psychiatric: Artifactual ulcers (often linear or bizarre geographic shapes)

Assessment

- Consider the following:
  - **Character:** Does the ulcer have ill-defined, shaggy borders, or does it appear punched out with well-defined borders? Is associated edema present or not (arterial ulcers)? Are there associated areas of venous stasis (hyperpigmentation, fibrosis, dermatitis, venous varicosities [venous stasis ulcer])? Is the ulcer markedly painful? Is dependent rubor present? Is the ulcer surrounded by callus and painless (diabetic ulcer)?
  - **Location:** Is the ulcer on the medial malleolus or calf (stasis ulcer), or is it on the distal extremity (i.e., toes or foot: arterial ulcer)? Is it on pressure points (i.e., ball of foot, heel, or toe: diabetic ulcer)?
  - **Onset:** How did it start (sudden versus gradual)?

- **Radiation:** Does the patient have isolated or multiple ulcers? What is the extent of venous stasis changes?
- **Intensity:** How large are the ulcers? How severe are the associated symptoms?
- **Duration:** How long has this been going on (long-standing versus recent ulceration)?
- **Events associated:**
  - A history of chronic edema or venous varicosities
  - Any recent signs of infection or symptoms of associated cellulitis
  - Recent injury
  - History of peripheral vascular disease with claudication
  - Diabetic neuropathy
- **Frequency:** Has the patient had any previous leg ulcers?
- **Palliative factors:** Does dependent position (e.g., hanging leg over bed) make the ulcer *less* painful (arterial ulcer) or *more* painful (venous ulcer)?
- **Provocative factors:** Could the ulcer have been induced by pressure, trauma, local infection, or edema?
- **PMH:** Diabetes, associated neuropathy, peripheral vascular disease, chronic lymphedema
- **MEDS:** Recent antibiotics to manage infection
- **SH:** Smoking, use of EtOH, and use of street drugs

Pearls
- Ill-defined ulcers on one or both ankles with shaggy borders, against a background of pitting edema, erythema, and hyperpigmentation with preserved peripheral pulses, represent venous stasis ulceration.
- Punched-out ulcers on one or more distal extremities (e.g., toe, lateral surface of fifth metatarsal) with no edema, reduced or absent peripheral pulses, and dependent rubor with risk factors for peripheral vascular disease are arterial ulcers.
- A painless or calloused ulcer or hematoma on a weight-bearing surface (e.g., plantar toe surfaces, metatarsal heads, heels) in a diabetic patient with known neuropathy is a diabetic or neuropathic ulcer.
- Unilateral ill-defined painful erythema with fever, chills, or malaise is suggestive of concurrent cellulitis.
- Note that some patients may have combined risk factors for ulceration (e.g., arterial and venous disease).

DRUG RASH: HISTORY AND FINDINGS

> **INSTRUCTIONS TO CANDIDATE: A 65-year-old woman presents with a widespread eruption of 3 days' duration. For a recent illness of the upper respiratory tract, she was prescribed an oral aminopenicillin antibiotic, which she stopped taking 1 week ago. Obtain an appropriate history to delineate the underlying cause of this eruption, and describe the eruption.**

DD$_X$: VITAMINS C
- **Infectious:** Viral eruption, toxin-mediated exanthem (e.g., scarlet fever, staphylococcal scalded skin syndrome [SSSS], toxic shock syndrome)
- **Autoimmune/allergic:** Allergic contact dermatitis, spectrum of Stevens-Johnson syndrome to toxic epidermal necrolysis
- **Idiopathic/iatrogenic:** Drug eruption (Figure 7-25)
- **Note:** The words *exanthem* and *eruption* may be used interchangeably.

Assessment
- Consider the following:
    - **Character:** Does the patient have urticarial (edematous or raised) erythema? Does this eruption partially or completely blanch with pressure? (Early drug eruptions usually blanch completely with pressure; contact dermatitis does not.) Is it macular and confluent (drug exanthem)? Does it have a palpable or "sandpaper" quality (scarlet fever)? Is the skin blistering or peeling (spectrum of Stevens-Johnson syndrome to toxic epidermal necrolysis, SSSS)? Does the eruption have an eczema-like quality with scale and vesicles (allergic contact dermatitis)? Are target lesions present (i.e., central dusky necrosis with surrounding erythema and edema [spectrum of Stevens-Johnson syndrome to toxic epidermal necrolysis])?
    - **Location:** Is the eruption generalized (all skin affected) or only on truncal areas and extremities? (Isolated regional involvement—e.g., extremities only—is unlikely to be a drug eruption.) Is any mucosal membrane involved (ulceration, blistering, and crusting of Stevens-Johnson syndrome or toxic epidermal necrolysis)? Is there peeling of palms and soles (which follows scarlet fever and toxic shock syndrome; drug and viral eruptions often spare palms)?
    - **Onset:** Was the onset sudden? Did it occur *before* or *after* the patient took new medications or had infectious symptoms?
    - **Radiation:** Is the involvement symmetric and bilateral with confluence of erythema over large areas (but most often truncal areas and proximal extremities), and did it later spread to distal extremities (drug or viral exanthem)? Was involvement predominantly in folds (neck, axilla, groin) with erythema and peeling seen in SSSS? Was regional involvement asymmetric (e.g., neck, chest, or face) with eczema-like eruption (allergic contact dermatitis)?
    - **Intensity:** Is the eruption *itchy* (drug, viral, allergic contact dermatitis) or *painful* (Stevens-Johnson syndrome, SSSS)?
    - **Duration:** How long have the current skin findings been present?
    - **Events associated:**
        - Has the patient had any upper respiratory tract or gastrointestinal symptoms? Did she take any new medications for either of these?
        - Does the patient feel systemically unwell (spectrum of Stevens-Johnson syndrome to toxic epidermal necrolysis; toxin-mediated illness)?
        - Has the patient had fever, hemodynamic instability, and visceral involvement (toxic shock syndrome)?
        - Has the patient had recent pharyngitis, systemic symptoms, and strawberry tongue (scarlet fever)?
    - **Frequency:** Has the patient had any previous reactions to drugs?
    - **Palliative factors:** Has the patient used any OTC or prescription topical therapy? (Some may cause allergic contact dermatitis.)
    - **Provocative factors:** After firm stroking of affected skin, does blistering spread (positive Nikolsky's sign, as seen in SSSS and in the spectrum of Stevens-Johnson syndrome to toxic epidermal necrolysis)?
- **PMH:** Previous drug hypersensitivity or medication-induced life-threatening skin eruptions
- **MEDS** (including OTC medications): Detailed account of all medications

Pearls
- Onset of drug eruption with medication is delayed and may occur from 1 to 2 weeks after primary exposure; patients may neglect to mention ingestion of medication that they are no longer taking, erroneously assuming that it could not be causing the eruption.
- A drug eruption evolves and spreads during 2 weeks, regardless of intervention (including discontinuation of implicated medication), and patients must be reassured

that the eruption is not "getting worse." However, new development of blisters may indicate development of a more serious drug reaction (i.e., Stevens-Johnson syndrome).
- In the absence of a history implicating a specific medication, drug eruptions and viral eruptions are often clinical and histologically indistinguishable.

NONMELANOMA SKIN MALIGNANCY: HISTORY AND FINDINGS

> **INSTRUCTIONS TO CANDIDATE: A 65-year-old man presents with a bump on his face of 6 months' duration that bleeds when he shaves. Obtain an appropriate history for a suspected sun-exposed skin malignancy, and accurately describe the lesion.**

DD$_X$: VITAMINS C
- **Vascular:** Rosacea, benign hemangioma
- **Infectious:** Folliculitis
- **Traumatic:** Excoriated nevus (mimics malignancy)
- **Neoplastic:** Basal cell carcinoma (BCC; Figure 7-26), squamous cell carcinoma (SCC), or other tumor (e.g., keratoacanthoma, atypical fibroxanthoma)
- **Congenital/genetic:** Nevus
- Seborrheic keratosis (Figure 7-27)
- Actinic keratosis
- Irritated nevus
- Sebaceous gland hyperplasia (Figure 7-28)

History
- Consider the following:
  - **Character:** Is the lesion a papule, ulcer (BCC, SCC), or scaly plaque (actinic keratosis, seborrheic keratosis)? Does it have a shiny, pearly quality with associated telangiectasia (BCC)? Does the lesion bleed easily (BCC, SCC)? Does the lesion have a warty, brown, stuck-on appearance (seborrheic keratosis)? Is the lesion flat, rough, and scaly with ill-defined borders (actinic keratosis)? Is a flesh-colored papule present with associated inflammation of surrounding skin (suggestive of irritated nevus)? Are multiple soft, yellow, umbilicated (indented) papules present (sebaceous hyperplasia)?
  - **Location:** Has any part of the skin been exposed extensively to the sun?
  - **Onset:** How did the lesion appear when the patient first noticed it?
  - **Radiation:** What is the size of the lesion? Are multiple lesions present (more suggestive of a benign process: seborrheic keratosis, sebaceous hyperplasia, and actinic keratosis)?
  - **Intensity:** Is the lesion painful (which may not help differentiate cause)?
  - **Duration:** Is the lesion new (i.e., weeks to months; more likely to represent BCC, SCC) or long-standing (i.e., years; more likely to represent noncancerous cause such as seborrheic keratosis, irritated nevus, sebaceous hyperplasia)? New-onset lesions are more likely to be cancerous.
  - **Events associated:**
    - Does the patient have a tendency to sunburn easily?
    - Does the patient have a history of significant sun exposure or blistering sunburns?
  - **Frequency:** Has the patient previously had any similar problem? If so, what type of surgical excision was used to manage it?
  - **Palliative factors:** Has the patient attempted any treatment for it to date (e.g., antibiotics, liquid nitrogen, excision)?
  - **Provocative factors:** Does trauma induce bleeding (suggestive of BCC and SCC but may also occur with other causes)?
- **PMH:** Previous skin malignancy, immunosuppression (SCC more common than BCC in this setting; also, multiple actinic keratosis may be present)
- **MEDS:** Acetylsalicylic acid (ASA; may enhance bleeding tendency), immunosuppressants

Pearl

- Although actinic keratoses are considered precancerous, they may be present for years and not develop into cancer.

MELANOMA: HISTORY AND FINDINGS

> **INSTRUCTIONS TO CANDIDATE: A 63-year-old man presents with a changing pigmented lesion on his back. Obtain an appropriate history, and describe the lesion, using accurate terminology.**

DD$_X$: VITAMINS C

- **V**ascular: Pyogenic granuloma, thrombosed or irritated hemangioma
- **N**eoplastic: Malignant melanoma (Figure 7-29), pigmented BCC, dysplastic nevus (Figure 7-30), seborrheic keratosis (Figure 7-31)
- **C**ongenital/genetic: Irritated congenital or compound nevus

Assessment

- Consider the following:
  - **Ch**aracter: Is the lesion pigmented? What is the predominant color (black, brown, pink, gray), or are there multiple colors? Is the lesion asymmetric? Does it have an irregular border? Is the lesion >0.5 cm in diameter? Is it ulcerated? Are other pigmented lesions present, and if so, do they look irregular or dysplastic?
  - **L**ocation: Is the lesion on an area of skin that has been exposed to the sun or not? What are the locations of other pigmented lesions, including the scalp, palms, soles, nails, and mucosal surfaces?
  - **O**nset: Is the lesion of new onset? Has it changed recently in size, shape, or color?
  - **R**adiation: How big is the lesion (broadest diameter in millimeters)?
  - **I**ntensity: Is any pain or itch associated with the lesion?
  - **D**uration: How long has the lesion been present? If there has been change in the lesion, how long has the original lesion been present?
  - **E**vents associated:
    - Has there been any bleeding of the lesion?
    - Has there been any ulceration?
    - Is there any lymph node involvement or other related symptoms (metastases)?
    - Are multiple nevi, typical or atypical, present (increased risk of melanoma)?
    - Does the patient have a history of excess sun exposure or blistering sunburns?
    - Does the patient have a history of tanning bed use?
    - Does the patient sunburn easily? Is his hair blond or red?
  - **F**requency: Has the patient had any other lesions like this? If so, when? How many?
- **PMH**: Previous skin biopsies for pigmented lesions, previous malignancy, or immunosuppression
- **FH**: Multiple atypical nevi, melanoma

Evidence

- In evaluations of a lesion to determine whether it is benign or a melanoma, the most widely used tool in North America remains the ABCD checklist: **a**symmetry (A), uneven **b**order (B), variegation in **c**olor (C) (i.e., more than one shade of pigment present), and >6-mm **d**iameter (D). The sensitivity for diagnosing melanoma is 92% if a positive test result means only one criterion is noted.[1] As the number of criteria present increases, the sensitivity decreases and the specificity increases, so that a lesion with all four criteria has a 54% sensitivity and 94% specificity.[2] Limitations of this approach include the potential to miss early, small melanomas; no accounting for ulceration; inapplicability to nodular melanoma or amelanotic melanoma; and the potential for benign lesions that fit these criteria to be counted. It is also proposed that "E" be added to ABCD to denote "evolution," which would indicate change in a lesion over time in size, shape, symptoms (itch, tenderness), or color. A nodular melanoma would be better detected with this criterion, inasmuch as lesion change is noted in 78% of nodular melanomas. Thomas and colleagues[3] found evolution to be the most specific of the five criteria (90%); the others have fewer specificities: 72% for asymmetry, 71% for border, 59% for color variegation, and 63% for diameter.

Pearl
- Patients with an abnormal or changing mole must undergo a complete examination of their skin, including palms, soles, scalp, genital skin, and mucosal surfaces. A patient's modesty must be respected; however, failure to perform a complete examination may result in overlooking lesions, with significant adverse consequences for the patient. The lymph nodes, liver, and spleen should also be examined in patients with suspected melanoma.

SAMPLE CHECKLISTS

Psoriasis: Physical Examination and Findings

> **INSTRUCTIONS TO CANDIDATE: A 25-year-old man with psoriasis is referred to your clinic for follow-up evaluation (Figure 7-32). Perform a focused physical examination, and describe your findings.**

Key Points	Satisfactorily Completed
Introduces self to the patient	❏
Determines how the patient wishes to be addressed	❏
Washes hands	❏
Explains nature of the examination to the patient	❏
Drapes the patient properly during the examination, and ensures the patient's comfort	❏
Examines the patient in a logical manner	❏
Inspection:	
• Examines the entire skin surface, including palms and soles, scalp, anogenital area, and nails	❏
• Notes any excoriations	❏
• Examines nails for pitting, onycholysis, and the oil drop sign (yellow to red discoloration of nail bed, a sign specific for psoriasis)	❏
• Examines scalp for lesions that predominate along hair line with silvery scales	❏
• Looks for Köebner's phenomenon (inspection only: linear or traumatized areas involved)	❏
• Looks for sausage digits (diffuse swelling of digit that is associated with seronegative arthropathies such as psoriatic arthritis)	❏
Palpation:	
• Looks for raised plaques versus erythema only (treated psoriasis)	❏
• Looks for Auspitz's sign (pinpoint bleeding that occurs on a psoriatic plaque with physical removal of scale; however, should be described only and not tested)	❏
• Examines large joints (hips, lumbosacral area) for range of motion (ROM), tenderness	❏
• Examines large tendinous insertions for swelling and tenderness	❏
• Examines hands for ROM, swelling, and tenderness (sausage digits)	❏
Description of findings:	
• Describes location and amount of skin involvement	❏
• Notes involvement predominantly of extensor surfaces and scalp (guttate psoriasis involves the trunk and proximal extremities)	❏
• Notes salmon-pink or beefy red plaques with overlying silvery scales	❏
• Notes plaques that are well demarcated from surrounding normal skin	❏
• Notes presence of widespread pustules or erythroderma (both medical emergencies)	❏
• Describes scalp and nail findings	❏
• Notes associated arthritic features	❏
Makes appropriate closing remarks	❏

Erythema Nodosum: Physical Examination and Findings

> **INSTRUCTIONS TO CANDIDATE:** A 35-year-old woman presents with a 1-week history of painful nodules, swelling, and "bruising" localized to the shins with no ulceration. Perform a focused physical examination, and describe your findings.

Key Points	Satisfactorily Completed
Introduces self to the patient	❏
Determines how the patient wishes to be addressed	❏
Washes hands	❏
Explains nature of the examination to the patient	❏
Drapes the patient properly during the examination, and ensures the patient's comfort	❏
Examines the patient in a logical manner	❏
Inspection:	
• Examines the entire skin surface, including palms and soles, scalp, anogenital area, and nails	❏
• Identifies typical distribution of findings on shins	❏
• Notes absence of ulceration	❏
• Notes absence of vasculitis findings such as extensive petechiae or purpura	❏
• Notes "bruiselike" changes	❏
• Inspects oropharynx for evidence of active or recent infection	❏
Palpation:	
• Palpates tender, deep, firm nodules over extensor aspect of lower extremities	❏
• Notes localized edema	❏
• Notes normal pulses in distal extremity	❏
• Comments on absence of visible or palpable thrombophlebitis	❏
Description of findings:	
• Describes bilateral location and extent of involvement	❏
• Notes distribution predominantly on lower extremity and extensor aspect	❏
• Comments on lack of ulceration, livedo reticularis, or purpura that would help rule out vasculitis	❏
• Notes lack of involvement in other areas (erythema nodosum is rarely seen anywhere but shins)	❏
• Considers further examination for extraintestinal manifestations of IBD and extrapulmonary manifestations of sarcoidosis	❏
Makes appropriate closing remarks	❏

Melanoma: History, Physical Examination, and Findings

INSTRUCTIONS TO CANDIDATE: A 63-year-old man presents with a changing pigmented lesion on his back (see Figure 7-27). He estimates its duration to be 1 year or more, and his wife had noticed that it was getting larger and darker. Obtain a brief history, and perform a focused physical examination. Describe your findings.

Key Points	Satisfactorily Completed
Introduces self to the patient	❏
Determines how the patient wishes to be addressed	❏
Washes hands	❏
Explains nature of the encounter to the patient	❏
Key historical features:	
• Asks about recent changes in the mole (size, shape, color, bleeding)	❏
• Ascertains history of previous sunburns, especially blistering burns	❏
• Inquires about use of tanning beds	❏
• Asks about family history of melanoma or atypical nevi	❏
• Asks about previous mole excision or personal history of skin cancers	❏
Drapes the patient properly during the examination, and ensures the patient's comfort	❏
Examines the patient in a logical manner	❏
Inspection:	
• Examines the entire skin surface, including palms and soles, scalp, anogenital area (appropriate to inquire about noted change and to defer the anogenital examination), and nails	❏
• Identifies the abnormal or atypical pigmented lesion among other normal moles	❏
• Notes skin type (e.g., fair skin)	❏
• Notes associated sun damage, including multiple lentigines (sun spots) and wrinkles	❏
• Scalp: notes hair color (particularly blond or red)	❏
• Notes absence of pigment in nails	❏
• Notes number and type of moles (e.g., congenital, compound, atypical, or dysplastic)	❏
Palpation:	
• Palpates lesion to determine whether it is elevated	❏
• Palpates surface of lesion, noting irregularities or ulcerations	❏
Description of findings:	
• Describes location of mole or moles	❏
• Comments on the ABCDE features of the lesion that elevate concern:	❏
• **A**symmetry	❏
• **B**order: irregularity	❏
• **C**olor: variegated color (mix of gray, dark black or brown, pink, and tan)	❏
• **D**iameter: size greater than a pencil eraser (≈0.6 cm)	❏
• **E**levation or enlargement	❏
• Identifies the abnormal or atypical pigmented lesion among other normal moles	❏
Makes appropriate closing remarks	❏

REFERENCES

1. Whited JD, Grichnik JM. The rational clinical examination: does this patient have a mole or a melanoma? *JAMA*. 279:696-701.
2. Abbasi NR, Shaw HM, Rigel DS, et al. Early diagnosis of cutaneous melanoma: revisiting the ABCD criteria. *JAMA*. 2004;292:2771-2776.
3. Thomas L, Tranchand P, Berard F, et al. Semiological value of ABCDE criteria in the diagnosis of cutaneous pigmented tumors. *Dermatology*. 1998;197:11-17.

Hematology

ANATOMY

- Active marrow in normal adults is confined to ends of long bones, pelvis, ribs, and vertebral bodies. In some situations, other regions of bone marrow are recruited.
- Lymph nodes are oval or bean-shaped, vary in size, and may not be palpable (Figure 8-1). Inguinal lymph nodes are relatively large (often 1 to 2 cm in area in an adult). The central nervous system contains no lymphatic nodes.
- Axillary lymph (central, humeral, pectoral, infraclavicular, subscapular) nodes drain most of the arm and breast (Figure 8-2). The ulnar surface of the forearm and hand drain first to the epitrochlear nodes, which are proximal to the medical epicondyle.
- Only the superficial system of lymphatic nodes is palpable in the lower limb (Figure 8-3). The superficial inguinal nodes constitute two groups: horizontal and vertical (see Figure 8-1). The horizontal group lies below the inguinal ligament and drains the superficial portions of the lower abdomen and buttock, external genitalia (not the testes), anal area, and lower third of the vagina. The vertical group clusters near the great saphenous vein and drains the portion of the leg drained by the small saphenous vein.

Pearls
- Whenever a node is enlarged or tender, look for a source such as infection in the area that it drains.
- Whenever a malignant or inflammatory lesion is observed, look for involvement of the regional lymph nodes to which it drains.

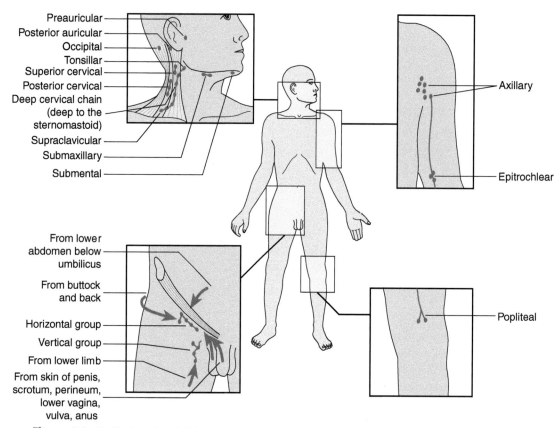

Figure 8-1 Distribution of palpable lymph nodes. (From Munro JF, Campbell IW, eds. *Macleod's Clinical Examination.* 10th ed. Edinburgh: Churchill Livingstone; 2000 [p. 59, Figure 2.42].)

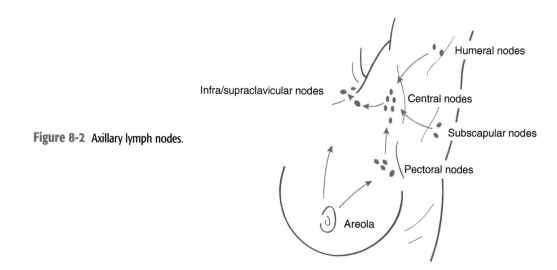

Figure 8-2 Axillary lymph nodes.

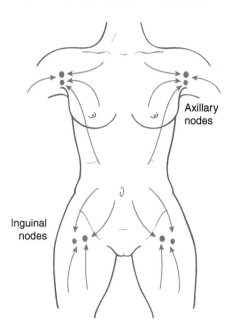

Figure 8-3 Superficial routes of lymphatic drainage. (Courtesy Dr. Tom Scott, Memorial University of Newfoundland, St. John's, Newfoundland.)

Axillary nodes

Inguinal nodes

GLOSSARY OF SIGNS AND SYMPTOMS

Constitutional Symptoms
- **Anorexia** is a loss of or lack of appetite.
- **Cachexia** is a profound state of debility; the term usually refers to wasting, malnutrition, and functional decline.
- **Asthenia** is a profound state of fatigue that patients describe as weakness or significant loss of energy.

Skin Lesions Associated with Bleeding
- **Petechiae** are pinpoint, nonblanching purple-red spots caused by intradermal or submucosal hemorrhage. The cause may be related to disorders of platelet quantity or quality or to the integrity of the vasculature.
- **Purpura** are palpable, nonblanching purple-red lesions caused by intradermal or submucosal hemorrhage.
- **Ecchymosis** is a medical term that refers to a bruise.

Findings Associated with Anemia
- **Angular cheilosis** is fissuring at the angles of the mouth.
- **Stomatitis** is mucosal inflammation in the mouth, whereas **glossitis** is inflammation specifically of the tongue. Features may include erythema, swelling and erosions, or ulcerations.
- **Koilonychia,** also called *spoon nails,* is a condition in which the nails are thinned and concave.

ESSENTIAL SKILLS

LYMPH NODES OF THE HEAD AND NECK: EXAMINATION

DD$_X$: VITAMINS C (Lymphadenopathy)
- **Infectious:** Regional infection, cat-scratch disease
- **Autoimmune/allergic:** Collagen vascular disease, infiltration with sarcoid/amyloid, and serum sickness
- **Metabolic:** Drug hypersensitivity
- **Neoplastic:** Lymphoma, leukemia, and metastatic disease

Patient Positioning
- Seat the patient in a chair and stand behind him or her. Flex the patient's neck slightly.

Inspection
- Observe any asymmetry, lumps, swelling, discoloration, or visible pulsations (carotid arteries and jugular vein).
- Continue to inspect while the patient sips water and swallows. Observe for any movement of a neck lump or mass (thyroid). Ask the patient to stick out his or her tongue, and similarly note any movement of a neck lump or mass (thyroglossal cyst).

Palpation
- Use the pads of your fingers to palpate in a rotatory motion (moving the skin over the underlying tissues). You may examine both sides of the head and neck simultaneously.
- Palpate the following nodes (see Figure 8-1):
  - Occipital: Base of skull posteriorly
  - Postauricular: Superficial to mastoid process
  - Preauricular: Anterior to ear
  - Tonsillar: Angle of mandible
  - Submandibular: Midway between the angle and the tip of the mandible
  - Submental: Midline under the chin (it is helpful to palpate with one hand while bracing the top of the head with the other hand)
  - Anterior cervical: Along the anterior border of the sternocleidomastoid muscle
  - Posterior cervical: Along anterior edge of trapezius muscle
  - Deep cervical: Deep to the sternocleidomastoid muscle and often inaccessible (hook your thumb and fingers around the sternocleidomastoid muscle, and roll the muscle between your fingers)
  - Supraclavicular: Deep in the angle between clavicle and sternocleidomastoid muscle
  - Infraclavicular: Inferior to the clavicle
- The mnemonic "**P**rofessors **T**each **S**lick **M**ed **S**tudents to **C**orrectly **D**efine **N**e**W** **L**umps" may be helpful:
  - **P**ulsatility
  - **T**enderness: Tenderness on palpation, as opposed to constant pain
  - **S**hape
  - **M**obility: Fixed versus mobile
  - **S**ize: Estimated measurement in centimeters
  - **C**onsistency: Hard versus soft; firm versus rubbery; compressible, fluctuant
  - **D**efinition: Well-defined or irregular margins
  - **N**umber: Solitary versus multiple, and **n**odularity: lumpy versus smooth
  - **W**armth
  - **L**ocation

Pearls
- The supraclavicular, submandibular, and submental nodes drain the mouth, throat, and part of the face.
- Enlargement of a supraclavicular node, especially on the left (Virchow's node), is suggestive of possible metastasis from a thoracic or abdominal malignancy.
- The submandibular nodes are smaller and smoother than the underlying submandibular salivary gland.
- Tender nodes are suggestive of inflammation; hard or fixed nodes are suggestive of malignancy.

AXILLARY LYMPH NODES: EXAMINATION

Patient Positioning
- Drape the patient appropriately with the axilla exposed. Position the patient with his or her arm raised above the head or with the hand resting behind the head.

Inspection
- Compare one axilla with the other to observe for any asymmetry.
- Inspect for any obvious lumps, swelling, or discoloration.

Palpation
- When examining the patient's right axilla, use your left hand to support the patient's right upper limb. Use your right hand to deeply palpate the axilla, including the apex and the medial, lateral, anterior, and posterior aspects. Using the pads of your fingers, palpate in a rotatory motion (moving the skin over the underlying tissues). Using the same technique, repeat the examination for the left axilla.
- Palpate the following nodes (see Figure 8-2):
  - Central group
  - Humeral group (lateral)
  - Pectoral group (anterior)
  - Infraclavicular group (apical)
  - Subscapular group (posterior)

Pearl
- Because of the pattern of lymph drainage to the axillary lymph nodes, a complete assessment of axillary lymphadenopathy must include an assessment of the corresponding upper limb and breast (see Figure 8-3).

BLEEDING DISORDER: HISTORY

> **INSTRUCTIONS TO CANDIDATE: A 19-year-old student visits the university health clinic for the first time. When disclosing his past medical history, he notes that he has "some kind of bleeding problem." Obtain a detailed history, exploring possible causes.**

Pathophysiology
- Three processes act to achieve hemostasis: vasoconstriction, formation of a platelet plug, and the coagulation cascade. The manifestations of disease vary according to the pathophysiologic processes (Table 8-1).

Table 8-1   Characteristics of Bleeding Disorders

Characteristic	Vascular and Platelet Disorders	Coagulation Disorders
Onset of bleeding	Immediate prolonged bleeding	Delayed bleeding after injury
Petechiae	Characteristic	Rare
Intramuscular hematomas	Rare	Characteristic
Superficial ecchymosis	Common (small and multiple)	Common (large and solitary)
Bleeding from superficial cuts and scratches	Persistent, often profuse	Minimal
Hemarthrosis	Rare	Characteristic
Mucosal bleeding (e.g., epistaxis, menorrhagia, GI bleeding	Common	Uncommon
Hematuria	Uncommon	More common
Sex	Relatively more common in girls and women	Most patients with hemophilia are male
Family history	Rarely positive	Commonly positive

GI, Gastrointestinal.

History

- Ask the patient the following questions:
  - **Character:** "Do you bleed or bruise easily? Are bruises unexplained or associated with injury?"
  - **Location:** "Where do you note bruises or bleeding (if at all)?"
    - Petechiae
    - Mucous membranes (epistaxis, gingival bleeding in association with tooth brushing)
    - Bleeding scratches
    - Joint bleeding or swelling (hemarthrosis)
    - Ecchymosis: torso, points of trauma (e.g., knee, shin, or elbow)
    - Hemoptysis
    - Hematuria
    - Melena, hematemesis, or hematochezia
  - **Onset:** "How soon does bleeding start in relation to injury (delayed versus immediate)?"
  - **Radiation:** "Do you have any other bleeding (bleeding from another location)?"
  - **Intensity:** "How severe is your bleeding problem? How large are the bruises (if any)? Is it getting better, getting worse, or staying the same? Does it limit your activities? Have you ever required a blood transfusion?"
  - **Duration:** "How old were you when this became a problem (hereditary versus acquired)?"
  - **Events associated:**
    - Hemorrhages: "Have you had excessive bleeding with tooth extraction, surgery, cutting of the umbilical cord, or at venipuncture sites?"
    - "Have you had left upper quadrant pain (splenomegaly) or enlarged lymph nodes (lymphadenopathy)?"
    - Headache: "Have you ever had bleeding in the brain (intracerebral hemorrhage)?"
    - Visual changes: "Have you ever had retinal bleeding?"
    - Henoch-Schönlein purpura: "Have you recently had an upper respiratory tract infection, bruised skin, abdominal pain, or joint pain (arthralgia)?"
    - Anemia: "Have you noticed pallor, weakness, fatigue, or palpitations?"
    - Constitutional symptoms: "Have you had fever, chills, night sweats, weight loss, anorexia, or asthenia (leukemia, lymphoma)?"
    - Diet: "Do you have vitamin K, C, or B_{12} deficiency; iron deficiency; or folate deficiency?"
  - **Frequency:** "How often does the bleeding happen (intermittent versus constant)?"
  - **Palliative factors:** "Does anything make it better? If so, what? Have you required treatment for bleeding in the past? If so, have you responded well to these treatments?"
  - **Provocative factors:** "Does anything make it worse? If so, what?"
- **Past medical history (PMH)/past surgical history (PSH):** Liver disease, renal disease, collagen vascular disease, malabsorption, human immunodeficiency virus (HIV) status, infectious hepatitis, or blood transfusions
- **Medications (MEDS):** Steroids, acetylsalicylic acid (ASA), anticoagulation therapy, chemotherapy, or radiation
- **Social history (SH):** Smoking, use of alcohol (EtOH), use of street drugs, diet, travel, and sexual practices
- **Family history (FH):** Bleeding diathesis (hemophilia, von Willebrand disease), collagen vascular disease, infant deaths, or infectious hepatitis

EASY BRUISING AND NOSEBLEEDS: HISTORY

INSTRUCTIONS TO CANDIDATE: A 36-year-old man presents with recent onset of easy bruising and nosebleeds. Obtain a detailed history, exploring possible causes.

DD$_X$: VITAMINS C
- **I**nfectious: Hypersplenism (e.g., mononucleosis), hemolytic uremic syndrome
- **A**utoimmune/**a**llergic: Idiopathic thrombocytopenic purpura, thrombotic thrombocytopenic purpura, Henoch-Schönlein purpura, and Wegener granulomatosis
- **M**etabolic: Disseminated intravascular coagulation (DIC), vitamin K deficiency (malabsorption syndromes, malnutrition), and Cushing syndrome (endogenous/exogenous)
- **I**diopathic/**i**atrogenic: Hypersplenism caused by portal hypertension
- **N**eoplastic: Leukemia, lymphoma

History
- Ask the patient the following questions:
  - **C**haracter: "How would you describe the bleeding? Are bruises unexplained or associated with injury?"
  - **L**ocation: "Where is the blood coming from? Where are the bruises?"
    - Petechiae
    - Ecchymosis
    - Joint bleed/swelling (hemarthrosis)
    - Mucous membranes (epistaxis, gingival bleeding associated with tooth brushing)
    - Hemoptysis
    - Hematuria
    - Melena, hematochezia, or hematemesis
  - **O**nset: "When did the bleeding start (hereditary versus acquired)?"
  - **R**adiation: "Any other bleeding (bleeding from another location)?"
  - **I**ntensity: "How severe is the bleeding (quantify)? Has it gotten worse?"
  - **D**uration: "How long has the bleeding been going on?"
  - **E**vents associated:
    - "Do you have left upper quadrant pain (splenomegaly) or enlarged lymph nodes (lymphadenopathy)?"
    - Henoch-Schönlein purpura: "Have you recently had an upper respiratory tract infection, bruised skin, abdominal pain, or joint pain (arthralgia)?"
    - Vitamin K deficiency: "Do you have problems with malabsorption (steatorrhea, weight loss)?"
    - Cushing syndrome (endogenous/exogenous): "Have you noticed a change in the shape of your face or body (moon facies, truncal obesity) or stretch marks (striae)?"
    - Thrombotic thrombocytopenic purpura: "Have you had jaundice, fever, or confusion (neurologic findings), or blood in the urine (renal disease)?"
    - Wegener granulomatosis: "Have you had nose bleeds, blood in the urine, or skin lesions?"
    - Constitutional symptoms: "Have you had fever, chills, night sweats, weight loss, anorexia, or asthenia (leukemia, lymphoma)?"
    - Anemia: "Have you noticed pallor, weakness, fatigue, and palpitations?"
  - **F**requency: "How often does the bleeding happen (intermittent versus constant)?"
  - **P**alliative factors: "Does anything make the bleeding lessen? If so, what?"
  - **P**rovocative factors: "Does anything make the bleeding worse? If so, what?"
- **PMH/PSH:** Liver disease, renal disease, collagen vascular disease, bleeding diathesis (hemophilia, von Willebrand disease), HIV status, or blood transfusions; history of hemorrhage in association with surgery
- **MEDS:** Nonsteroidal anti-inflammatory drugs (NSAIDs), ASA, warfarin, steroids, antibiotics, or chemotherapy
- **SH:** Smoking, use of EtOH, use of street drugs
- **FH:** Bleeding diathesis (hemophilia, von Willebrand disease), collagen vascular disease

CONSTITUTIONAL SYMPTOMS: HISTORY

> **INSTRUCTIONS TO CANDIDATE:** A 27-year-old man presents to his family physician complaining of weight loss and night sweats. Obtain a detailed history of his symptoms, exploring possible causes.

DD$_X$: VITAMINS C
- **Infectious:** Tuberculosis, HIV infection
- **Autoimmune/allergic:** Collagen vascular disease
- **Neoplastic:** Lymphoma (Hodgkin's and non-Hodgkin's types), leukemia, and other malignancy

History
- Ask the patient the following questions:
  - **Character:** "Can you describe how you are feeling?"
  - **Onset:** "When did you first notice the weight loss? When did you first notice the night sweats?"
  - **Intensity:** "How much weight have you lost? How severe are the night sweats? Do you soak your pajamas? Your sheets?"
  - **Duration:** "Over what period of time has this weight loss occurred?"
  - **Events associated:**
    - Other constitutional symptoms: "Have you had fever, chills, anorexia, pruritus, or asthenia?"
    - Lymphadenopathy: "Have you experienced 'gland' enlargement (neck, armpit, or groin), cough or shortness of breath (mediastinal enlargement), or alcohol-induced pain (rare)?"
    - Pel-Ebstein fever: "Have you had fever alternating with periods of 15 to 28 days of normal or low temperature?"
    - Anemia (caused by bone marrow infiltrate, hypersplenism): "Have you noted pallor, weakness, or fatigue?"
    - Pain caused by bony infiltration or nerve root compression: "Do you have pain?"
    - Pancytopenia: "Have you experienced easy bruising and infections?"
    - Lymphatic obstruction in the pelvis or groin: "Do you have leg swelling (edema)?"
    - Compression of the stomach by enlarged spleen: "Have you experienced early satiety or nausea or vomiting?"
    - Cervical sympathetic chain compression: "Do you have Horner's syndrome?"
    - Recurrent laryngeal nerve compression: "Have you experienced hoarseness?"
    - Tuberculosis: "Do you have a history of exposure to tuberculosis, fever, cough, shortness of breath, and hemoptysis?"
    - HIV: "Do you have multiple sexual partners? Do you use intravenous drugs? Have you had blood transfusions? Have you experienced diarrhea or opportunistic infection?"
  - **Frequency:** "How often do the night sweats happen (intermittent versus every night)?"
  - **Palliative factors:** "Does anything make the night sweats better? If so, what?"
  - **Provocative factors:** "Does anything make the night sweats worse? If so, what?"
- **PMH/PSH:** Malignancy, past surgery, organ transplantation, or HIV infection; history of exposure to radiation (therapeutic, occupational)
- **MEDS:** Immunosuppressants, allopurinol or phenytoin (hypersensitivity to these two may cause lymphadenopathy)
- **FH:** Lymphoma, familial malignancies

ANEMIA: HISTORY AND PHYSICAL EXAMINATION

> **INSTRUCTIONS TO CANDIDATE:** A 60-year-old woman presents to the emergency department, complaining of fatigue and weakness. She visited her family doctor 3 days ago with the same concern, and he ordered some blood tests. The astute triage nurse checks for recent laboratory investigations and brings you the results of the patient's complete blood cell count (CBC): hemoglobin, 68 g/L; white blood cell count, 8.6×10^9/L; and platelet count, 150×10^9/L. The mean corpuscular volume is 66 fL. Obtain a detailed history, exploring possible causes, and perform a focused physical examination.

- This patient has a marked microcytic anemia (Table 8-2).

History
- Ask the patient the following questions:
  - **Character:** "How are you feeling? Tell me about your weakness and fatigue."
  - **Location:** "Are you aware of any possible blood loss?"
    - Gastrointestinal blood loss: melena, hematochezia, or hematemesis
    - Hemoptysis
    - Hematuria
    - If the patient is still menstruating, inquire about menorrhagia: presence of clots, number of sanitary pads or tampons needed per day
    - Trauma
  - **Onset:** "How did this problem start?"
  - **Intensity:** "Has the problem gotten worse (ask about symptom progression)?"
  - **Duration:** "How long have you been feeling unwell?"
  - **Events associated:**
    - "Do you have shortness of breath, palpitations, or chest pain on exertion?"
    - Pica: "Do you have a craving for dirt, paint, or ice?"
    - Iron deficiency: "Do you have brittle nails, smooth tongue, or mouth sores (angular cheilosis)?"
    - Plummer-Vinson syndrome (associated pharyngeal web): "Do you have trouble swallowing (dysphagia)?"
    - Malnutrition: "Are you getting enough dietary iron or vitamin C?"
    - Constitutional symptoms: "Have you had fever, chills, night sweats, weight loss, anorexia, or asthenia (malignancy)?"
  - **Frequency:** "Have you ever experienced this problem before?"
  - **Palliative factors:** "Does anything make you feel better? If so, what?"
  - **Provocative factors:** "Does anything make you feel worse? If so, what?"
    - Exertional symptoms

Table 8-2 Classification of Anemia

Microcytic (MCV, <80 fL)	Normocytic (MCV, 80–95 fL)	Macrocytic (MCV, >95 fL)
Iron deficiency	Acute blood loss	Vitamin B_{12} deficiency
Thalassemia	Hemolysis	Folate deficiency
Sideroblastic anemia	Hypoproduction of RBCs	Alcohol
	Anemia of chronic disease	

MCV, Mean corpuscular volume; RBC, red blood cell.

- **PMH/PSH:** Anemia, bleeding diathesis, malignancy, cardiovascular disease, liver or renal disease, or blood transfusions
- **MEDS:** NSAIDs, ASA, iron supplements, or anticoagulants
- **SH:** Smoking, use of EtOH, use of street drugs
- **FH:** Thalassemia, familial malignancy (e.g., colon cancer), or bleeding diathesis

Physical Examination
- **Vital signs (Vitals):** Evaluate heart rate (HR), respiratory rate (RR), blood pressure (BP), and temperature.
- **General:** Evaluate for cachexia, jaundice.
- **Skin:** Check for pallor (lips, buccal mucosa, conjunctiva, palmar creases), koilonychia (brittle, ridged, or spoon nails).
- **Head, eyes, ears, nose, and throat (HEENT):** Note glossitis, angular cheilosis, frontal bossing, or abnormal facies.
- **Lymphatic system:** Examine lymph nodes in the head and neck, axillae, and groin (note size, shape, mobility, consistency, tenderness, warmth, and number of enlarged nodes).
- **Respiratory system (Resp):** Auscultate the lungs (breath sounds, adventitious sounds).
- **Cardiovascular system (CVS):** Palpate peripheral pulses. Note pulse volume, contour, and rhythm. Auscultate the heart, listening for extra heart sounds or flow murmurs. Look for signs of cardiac compromise: displaced apical impulse (cardiac dilatation), hyperdynamic precordium, bounding pulses, and aortic flow murmur.
- **Abdomen:** Inspect the abdomen. Auscultate for bowel sounds. Percuss lightly in all four quadrants. Perform light and deep palpation, and identify any masses or areas of tenderness. Check for rebound tenderness. Examine the liver and spleen (look for organomegaly). Perform a digital rectal examination, looking for a mass, gross blood, melena, or occult blood.

Evidence
- Pallor has been studied fairly extensively as a physical indicator of anemia, largely in the pediatric population of African nations.[1] In a study of patients older than 12 years in India, the usefulness of pallor was assessed in four sites: conjunctivae, which were considered pale if the anterior rim of the lower palpebral conjunctiva looked as pale as the deeper posterior rim; dorsal surface of the tongue; palmar creases; and nail beds. The interrater reliability was poor for all four sites. The tongue was superior to the conjunctivae, palmar, and nail bed sites for detecting severe anemia (hemoglobin <70 g/L) with a positive likelihood ratio (+LR) of 9.87 (95% confidence interval [CI] 2.81 to 34.6).[2]

DEEP VENOUS THROMBOSIS: HISTORY AND PHYSICAL EXAMINATION

> **INSTRUCTIONS TO CANDIDATE: A 47-year-old woman presents to the emergency department with a swollen and painful right leg. Obtain a detailed history, focusing on risk factors for thromboembolic disease, and perform a focused physical examination.**

DD$_X$: VITAMINS C
- **Vascular:** Deep venous thrombosis (DVT), thrombophlebitis, and arterial insufficiency
- **Infectious:** Cellulitis
- **Traumatic:** Traumatic injury, ruptured Baker cyst
- **Idiopathic/iatrogenic:** Neuropathy, referred pain

History
- Ask the patient the following questions:
  - **Character:** "Can you describe the pain in your leg?"
  - **Location:** "What part of your leg is swollen? What part of your leg is painful?"
  - **Onset:** "How did the leg pain start (sudden versus gradual)?"

- **Radiation:** "Does the pain move anywhere? Into your foot? Or up your leg?"
- **Intensity:** "How severe is your pain right now on a scale of 1 to 10, with 1 being mild and 10 being the worst? Has your pain gotten worse?"
- **Duration:** "How long has your leg been painful? Swollen?"
- **Events associated:**
  - "Have you had fever, localized redness and swelling, and heat (may be consistent with infection)?"
  - "Have you been injured recently?"
  - Rupture of Baker cyst: "Have you had knee effusion, sudden onset of pain and swelling, or a popliteal mass?"
  - Superficial thrombophlebitis: "Do you have a red, tender cord in the calf?"
- **Frequency:** "Have you ever experienced this problem before? If so, how often does it happen? When did you last have leg pain and swelling?"
- **Palliative factors:** "Does anything make your leg pain better? If so, what?"
- **Provocative factors:** "Does anything make your leg pain worse? If so, what?"
  - Calf pain that occurs with activity and resolves with rest is called *claudication* (arterial insufficiency).
- **PMH/PSH:** Thromboembolic disease, blood dyscrasias, polycythemia, recent surgery, pregnancy, diabetes mellitus, or obesity
- **MEDS:** Estrogens, anticoagulants (nonadherence to a medication regimen or addition of a new medication may alter efficacy)
- **FH:** Thromboembolic disease; antithrombin III deficiency; protein C or protein S deficiency, or both; or factor V Leiden mutation

Risk Factors for Thromboembolic Disease[3]
- **Virchow's triad:** Endothelial injury, hypercoagulability, and stasis
  - Injury: Vascular catheter insertion, injection of irritating substances, trauma (odds ratio 12.7; 95% CI 4.1 to 39.7), and surgery (odds ratio 21; 95% CI 9.4 to 49.9)
  - Hypercoagulability: Malignancy (with chemotherapy, odds ratio 6.5, 95% CI 2.1 to 20.2; without chemotherapy, odds ratio 4.1, 95% CI 1.9 to 8.5); polycythemia; estrogen administration (oral contraceptives: odds ratio 3.0, 95% CI 2.6 to 3.4); thrombophlebitis; dehydration; nephrotic syndrome; inflammatory bowel disease; infusion of prothrombin complex concentrates; factor V Leiden mutation; antithrombin III deficiency; protein C or protein S deficiency, or both; lupus anticoagulant; and antiphospholipid syndrome
  - Stasis: Myocardial infarction, heart failure, pregnancy (conducive to inferior vena cava compression), and prolonged immobility (e.g., hospitalization or nursing home residence: odds ratio 8.0; 95% CI 4.5 to 14.2), lower extremity paresis (odds ratio 3.0; 95% CI 1.3 to 7.4)
- Other: Smoking, use of EtOH, use of street drugs, age >60 years, history of thromboembolic disease, obesity, and diabetes mellitus

Physical Examination
- **Vitals:** Evaluate HR and heart rhythm, RR, BP, and temperature.
- **General:** Evaluate gait and patient's position on stretcher or chair.
- **Skin:** Check for peripheral edema, skin color, skin temperature over feet and legs (using the backs of your fingers), skin quality (atrophic changes, ulcers), and capillary refill.
- **Resp:** Auscultate the lungs (breath sounds, adventitious sounds, pleural friction rub).
- **CVS:** Palpate peripheral pulses (dorsalis pedis, posterior tibial, popliteal, femoral). Note pulse volume, contour, and rhythm. Auscultate the heart, listening for extra heart sounds or flow murmurs. Consider the "6Ps" of arterial occlusion:
  - Pain
  - Pulselessness
  - Pallor
  - Polar (cool temperature)
  - Paresthesia
  - Paralysis

Table 8-3 Wells Score for DVT

Clinical Feature	Score
Active cancer (treatment ongoing or within previous 6 months or palliative)	1
Paralysis, paresis, or recent plaster immobilization of the lower extremities	1
Recently bedridden for more than 3 days or major surgery within 4 weeks	1
Localized tenderness along the distribution of the deep venous system	1
Entire leg swollen	1
Calf swelling by more than 3 cm when compared with the asymptomatic leg (measured 10 cm below tibial tuberosity)	1
Pitting edema (greater in the symptomatic leg)	1
Collateral superficial veins (nonvaricose)	1
Alternative diagnosis as likely or greater than that of deep vein thrombosis (DVT)	−2

From Wells PS, Anderson DR, Bormanis J, et al. Value of assessment of pretest probability of deep-vein thrombosis in clinical management. *Lancet*. 1997;350:1795-1798.
High probability is a score ≥3, for which prevalence of DVT is 75% (95% confidence interval [CI] 63%–81%). Moderate probability is a score of 1–2, for which prevalence of DVT is 17% (95% CI 12%–23%). Low probability is a score of 0 or less, for which prevalence of DVT is 3% (95% CI 1.7%–5.9%).

- **Abdomen:** Inspect the abdomen. Auscultate for bowel sounds. Percuss lightly in all four quadrants. Perform light and deep palpation, and identify any masses or areas of tenderness. Examine the liver and spleen (look for organomegaly).
- **Musculoskeletal system:** Note any signs of trauma or varicose veins (dilated and tortuous veins).
  - Swelling: Measure circumference of the thigh and leg 10 cm below the tibial tuberosity. A difference of >3 cm is considered significant.
  - Look for knee effusion. Palpate the popliteal fossa for protrusion cyst of the knee, known as Baker cyst.

Evidence
- **Homans' sign:** Flex the patient's knee. Forcefully and abruptly dorsiflex the ankle. This produces pain in 11% to 56% of patients with DVT, but pain is also present in 11% to 61% of patients without DVT.[4] Some authorities believe that performing this examination may dislodge the clot and precipitate pulmonary embolism.
- Physical diagnosis of DVT through inspection of the lower limb, leg measurement, and elicitation of Homan's sign has proved problematic, generating +LRs of 1 to 2 with some Cls overlapping 1.[4] However, a combination of clinical symptoms and signs can be used to stratify patients' risk categories and plan further diagnostic evaluations (Table 8-3).

PULMONARY EMBOLISM: HISTORY AND PHYSICAL EXAMINATION

INSTRUCTIONS TO CANDIDATE: The patient previously described has a Doppler ultrasound evaluation of the right leg, which confirms a DVT that extends from the knee into the deep femoral venous system. She is discharged with appropriate treatment and follow-up evaluation. She returns to the emergency department the next day with shortness of breath and chest discomfort. Obtain an appropriate history, and perform a focused physical examination.

DD$_X$
- Pulmonary embolism until proved otherwise.

Definition

- Pulmonary embolism obstructs flow in the pulmonary arterial circulation and commonly arises from thrombi in deep leg or pelvic veins (less commonly from the arm or right side of the heart). If the embolism is not fatal, the clot will lyse, and symptoms will resolve (unless infarction occurs). Pulmonary infarction is rare because the lung has a dual blood supply (pulmonary and bronchial circulation). Symptoms of embolization occur abruptly; infarction develops over hours. Massive pulmonary embolism may manifest as cardiac arrest or shock.
- **First evaluate airway, breathing, and circulation (ABCs).** It may be necessary to perform an immediate intervention, such as administering supplemental O_2, establishing intravenous access, or initiating airway management.
    - Is the patient able to talk? Swallow? Cough?
    - Are both lungs ventilated? Is the patient oxygenating (check mentation, pulse oximetry)?
    - Are vital signs abnormal? Is the peripheral circulation (pulses, capillary refill) abnormal?
    - If no immediate interventions are required, proceed to obtain the history, and perform the physical examination.

History

- Ask the patient the following questions:
    - **Character:** "Can you describe the nature of your breathing difficulty?"
    - **Location:** "Where were you when you became short of breath?"
    - **Onset:** "How did the shortness of breath start (sudden versus gradual)? What were you doing when you became short of breath?"
    - **Intensity:** "How severe is your shortness of breath right now on a scale of 1 to 10, with 1 being mild and 10 being the worst? Has your shortness of breath gotten worse?"
    - **Duration:** "How long have you been short of breath?"
    - **Events associated:**
        - Pulmonary embolism triad (rare): "Did you experience sudden shortness of breath, chest pain with inspiration, and cough up blood (hemoptysis)?"
        - "Have you had fever, palpitations, or fainting?"
        - Pulmonary infarction: "Have you had bloody sputum and chest pain, fever (a pleural friction rub may be audible and physical findings compatible with consolidation or pleural effusion may be noted)?"
    - **Frequency:** "Have you ever experienced this problem before? If so, how often does it happen? When was the last time you became short of breath?"
    - **Palliative factors:** "Does anything make your shortness of breath better? If so, what?"
    - **Provocative factors:** "Does anything make your shortness of breath worse? If so, what?"
- **PMH/PSH:** Thromboembolic disease, ischemic heart disease, asthma, or pericardial disease
- **MEDS:** Anticoagulants

Physical Examination

- **Vitals:** Evaluate HR and heart rhythm (sinus tachycardia is common), RR (depth, effort, and pattern), BP, and temperature.
- **General:** Evaluate for respiratory distress, unilateral splinting of chest (pleuritic chest pain).
- **Skin:** Check for peripheral edema, cyanosis, clubbing, and capillary refill.
- **HEENT:** Check for central cyanosis, and observe tracheal position.
- **Resp:** Evaluate chest expansion (for symmetry), test tactile fremitus, and perform percussion and auscultation (breath sounds, adventitious sounds, pleural friction rub).

- **CVS:** Measure the jugular venous pressure. Palpate peripheral pulses. Note pulse volume, contour, and rhythm. Auscultate the heart, listening for loud P_2, S_3, or murmurs. Palpate the apical impulse. Consider the signs of cor pulmonale (increased jugular venous pressure, positive hepatojugular reflux, and right ventricular heave).
- **Neurologic (Neuro):** Check the patient's mental status (adequate brain oxygenation).

Evidence

- The Simplified Wells Score has been studied extensively and can be used to differentiate patients at high and low risk for pulmonary embolism (Table 8-4). Interestingly, the clinical gestalt of experienced clinicians is also reasonably accurate for risk stratification of patients suspected to have pulmonary embolism.[3]

Table 8-4   The Simplified Wells Score

Clinical Feature	Score
Clinical signs/symptoms of DVT	3.0
No alternate diagnosis likely or more likely than a PE	3.0
Heart rate >100	1.5
Immobilization or surgery in the last 4 weeks	1.5
Previous history of DVT or PE	1.5
Hemoptysis	1.0
Cancer actively treated in the last 6 months	1.0

From Wells PS, Anderson DR, Rodger M, et al. Excluding pulmonary embolism at the bedside without diagnostic imaging: management of patients with suspected pulmonary embolism presenting to the emergency department by using a simple clinical model and D-dimer. *Ann Intern Med.* 2001;135:98-107.

High probability is a score >6, for which posttest probability of pulmonary embolism is 40.6% (95% confidence interval [CI] 28.7%–53.7%). Moderate probability is a score of 2–6, for which posttest probability of pulmonary embolism is 16.2% (95% CI 12.5%–20.6%). Low probability is a score of <2, for which posttest probability of pulmonary embolism is 1.3% (95% CI 0.5%–2.7%). DVT, Deep venous thrombosis; PE, pulmonary embolism.

SAMPLE CHECKLIST

Lymph Nodes of the Head and Neck: Examination

INSTRUCTIONS TO CANDIDATE: Examine the lymph nodes of the head and neck. Describe your findings.

Key Points	Satisfactorily Completed
Introduces self to the patient	❏
Determines how the patient wishes to be addressed	❏
Washes hands	❏
Explains nature of the examination to the patient	❏
Examines the patient in a logical manner	❏
Inspects for the following:	
• Symmetry	❏
• Visible masses	❏
Examines lymph nodes:	
• Occipital	❏
• Postauricular	❏
• Preauricular	❏
• Tonsillar	❏
• Submandibular	❏
• Submental	❏
• Anterior cervical	❏
• Posterior cervical	❏
• Supraclavicular	❏
• Infraclavicular	❏
Describes palpable lymph nodes:	
• Location and number	❏
• Size and shape	❏
• Mobility	❏
• Consistency	❏
• Tenderness	❏
• Warmth	❏
Drapes the patient appropriately	❏
Makes appropriate closing remarks	❏

ADVANCED SKILLS

LYMPHOMA: PHYSICAL EXAMINATION

> **INSTRUCTIONS TO CANDIDATE:** You are doing a rotation in hematology and are asked to see a 22-year-old man referred with a tentative diagnosis of lymphoma. Examine the patient, and describe your findings.

Physical Examination
- **Vitals:** Evaluate HR, RR, BP, and temperature (low-grade fever may be present).
- **General:** Evaluate for cachexia and diaphoresis.
- **Skin:** Look for jaundice, pallor (lips, buccal mucosa, conjunctiva, palmar creases), petechiae, and ecchymosis.
- **Lymphatic system:** Examine lymph nodes in the head and neck, axillae, and groin (note size, shape, mobility, consistency, tenderness, warmth, and number of enlarged nodes). Enlarged lymph nodes are rubbery and discrete and later, with disease progression, become matted.
- **Resp:** Auscultate the lungs (breath sounds, adventitious sounds). Note any signs of infection, pleural effusion, or tracheobronchial compression.
- **CVS:** Palpate peripheral pulses. Note pulse volume, contour, and rhythm. Auscultate the heart, listening for extra heart sounds or flow murmurs. Look for signs of severe anemia (hyperdynamic precordium, bounding pulses, and aortic flow murmur). Also look for signs of superior vena cava (SVC) syndrome (congestion and edema of the face and neck caused by compression of the SVC).
- **Abdomen:** Inspect the abdomen. Auscultate for bowel sounds. Percuss lightly in all four quadrants. Perform light and deep palpation, and identify any masses or areas of tenderness. Significantly enlarged para-aortic lymph nodes may be palpable as a deep central mass. Examine the liver and spleen (looking for organomegaly).
- Note any signs and sources of infection.

Pearl
- Two problems commonly associated with non-Hodgkin's lymphoma and, in rare cases, with Hodgkin's lymphoma are SVC syndrome and renal failure (caused by ureteral compression from large pelvic lymph nodes).

LEUKEMIA: HISTORY AND PHYSICAL EXAMINATION

> **INSTRUCTIONS TO CANDIDATE:** A 55-year-old woman presents to the emergency department feeling generally unwell. She has a low-grade fever (temperature 38° C). Her CBC results reveal a hemoglobin level of 95 g/L, a white blood cell count of 100×10^9/L, and a platelet count of 40×10^9/L. Obtain a detailed history, exploring possible causes, and perform a focused physical examination.

DD$_X$: VITAMINS C
- **Idiopathic/iatrogenic:** Myeloproliferative disorders
- **Neoplastic:** Acute leukemia

History
- Ask the patient the following questions:
  - **Character:** "How are you feeling? Have you had constitutional symptoms (fever, chills, night sweats, weight loss, anorexia, or asthenia)?"
  - **Onset:** "How did this problem start?"

- ▪ **Intensity:** "Has this problem gotten worse (ask about symptom progression)?"
- ▪ **Duration:** "How long have you been feeling unwell?"
- ▪ **Events associated:**
  - ◆ Infection: "Have you had fever, productive cough (pneumonia), painful urination (dysuria) or urinary frequency (urinary tract infection), or diarrhea?"
  - ◆ Anemia: "Are you experiencing fatigue, weakness, shortness of breath on exertion (SOBOE), chest pain, or palpitations?"
  - ◆ Thrombocytopenia: "Have you noticed easy bruising or bleeding from gums?"
  - ◆ Compression of stomach by hepatosplenomegaly: "Have you experienced early satiety or nausea or vomiting?"
  - ◆ Pleural effusion or mediastinal enlargement: "Are you short of breath?"
  - ◆ Infiltration of normal tissues by leukemic cells: "Do you have bone pain; leg weakness (cord compression); swollen gums; swollen glands in neck, groin or armpit; joint pain; or shortness of breath?"
- ▪ **Frequency:** "Have you ever experienced this problem before?"
- ▪ **Palliative factors:** "Does anything make you feel better? If so, what?"
- ▪ **Provocative factors:** "Does anything make you feel worse? If so, what?"
- **PMH/PSH:** Malignancy, history of exposure to radiation (therapeutic, occupational)?
- **MEDS**
- **Allergies**
- **SH:** Use of EtOH, use of street drugs
- **FH:** Hematologic malignancy

Physical Examination
- **Vitals:** Evaluate HR, RR, BP, and temperature.
- **General:** Evaluate for cachexia and diaphoresis.
- **Skin:** Look for pallor (lips, buccal mucosa, conjunctiva, palmar creases) and petechiae.
- **HEENT:** Assess the gingivas for hypertrophy or bleeding. Inspect the eyes for proptosis.
- **Lymphatic system:** Examine lymph nodes in the head and neck, axillae, and groin (note size, shape, mobility, consistency, tenderness, warmth, and number of enlarged nodes).
- **Resp:** Auscultate the lungs (breath sounds, adventitious sounds). Note any signs of infection, pleural effusion, or tracheobronchial compression.
- **CVS:** Palpate peripheral pulses. Note pulse volume, contour, and rhythm. Auscultate the heart, listening for extra heart sounds or flow murmurs. Look for signs of severe anemia (hyperdynamic precordium, bounding pulses, and aortic flow murmur).
- **Abdomen:** Inspect the abdomen. Auscultate for bowel sounds. Percuss lightly in all four quadrants. Perform light and deep palpation, and identify any masses or areas of tenderness. Significantly enlarged para-aortic nodes may be palpable as a deep central mass. Examine the liver and spleen (looking for organomegaly).

Pearl
- Look for signs and sources of infection. Although the patient has a profound leukocytosis (100×10^9/L), these cells are probably not functioning appropriately and thus leave the patient vulnerable to infection.

SAMPLE CHECKLIST

Monoclonal Gammopathy of Unknown Significance: History and Physical Examination

> **INSTRUCTIONS TO CANDIDATE: A 67-year-old man presents to your office for a yearly follow-up visit. A number of years ago, he received a diagnosis of monoclonal gammopathy of unknown significance. Obtain a detailed history, focusing on symptoms of multiple myeloma, and perform a focused physical examination.**

Key Points	Satisfactorily Completed
Introduces self to the patient	❏
Determines how the patient wishes to be addressed	❏
Washes hands	❏
Explains the purpose of the encounter	❏
Performs a review of systems, including the following:	
• Bone pain	❏
• Pain with movement	❏
• Night pain	❏
• Symptoms associated with infections, such as urinary tract infection, pneumonia, or cellulitis	❏
• Fatigue, pallor, and weakness (anemia)	❏
• Petechiae, mucosal bleeding (platelet dysfunction)	❏
• Nausea or vomiting, lethargy, chest pain (pericarditis, pleuritis), yellowish skin (uremia)	❏
• "Moans, bones, stones, and psychiatric overtones" (hypercalcemia): Weakness, fatigue, myalgias Bone pain Kidney stones Depression, cognitive impairment	❏
• Flank pain, hematuria (nephrolithiasis related to hypercalcemia, hyperuricemia)	❏
Assesses mental status	❏
Asks about past medical and surgical histories	❏
Asks about medications	❏
Asks about social history	❏
Asks about family history	❏
Explains nature of the examination to the patient	❏
Examines the patient in a logical manner	❏
Inspects for the following:	
• Cachexia	❏
• Skin: pallor, petechiae, uremic frost	❏
• Kyphosis	❏
• Gait	❏
Examines the lymphatic system:	
• Lymph nodes in the head and neck	❏
• Lymph nodes in the axillae and groin	❏
• Liver and spleen	❏

Key Points	Satisfactorily Completed
Evaluates musculoskeletal system:	
• Palpates the spine for tenderness and deformity	❏
• Assesses reflexes, strength, and sensation in the lower extremities	❏
• Performs a digital rectal examination for rectal tone	❏
• Assesses perineal sensation	❏
Drapes the patient appropriately	❏
Makes appropriate closing remarks	❏

REFERENCES

1. Chalco JP, Huicho L, Alamo C, et al. Accuracy of clinical pallor in the diagnosis of anaemia in children: a meta-analysis. *BMC Pediatr.* 2005;5:46.
2. Kalantri A, Karambelkar M, Joshi R, et al. Accuracy and reliability of pallor for detecting anaemia: a hospital-based diagnostic accuracy study. *PLoS One.* 2010;5(1):e8545.
3. Chunilal SD, Eikelboom JW, Attia J, et al. Does this patient have pulmonary embolism? *JAMA.* 2003;290:2849-2858.
4. Anand SS, Wells PS, Hunt D, et al. Does this patient have deep vein thrombosis? *JAMA.* 1998;279:1094-1099.

Endocrinology

ANATOMY

- In terms of embryology, the **thyroid** develops from the floor of the pharynx. The primitive thyroid gland migrates caudally to rest anterior to the trachea. If migration fails to stop anterior to the second or third tracheal ring, the thyroid may become partially or wholly substernal. If the migratory tract fails to obliterate, a thyroglossal cyst may develop.
- The normal thyroid gland is inferior to the cricoid cartilage, anterior and lateral to the trachea, in the anterior triangle of the neck (Figure 9-1). The two lateral lobes are connected by an **isthmus,** which extends across the trachea, anterior to the second tracheal ring. The thyroid gland is often not palpable (the isthmus may be palpable).
- The thyroid is firmly embedded in the pretracheal fascia, so it ascends with swallowing. This movement helps distinguish the thyroid from other masses in the neck.
- The recurrent laryngeal nerve lies deep to the medial aspect of the thyroid and may be damaged during thyroid surgery or in invasive malignant disease; damage causes hoarseness.
- The thyroid hormone produced by the thyroid gland influences cellular metabolism (Figure 9-2).

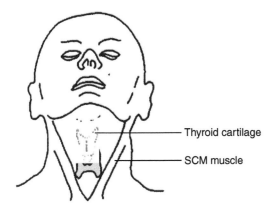

Figure 9-1 Surface anatomy of the thyroid. SCM, sternocleidomastoid. (Used with permission of Dr. Tom Scott, Memorial University of Newfoundland, St. John's, Newfoundland.)

Thyroid cartilage

SCM muscle

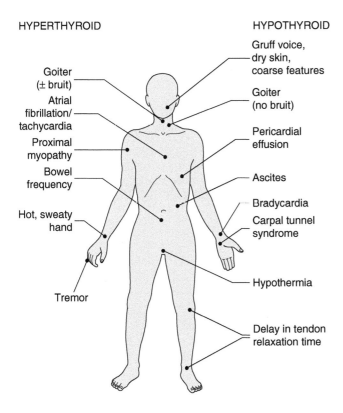

HYPERTHYROID

Goiter (± bruit)
Atrial fibrillation/ tachycardia
Proximal myopathy
Bowel frequency
Hot, sweaty hand
Tremor

HYPOTHYROID

Gruff voice, dry skin, coarse features
Goiter (no bruit)
Pericardial effusion
Ascites
Bradycardia
Carpal tunnel syndrome
Hypothermia
Delay in tendon relaxation time

Figure 9-2 Features of hyperthyroidism and hypothyroidism. (From Munro JF, Campbell IW, eds. *Macleod's Clinical Examination*. 10th ed. Edinburgh: Churchill Livingstone; 2000 [p. 63, Figure 2.47].)

GLOSSARY OF SIGNS AND SYMPTOMS

- **Alopecia** is hair loss. **Queen Anne's eyebrow** is the lateral truncation of the eyebrows. Loss of the lateral third of the eyebrows is associated with hypothyroidism.
- **Amenorrhea** is absence of menses (**primary amenorrhea**) or abnormal cessation of menses (**secondary amenorrhea**).
- **Exophthalmos** is the protrusion of one or both eyeballs.
- **Galactorrhea** is the abnormal presence of lactation, specifically lactation that is persistent and takes place outside the context of breastfeeding or during the peripartum period.
- A **goiter** is a non-neoplastic enlargement of the thyroid gland. It is an endemic condition in areas where iodine deficiency is prevalent. The physical characteristics of the thyroid gland, such as size and consistency, do not reflect its function: Patients with a goiter can have hyperthyroidism, hypothyroidism, or normal thyroid function.

- **Gynecomastia** is excessive development of one or both male mammary glands, resulting in breast enlargement.
- **Hirsutism** is the presence of excessive body and facial hair in androgen-stimulated locations such as the face, chest, and areolae (male-patterned hair growth) in girls and women. **Hypertrichosis** also refers to excessive hair growth, but it is generally used to refer to growth in areas that are not androgen dependant.
- **Moon facies** is the full, rounded appearance of the face of a patient with Cushing syndrome.
- **Polydipsia** is excessive and prolonged thirst.
- **Polyuria** is excessive volume of urination. Polyuria should be differentiated from urinary frequency.
- **Myxedema** refers to nonpitting, waxy dermal edema caused by deposition of mucopolysaccharides.
- **Thyroid acropachy** is an unusual manifestation of thyroid disease. It is morphologically similar to clubbing, with soft tissue swelling and periosteal reaction.

ESSENTIAL SKILLS

THYROID GLAND: EXAMINATION

Inspection
- Ask the patient to extend the neck slightly. Use tangential lighting to inspect the region below the cricoid cartilage for the thyroid gland. Ask the patient to take a sip of water, slightly extend the neck, and swallow. Watch for movement of the thyroid, noting contour and symmetry. Normally the thyroid gland, thyroid cartilage, and cricoid cartilage rise with swallowing. Ask the patient to stick out the tongue; a thyroglossal cyst should move on protrusion of the tongue.

Palpation
- **Posterior approach:** Palpation yields the most precise findings when performed from behind the patient. Slightly extend the patient's neck. Overextending interferes with palpation (taut muscles). Palpate the lateral lobes of the thyroid (Figure 9-3). The isthmus is more often palpable than the lateral lobes. Ask the patient to sip and swallow as necessary. Feel for any glandular tissue rising under your finger pads. Note size, shape, consistency, nodularity, and tenderness of the gland. The physical characteristics of the thyroid gland do *not* reflect its function.

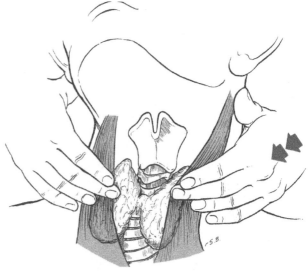

Figure 9-3 Posterior approach to examination of the thyroid. (From Barkauskas VH, Baumann LC, Darling-Fisher CS. *Health and Physical Assessment.* 3rd ed. St. Louis: Mosby; 2002 [p. 238, Figure 11-16(1)].)

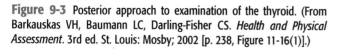

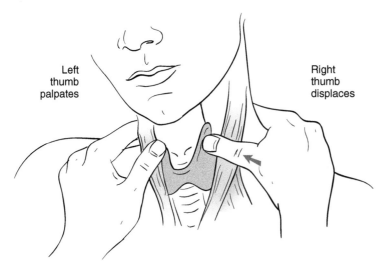

Figure 9-4 Anterior approach to examination of the thyroid. (From Jarvis CJ. *Physical Examination and Health Assessment.* 2nd ed. Philadelphia: Saunders; 1996 [p. 284, Figure 11-15].)

Left thumb palpates

Right thumb displaces

- **Anterior approach:** Sit in front of the patient. To palpate the right lobe, slightly flex the patient's neck, and turn the chin toward the right side. Displace the left lobe with your right hand, and palpate the right lobe with your left hand (Figure 9-4). Ask the patient to swallow, and feel the tissue rising under your fingers.

Auscultation
- If the thyroid gland is enlarged, auscultate over the lateral lobes with the bell of your stethoscope to detect a bruit (hyperdynamic circulation).

Evidence
- Inspection and palpation of the thyroid gland are useful for detecting goiter (i.e., thyroid gland size >20 g (positive likelihood ratio [+LR] 3.8, 95% confidence interval [CI] 3.3 to 4.5; negative likelihood ratio [−LR] 0.37, 95% CI 0.33 to 0.40).[1] The interobserver precision as measured by the κ statistic was "substantial" in most studies (0.59 to 0.77).[1]

NECK LUMP: HISTORY

INSTRUCTIONS TO CANDIDATE: A 62-year-old man presents for surgical consultation. He has a "lump" in his neck anteriorly. Obtain a detailed history, focusing on risk factors for malignancy.

DD$_X$: VITAMINS C
- **Vascular:** Carotid aneurysm
- **Infectious:** Lymphadenitis
- **Neoplastic:** Thyroid nodule, hematologic malignancy, salivary gland tumor
- **Idiopathic/iatrogenic:** Benign enlargement of the salivary gland (e.g., sialolithiasis)
- **Congenital/genetic:** Thyroglossal cyst

History
- Ask the patient the following questions:
  - **Character:** "What does the lump feel like?"
  - **Location:** "Where is the lump (point to it with one finger)?"
  - **Onset:** "When did you first notice it? How did you first come to notice it?"
  - **Intensity:** "How large is the lump? Is the size changing (getting larger or smaller or staying the same)?"
  - **Duration:** "How long has the lump been there?"

> **Box 9-1**   Features of a Thyroid Nodule Suspected for Malignancy
>
> - Age <20 or >60 years
> - Male sex
> - Rapid growth
> - Associated hoarseness or dysphagia
> - History of radiation delivered to the head or neck
> - Firm and fixed, nontender nodule
> - Nodule >2 cm
> - Associated lymphadenopathy
> - "Cold" nodule on thyroid scan
> - Complex cystic nodule
> - Family history of medullary cancer of thyroid, multiple endocrine neoplasia (MEN) type II

- Events associated (Box 9-1):
  - "Have you experienced any pain?"
  - "Have you recently had any infections?"
  - "Do you have difficulty swallowing (dysphagia)? Hoarseness?"
  - Hyperthyroidism: "Have you experienced weight loss despite increased appetite? Have you also noted heat intolerance, diarrhea, or protrusion of your eyes (exophthalmos)?"
  - Hypothyroidism: "Have you experienced weight gain despite decreased appetite? Have you also noted cold intolerance or constipation?"
  - Constitutional symptoms: "Have you had fever, chills, night sweats, weight loss, anorexia, or asthenia?"
- Frequency: "Have you ever had a lump before? If so, how many?"
- Palliative factors: "Does anything make the lump better? If so, what?"
- Provocative factors: "Does anything make the lump worse? If so, what?"
  - Eating (obstructed salivary duct)
- **Previous investigations:** Thyroid scan, biopsy
- **Past medical history (PMH)/past surgical history (PSH):** Any previous irradiation of neck, thyroid disease, lymphoma, leukemia, other malignancy, or multiple endocrine neoplasia (MEN)
- **Social history (SH):** Smoking, use of alcohol (EtOH), use of street drugs
- **Family history (FH):** Thyroid disease, medullary thyroid cancer, MEN type II (pheochromocytoma, hyperparathyroid hormone, thyroid cancer)

OSTEOPOROSIS: HISTORY

INSTRUCTIONS TO CANDIDATE: An 85-year-old woman presents after a "broken arm" with concerns about osteoporosis. Obtain a detailed history, focusing on risk factors.

Definition
- **Osteoporosis** is a disorder characterized by markedly decreased bone density or bone mass, which increases the risk of fracture (Figure 9-5).
- A **fragility fracture** is most commonly considered to be one of the wrist, hip, humerus, or vertebra. The following factors increase the risk of fragility fractures:
  - Poor overall health
  - Residence in a nursing home, especially with dementia
  - Being bed-bound or immobilized
  - Poor eyesight
  - Poor balance
  - Falls

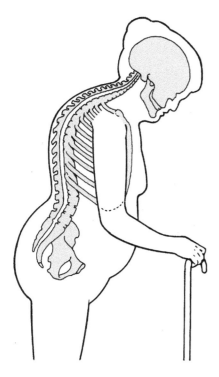

Figure 9-5 Posture of osteoporosis: dowager hump. (From Seidel HM, Ball JW, Dains JE, et al. *Mosby's Guide to Physical Examination.* 5th ed. St. Louis: Mosby; 2003 [p. 764, Figure 20-77].)

Risk Factors

- Primary osteoporosis is almost always diagnosed clinically and can be confirmed with bone densitometry. A complete assessment of the patient's risk factors is essential when the history is obtained:
  - Age: Postmenopausal
  - Female sex
  - Estrogen status: Decreased production or any postpubertal deficiency
  - Low peak bone mass: Malnutrition, genetic (multifactorial)
  - Race: White, East Asian
  - Family history: Osteoporosis or a fragility fracture in a first-degree relative
  - History of a fragility fracture as an adult
  - Lifestyle: Smoking, alcoholism
  - Diet: Inadequate calcium intake, inadequate vitamin D intake, or both
  - Physical activity: Sedentary
  - Body habitus: Low body weight, with the highest risk in thin women
- Secondary causes of osteoporosis may be approached with a "review of systems" assessment, focusing on nephrologic, hepatic, endocrine, gastrointestinal, and malignant causes.
  - Renal disease: Chronic renal failure, which impairs metabolism of vitamin D (renal osteodystrophy)
  - Hepatic disease: Chronic liver disease impairs metabolism of vitamin D
  - Endocrine disease: Hyperparathyroidism, hyperthyroidism, Cushing syndrome (endogenous or exogenous corticosteroid intake), hypogonadism, and acromegaly
  - Gastrointestinal disease: Malabsorption states (e.g., inflammatory bowel disease, celiac disease, pancreatic insufficiency), bowel resection, and long-term total parenteral nutrition (TPN)
  - Malignancy: Multiple myeloma, leukemia, lymphoma, and solid tumors (breast, thyroid, lung, colorectal)
- Medications: Corticosteroids, anticonvulsants, aluminum-containing antacids, immunosuppressants (e.g., methotrexate and cyclosporine), long-term heparin therapy

DIABETES: HISTORY AND FUNDUSCOPY

> **INSTRUCTIONS TO CANDIDATE:** A 38-year-old man with type 1 diabetes mellitus presents to his family doctor for routine evaluation. Obtain a focused history, and perform funduscopy on this patient. Describe your findings.

History
- Ask the patient the following questions:
  - **Character:** "What type of diabetes do you have (type 1, or 'juvenile diabetes')? Have you ever been admitted to the hospital for diabetes? If so, why, and what happened?"
  - **Onset:** "How old were you when you received the diagnosis of diabetes mellitus? How was it diagnosed (how did you find out)?"
  - **Intensity:** "How often do you monitor your 'blood sugars'? What are the levels? How does diabetes affect your life?"
  - **Duration:** "How long have you had diabetes?"
  - **Events associated:**
    - "Do you have episodes of hypoglycemia? How often?"
    - Symptoms of hypoglycemia: "Have you had pallor, sweating, palpitations, tremor, headache, hunger or abdominal pain, decreased level of consciousness, or fainting (syncope)?"
    - Symptoms of hyperglycemia: "Have you experienced increased urination (polyuria), increased thirst (polydipsia), fatigue, or blurred vision?"
    - Foot care: "Do you wear properly fitting shoes? Do you perform self-inspection for wounds or ulcers on your feet?"
    - "Have you ever had an episode of diabetic ketoacidosis, or 'diabetic coma'?"
    - "When did you last have a test of your hemoglobin A_{1c} (HbA_{1c})? When did you last have your lipid profile tested? When did you last have a urine screen for microalbuminuria?"
    - "When were you last assessed by an ophthalmologist, a nephrologist, or an endocrinologist?"
    - "Have you received education with a diabetes educator and a nutritionist? Do you participate in support groups?"
- Use the mnemonic **BEANN** to remember the complications of diabetes mellitus:
  - **Bugs:** Infections
  - **Eyes:** Retinopathy, cataracts, and glaucoma
  - **Arteries:** Hypertension, ischemic heart disease, peripheral vascular disease, and stroke/transient ischemic attack
  - **Nephropathy:** Microalbuminuria, renal failure
  - **Nerves:** Altered proprioception, mononeuropathies (cranial nerves III, IV, and VI), peripheral neuropathy, and autonomic neuropathy (postural hypotension, gastroparesis, impotence, urinary retention)
- **PMH/PSH:** Hypertension, nephropathy, increased cholesterol, or retinopathy
- **Medications (MEDS):** Insulin (dosage, frequency and means of delivery), angiotensin-converting enzyme (ACE) inhibitors, lipid-lowering agents, or glucocorticoids
- **SH:** Smoking, use of EtOH, use of street drugs, diet, exercise, and family/peer support
- **FH:** Diabetes mellitus, vascular disease, or endocrinopathies

Funduscopic Examination
- Patients with type 1 diabetes mellitus should be examined by an ophthalmologist within 3 to 5 years of the initial diagnosis, although it is not necessary before 10 years of age. Patients with type 2 diabetes mellitus should be examined by an ophthalmologist shortly after the initial diagnosis. Subsequent examinations should be completed yearly.

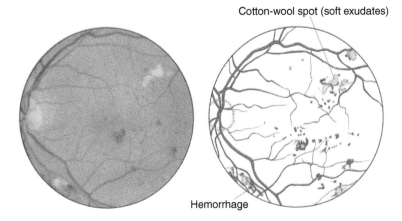

Cotton-wool spot (soft exudates)

Hemorrhage

Figure 9-6 Background retinopathy. (From Seidel HM, Ball JW, Dains JE, et al. *Mosby's Guide to Physical Examination*. 5th ed. St. Louis: Mosby; 2003 [p. 310, Figure 11-42].)

- Darken the room. The examination may be aided by dilating the pupil. Use your left eye to examine the patient's left eye. Approach the patient from the temporal side on a 15-degree angle, eliciting the red reflex. Absence of the red reflex suggests corneal opacity (e.g., cataracts). Inspect the cornea, lens, and vitreous for opacities.
- Inspect the optic discs. Compare the discs for symmetry, and note the following:
  - Clarity of the disc outline.
  - Color: Normal is yellowish orange to creamy pink.
  - Cup-to-disc ratio: Normal is <0.4.
- Inspect the retina. Follow the vessels to each of four quadrants.
  - Arteries are light red, have a bright-light reflex, and are smaller than veins.
  - Veins are dark red and do not reflect light.
  - Note exudates, hemorrhages, or other lesions.
- Inspect the macula and fovea.

Findings in Diabetic Retinopathy
- **Background retinopathy** (Figure 9-6): Microaneurysms, dot and flame hemorrhages, hard and cotton-wool exudates
- **Proliferative retinopathy:** Neovascularization on retina and on vitreous and scarring (leads to vitreous hemorrhage and retinal detachment)

HYPERTHYROIDISM: HISTORY AND PHYSICAL EXAMINATION

> **INSTRUCTIONS TO CANDIDATE: A 36-year-old woman presents to her family physician with concerns about heat intolerance and weight loss despite increased appetite. Her thyroid-stimulating hormone level is 0.07 mU/L. Obtain a focused history, and perform a focused physical examination.**

DD$_X$: VITAMINS C
- **A**utoimmune/allergic: Subacute thyroiditis, Hashimoto thyroiditis, and Graves disease (diffuse toxic goiter)
- **M**etabolic: Exogenous thyroid hormone, excessive iodine ingestion
- **I**diopathic/iatrogenic: Plummer disease (nodular toxic goiter)

History
- Ask the patient the following questions:
  - **Character:** "Can you describe how you are feeling?"
  - **Onset:** "How has this problem come about (sudden versus gradual)? When did you first notice the weight loss? Increased appetite? Heat intolerance?"
  - **Intensity:** "How much weight have you lost? Do your clothes still fit you? How severe is the heat intolerance? Do you get sweaty? Does it soak your clothes? How often do you eat? Are your symptoms getting better, getting worse, or staying the same?"

- Duration: "Over what period of time have these symptoms occurred (acute versus chronic)?"
- Events associated:
  - "Have you noticed any change in bowel habit? Diarrhea?"
  - "Have you had palpitations? Irritability? Difficulty sleeping?"
  - "Have you had any tremor or shakes? Muscle weakness (e.g., difficulty standing from a sitting position)?"
  - "Have you noticed any change in your menstrual periods (e.g., decreased duration and frequency)? What was the date of your last menstrual period (LMP)? Are you pregnant?"
  - "Do you have any swelling in your legs (pretibial myxedema)? Itching? Any eye changes (e.g., bulging)?"
  - "Have you noticed any changes in vision? Diplopia (infiltration of eye muscles in Graves disease may lead to diplopia)?"
  - Constitutional symptoms: "Have you had fever, chills, night sweats, anorexia, or asthenia?"
- Frequency: "How often do you notice these symptoms (intermittent versus constant)?"
- Palliative factors: "Does anything make this problem better? If so, what?"
- Provocative factors: "Does anything make this problem worse? If so, what?"
- **PMH/PSH:** Thyroid disease, previous radiation delivered to the neck or known radiation exposure (occupational, therapeutic), or malignancy (thyroid, MEN)
- **MEDS:** Sources of exogenous thyroid such as propylthiouracil and thyroxine
- **SH:** Smoking, use of EtOH, use of street drugs, and diet (excessive iodine)
- **FH:** Thyroid disease, MEN

Physical Examination

- **Vital signs (Vitals):** Evaluate heart rate (HR) and heart rhythm, respiratory rate (RR), blood pressure (BP), and temperature.
  - Tachycardia or atrial fibrillation may be present. Note a widened pulse pressure or fever.
- **General:** Evaluate body habitus, and check for diaphoresis and anxiety.
- **Skin:** Document any nonpitting edema (lower limb), clubbing (thyroid acropachy), excoriations, and onycholysis (Plummer's nails).
- **Head, eyes, ears, nose, and throat (HEENT):** Inspect the eyes, noting any eye protrusion, lid retraction, or lid lag. Exophthalmos is unique to Graves disease. Inspect and palpate the thyroid gland. Note size, shape, consistency, nodularity, and any tenderness. Percuss for substernal extension. Auscultate over the lateral lobes with the bell of the stethoscope to detect a bruit (hyperdynamic circulation).
- **Respiratory (Resp):** Auscultate the lungs (breath sounds, adventitious sounds).
- **Cardiovascular system (CVS):** Palpate peripheral pulses. Note pulse volume, contour, and rhythm. Auscultate the heart, listening for extra heart sounds or flow murmurs associated with hyperdynamic circulation.
- **Abdomen:** Inspect the abdomen. Auscultate for bowel sounds (sounds may be increased in hyperthyroidism). Percuss lightly in all four quadrants. Perform light and deep palpation, and identify any masses or areas of tenderness. Check for rebound tenderness. Examine the liver and spleen.
- **Neurologic (Neuro):** Inspect for tremor. Examine the reflexes (hyperreflexia may be present). Test muscle strength, especially proximal muscles (e.g., ask the patient to rise from a seated position). Examine the extraocular eye movements, noting any ophthalmoplegia. Perform a funduscopic examination, and note any papilledema.

HYPOTHYROIDISM: HISTORY AND PHYSICAL EXAMINATION

INSTRUCTIONS TO CANDIDATE: A 49-year-old woman presents to the emergency department with facial swelling and weakness. When asked about past medical problems, she admits that she used to have "low thyroid." She stopped taking her medications several months ago when her drug plan expired. Obtain a focused history, and perform a focused physical examination.

DD$_X$: VITAMINS C
- **T**raumatic: Radioactive thyroid ablation, thyroidectomy
- **A**utoimmune/**a**llergic: Hashimoto thyroiditis
- **M**etabolic: Hypopituitarism
- **I**diopathic/**i**atrogenic: Idiopathic atrophy of the thyroid

History
- Ask the patient the following questions:
  - **Character:** "Can you describe your facial swelling? What do you mean by 'weakness'? Do you mean weakness of your muscles, or fatigue, or something else?"
  - **Location:** "Where have you noticed the swelling? Around your eyes? Your whole face? Where is the weakness? Arms? Legs?"
  - **Onset:** "How did this problem come about (sudden versus gradual)? When did you first notice the swelling? When did you first notice the weakness?"
  - **Intensity:** "How swollen is your face, in comparison with normal? How weak are you? Are you able to get around? Does the weakness limit your activities? Is it getting better, getting worse, or staying the same?"
  - **Duration:** "Over what period of time have these symptoms occurred (acute versus chronic)?"
  - **Events associated:**
    - "Have you noticed any change in bowel habit? Constipation? Weight gain? Decreased appetite?"
    - "Have you noticed any sleepiness? Slowed thought or speech? Difficulty with memory?"
    - "Have you experienced any fatigue? Muscle cramps? Cold intolerance?"
    - "Have you noticed any changes in your skin or hair, such as dryness or hair loss?"
    - "Have you noticed any change in your menstrual periods (e.g., increased duration, frequency)? What was the date of your LMP? Are you pregnant?"
    - "Do you have any hand numbness or weakness (carpal tunnel syndrome)?"
  - **Frequency:** "How often do you notice these symptoms (intermittent versus constant)?"
  - **Palliative factors:** "Does anything make these symptoms better? If so, what?"
  - **Provocative factors:** "Does anything make these symptoms worse? If so, what?"
- **PMH/PSH:** Thyroid disease, any previous radiation delivered to the neck or known radiation exposure (occupational, therapeutic), thyroidectomy, diabetes mellitus, Addison disease, or pernicious anemia
- **MEDS:** Amiodarone, lithium
- **SH:** Smoking, use of EtOH, and use of street drugs
- **FH:** Thyroid disease

Physical Examination
- **Vitals:** Evaluate HR and heart rhythm, RR, BP, and temperature.
  - Bradycardia may be present. Note a narrowed pulse pressure or low temperature.
- **General:** Evaluate body habitus, and observe for dulled facial expression.
- **Skin:** Note any dry, coarse skin; yellow-red pigmentation on palms and soles (carotenemia); or brittle nails.

- **HEENT:** Inspect the hair; it may be coarse and brittle. Note loss of the lateral third of the eyebrows (Queen Anne's eyebrows). Inspect the face, noting edema around the eyes and macroglossia. Inspect and palpate the thyroid gland. Note the size, shape, consistency, nodularity, and any tenderness. Percuss for substernal extension of the thyroid. Auscultate over the lateral lobes with the bell to detect a bruit (hyperdynamic circulation).
- **Resp:** Check chest expansion (symmetry), and percussion. Auscultate the lungs (breath sounds, adventitious sounds). Note signs consistent with pleural effusion.
- **CVS:** Palpate peripheral pulses. Note pulse volume, contour, and rhythm. Auscultate the heart, listening for extra heart sounds or murmurs. Muffled heart sounds and an elevated jugular venous pressure may be suggestive of pericardial effusion.
- **Abdomen:** Inspect the abdomen. Auscultate for bowel sounds (sounds may be decreased in hypothyroidism). Percuss lightly in all four quadrants. Perform light and deep palpation, and identify any masses or areas of tenderness. Check for rebound tenderness. Examine the liver and spleen.
- **Neuro:** Inspect for tremor. Examine the reflexes. Note a slow return phase of deep tendon reflexes. Test muscle strength, and examine for carpal tunnel syndrome.

Evidence

- In patients in whom hypothyroidism is suspected on the basis of history, the physical findings most useful for detecting hypothyroidism were bradycardia (+LR 3.88; 95% CI 1.91 to 7.87), abnormal ankle reflex (+LR 3.41; 95% CI 1.81 to 6.43), and coarse, thick skin on the hands, forearms, and elbows (+LR 2.3; 95% CI 1.47 to 3.67).[2] In a study of women presenting to an endocrinology clinic, the presence of a delayed ankle reflex had a sensitivity of 77% and a specificity of 93.5% for hypothyroidism (calculated +LR 11.8).[3]

CENTRAL OBESITY AND "STRETCH MARKS": HISTORY AND PHYSICAL EXAMINATION

> **INSTRUCTIONS TO CANDIDATE:** A 53-year-old woman is referred with central obesity and "stretch marks" on her abdomen and torso. Obtain a focused history, and perform a focused physical examination.

DD$_X$: VITAMINS C

- **Metabolic:** Cushing disease (overproduction of adrenocorticotropic hormone [ACTH] by the pituitary gland), ectopic ACTH production, and exogenous corticosteroid therapy
- **Neoplastic:** Cortisol-secreting tumor or nodule

History

- Ask the patient the following questions:
  - **Character:** "What do the stretch marks look like? What color are they?"
  - **Location:** "Do you feel that you carry your weight on your midriff? What about your arms and legs? Where do you notice the stretch marks? Abdomen? Axilla?"
  - **Onset:** "When did you first notice a change in your weight or its distribution? When did you first notice the stretch marks? Under what circumstances did this come about?"
  - **Intensity:** "How much weight have you gained? How large are the stretch marks? Length? Width? Are they getting better, getting worse, or staying the same? Do they limit your activities?"
  - **Duration:** "How long have you had the stretch marks (acute versus chronic)?"
  - **Events associated:**
    - "Have you experienced muscle weakness (e.g., difficulty standing from a sitting position)?"
    - "Have you noticed any skin changes? Acne? Easy bruising? Any change in wound healing?"

- ◆ "Have you noticed any change in your menstrual periods (e.g., decreased duration, frequency)? What was the date of your LMP?"
  - ◆ "Are you more emotional than usual? Do you have increased anxiety?"
  - ◆ "Do you have any difficulty sleeping? Difficulty with memory or concentration?"
  - ◆ Symptoms of hyperglycemia: "Do you have increased urination (polyuria), increased thirst (polydipsia), fatigue, or blurred vision?"
  - ◆ "Have you had headaches? Visual disturbance (bitemporal hemianopsia)?"
  - ■ Palliative factors: "Does anything make the stretch marks better? If so, what?"
    - ▨ Provocative factors: "Does anything make the stretch marks worse? If so, what?"
- **PMH/PSH:** Pituitary adenoma, hypertension, renal colic, osteoporosis, diabetes mellitus, adrenal nodules, or steroid-dependent disease
- **MEDS:** Corticosteroids
- **SH:** Smoking, use of EtOH, use of street drugs, and diet
- **FH:** Endocrinopathy

Physical Examination
- **Vitals:** Evaluate HR and heart rhythm, RR, BP, and temperature.
  - ■ Hypertension may be present.
- **General:** Evaluate body habitus (truncal obesity, supraclavicular fat pads, "buffalo hump," wasting of arms and legs).
- **Skin:** Document hair growth (hirsutism, hypertrichosis), violaceous striae (abdomen, axilla), skin atrophy, hyperpigmentation, acne, ecchymosis, or poor wound healing.
- **HEENT:** Inspect the hair. Note any temporal balding. Inspect the face (plethoric "moon" facies).
- **Resp:** Auscultate the lungs (breath sounds, adventitious sounds).
- **CVS:** Palpate peripheral pulses. Note pulse volume, contour, and rhythm. Auscultate the heart, listening for extra heart sounds or murmurs.
- **Abdomen:** Inspect the abdomen, noting any striae. Auscultate for bowel sounds. Percuss lightly in all four quadrants. Perform light and deep palpation, and identify any masses or areas of tenderness. Check for rebound tenderness. Examine the liver and spleen.
- **Neuro:** Examine the reflexes. Inspect for muscle wasting in the thighs and arms. Test muscle strength, especially proximal muscles (e.g., ask the patient to rise from a seated position). Perform a cranial nerve examination. A macroadenoma of the pituitary gland may cause bitemporal hemianopsia as a result of compression of the optic chiasm. Perform a funduscopic examination, and note any papilledema.

SAMPLE CHECKLISTS

Thyroid Gland: Examination

INSTRUCTIONS TO CANDIDATE: Perform a physical examination of the thyroid gland.

Key Points	Satisfactorily Completed
Introduces self to the patient	❏
Determines how the patient wishes to be addressed	❏
Explains nature of the examination to the patient	❏
Examines the patient in a logical manner	❏
Inspects the thyroid gland:	
• Static	❏
• On swallowing	❏
• On tongue protrusion	❏
Palpates the thyroid gland:	
• Isthmus	❏
• Lobe margins	❏
• Movement on swallowing	❏
• Movement on protrusion of the tongue	❏
• Relaxation of sternocleidomastoid muscle	❏
• Size and symmetry	❏
• Consistency	❏
• Presence of nodules	❏
• Tenderness	❏
Uses one of the following examination techniques:	
• Bimanual technique: Anterior approach	❏
• Bimanual technique: Posterior approach	❏
Percusses for substernal thyroid	❏
Auscultates the gland for bruits	❏
Drapes the patient appropriately	❏
Makes appropriate closing remarks	❏

Extrathyroid Manifestations of Hyperthyroidism: Physical Examination

INSTRUCTIONS TO CANDIDATE: A 21-year-old woman is undergoing a workup for thyroid dysfunction. Assess this patient for extrathyroid manifestations of hyperthyroidism, and describe your findings.

Key Points	Satisfactorily Completed
Introduces self to the patient	❑
Determines how the patient wishes to be addressed	❑
Explains nature of the examination to the patient	❑
Examines the patient in a logical manner	❑
Evaluates vital signs:	
• Requests a complete set of vital sign measurements	❑
• Notes any abnormalities such as tachycardia, rhythm irregularity (atrial fibrillation), hypertension, or widened pulse pressure	❑
Evaluates eyes:	
• Conjunctival injection, chemosis (conjunctival edema)	❑
• Proptosis or exophthalmos	❑
• Periorbital edema	❑
• "Thyroid stare"	❑
• Lid lag	❑
• Asymmetry of extraocular movements (gaze palsies)	❑
Assesses skin, nails, and hair:	
• Warm, sweaty	❑
• Smooth skin (decreased keratin)	❑
• Hives (Graves disease—uncommon)	❑
• Pretibial myxedema (Graves disease—uncommon)	❑
• Onycholysis	❑
• Thyroid acropachy	❑
• Thinning of hair and vitiligo (autoimmune)	❑
Assesses mental status	❑
Drapes the patient appropriately	❑
Makes appropriate closing remarks	❑

ADVANCED SKILLS

HIRSUTISM: HISTORY

> **INSTRUCTIONS TO CANDIDATE:** A 37-year-old woman presents with concerns about increased hair growth on her body. Obtain a detailed history, exploring possible causes (Figure 9-7).

DD$_X$: VITAMINS C
- **Metabolic:** Cushing syndrome, androgen-secreting ovarian tumors, polycystic ovarian syndrome (PCOS), congenital adrenal hyperplasia (CAH), acromegaly, and drug reactions
- **Idiopathic/iatrogenic:** Obesity
- **Congenital/genetic:** Familial conditions (especially in families of Mediterranean origin)

History
- **ID:** ethnic origin
- Ask the patient the following:
  - **Character:** "What does the hair look like (coarse versus fine, pigmented versus light)?"
  - **Location:** "Where is the hair growth (face, upper arms, chest, upper abdomen, back, inner thighs, buttocks)?"
  - **Onset:** "When did the hair growth start? How has it progressed (rapid versus insidious)?"
  - **Intensity:** "How much hair is present, and how severe is it? How is it affecting your life?"
  - **Duration:** "How long has this hair growth been going on?"
  - **Events associated:**
    - Virilization (e.g., PCOS, androgen-secreting tumor): "Have you had acne, decreased frequency or cessation of menstrual periods, deepened voice, decreased breast size, male muscle pattern, temporal balding, or clitoral enlargement?"

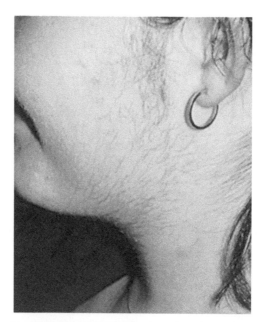

Figure 9-7 Facial hirsutism. (From Seidel HM, Ball JW, Dains JE, et al. *Mosby's Guide to Physical Examination.* 5th ed. St. Louis: Mosby; 2003 [p. 217, Figure 8-59].)

- Pituitary adenoma: "Have you had headaches, milk leaking from breasts, or changes in vision (bitemporal hemianopsia)?"
- Cushing syndrome: "Do you have truncal obesity, menstrual irregularity, rounded face (moon facies), or stretch marks (striae)?"
- Acromegaly: "Have you noticed whether your skin is thick, coarse, and oily? Do you have acne? Does your jaw protrude (prognathism)? Have your noticed increased space between your teeth? Have you noticed increases in shoe, hat, glove, or ring sizes?"
- Constitutional symptoms: "Have you had fever, chills, night sweats, weight loss, anorexia, or asthenia?"
  - Frequency: "Has this hair growth ever happened to you before? When?"
- **PMH/PSH:** PCOS, pituitary tumor, adrenal tumor, ovarian cancer, or porphyria cutanea tarda
- **MEDS:** Steroids, antihypertensives, oral contraceptive pill, androgens, or cyclosporine
- **FH:** Hirsutism, ovarian cancer, or adrenal or pituitary tumors

GALACTORRHEA: HISTORY AND PHYSICAL EXAMINATION

INSTRUCTIONS TO CANDIDATE: A 25-year-old woman presents to her family doctor with "milk" leaking from her breasts intermittently during the past month. Obtain a focused history, and perform a focused physical examination.

DD$_X$: VITAMINS C
- **M**etabolic: Drug reactions, breastfeeding, acromegaly, hypothyroidism, and Cushing syndrome
- **I**diopathic/iatrogenic: Liver failure
- **N**eoplastic: Prolactinoma, breast malignancy, paraneoplastic syndrome (ectopic prolactin secretion)
- **S**ubstance abuse/psychiatric: Pseudocyesis (false pregnancy)
- **O**ther: Pregnancy, status postpartum

History
- Ask the patient the following questions:
  - **Character:** "What is the discharge like? Describe the color, odor, and consistency of the discharge."
  - **Location:** "From where does the discharge come? The areola? Another location? From one or both breasts?"
  - **Onset:** "How did the discharge begin (suddenly versus gradually)?"
  - **Intensity:** "How much discharge do you notice daily? Does it leak through your clothes? Is it getting better, getting worse, or staying the same? Does it limit your activities?"
  - **Duration:** "How long has this discharge been going on (acute versus chronic)?"
  - **Events associated:**
    - "Do you have any rashes or ulcers on the breasts? Any redness or pain?"
    - "Have you found any lumps on breast self-examination?"
    - "What was the date of your LMP? Are you pregnant? Have you recently had a baby?"
    - "Do you have decreased libido? Infertility?"
    - "Have you had headaches? Visual disturbance (bitemporal hemianopsia)?"
    - Constitutional symptoms: "Have you had fever, chills, night sweats, weight loss, anorexia, or asthenia?"
  - **Frequency:** "Have you ever had such discharge before? If so, when? Does it happen every day (intermittent versus constant)?"
  - **Palliative factors:** "Does anything lessen the discharge? If so, what?"
  - **Provocative factors:** "Does anything make the discharge worse? If so, what?"
    - Breast stimulation

- **PMH/PSH:** Breast or thoracic surgery, breast cancer, endocrine disease, pregnancy, or pseudocyesis
- **MEDS:** Hormones, antipsychotics, antidepressants, antihypertensives, methyldopa, herbs and "natural" medicines
- **SH:** Smoking, use of EtOH, use of street drugs, and sexual practices
- **FH:** Breast cancer, endocrine disease

Physical Examination
- **Vitals:** Evaluate HR, RR, BP, and temperature.
- **General:** Evaluate body habitus and distribution of body hair.
- **Skin:** Assess skin quality (dry/oily), and check for hyperpigmentation, acne, and hirsutism.
- **Lymphatic system:** Examine lymph nodes in the head, neck, and axilla. Note size, shape, mobility, consistency, tenderness, warmth, and number of enlarged nodes.
- **HEENT:** Examine the thyroid gland (see pp. 264-265).
- **Resp:** Auscultate the lungs (breath sounds, adventitious sounds).
- **CVS:** Palpate peripheral pulses. Note pulse volume, contour, and rhythm. Auscultate the heart, listening for extra heart sounds or flow murmurs associated with hyperdynamic circulation.
- **Abdomen:** Inspect the abdomen. Auscultate for bowel sounds. Percuss lightly in all four quadrants. Perform light and deep palpation, and identify any masses or areas of tenderness. Check for rebound tenderness. Examine the liver and spleen.
- **Neuro:** Perform a cranial nerve examination with attention to cranial nerves II, III, IV, and VI. A macroadenoma of the pituitary gland may cause bitemporal hemianopsia as a result of compression of the optic chiasm. Perform a funduscopic examination, and note any papilledema.
- **Gynecologic (Gyne):** Perform a thorough examination of the breasts (see pp. 304-306 in Chapter 11). Note any discharge, skin changes, masses, or tenderness.

SAMPLE CHECKLISTS

Hypocalcemia: Assessment

> **INSTRUCTIONS TO CANDIDATE:** A young woman with Graves disease opts to have a thyroidectomy. On her second postoperative day, you are called to her bedside to assess her for signs and symptoms of hypocalcemia. Perform a focused assessment, and describe your findings.

Key Points	Satisfactorily Completed
Introduces self to the patient	❑
Determines how the patient wishes to be addressed	❑
Explains nature of the examination to the patient	❑
Examines the patient in a logical manner	❑
Asks about the following:	
• Fatigue	❑
• Perioral numbness	❑
• Acral paresthesias	❑
• Muscle cramps	❑
• Muscle spasms	❑
• Seizures	❑
Evaluates vital signs:	
• Requests a complete set of vital sign measurements	❑
• Notes any abnormalities, particularly with respiratory rate	❑
Inspects for the following:	
• Diaphoresis	❑
• Posture of hands and feet	❑
Evaluates for Trousseau's sign:	
• Inflates sphygmomanometer above systolic blood pressure for 3 minutes	❑
• Observes for carpopedal spasm (Figure 9-8)	❑
Evaluates for Chvostek's sign:	
• Taps the facial nerve (anterior to the ear)	❑
• Observes for contraction of ipsilateral facial musculature	❑
Performs funduscopy, looking for papilledema	❑
Assesses mental status (anxiety, confusion, hallucinations)	❑
Drapes the patient appropriately	❑
Makes appropriate closing remarks	❑

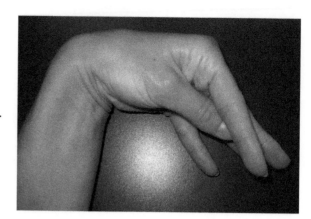

Figure 9-8 Carpopedal spasm.

Addison's Disease: Physical Examination

INSTRUCTIONS TO CANDIDATE: A 28-year-old man is referred for assessment of Addison's disease. Perform a focused physical examination, and describe your findings.

Key Points	Satisfactorily Completed
Introduces self to the patient	❏
Determines how the patient wishes to be addressed	❏
Explains nature of the examination to the patient	❏
Examines the patient in a logical manner	❏
Evaluates vital signs:	
• Requests a complete set of vital sign measurements, including postural heart rate and blood pressure	❏
• Notes any abnormalities such as tachycardia, hypotension, or postural variation	❏
Assesses for increased pigmentation in the following:	
• Sun-exposed areas (face, neck, dorsal surface of hands)	❏
• Pressure or friction areas (elbows, knees, spine, shoulders, knuckles, waist)	❏
• Palmar creases	❏
• Areolae, axillae, perineum, umbilicus	❏
• Scars (if acquired during untreated adrenal insufficiency)	❏
• Mucous membranes	❏
Assesses for vitiligo (present in autoimmune adrenal insufficiency)	❏
Assesses mental status	❏
Drapes the patient appropriately	❏
Makes appropriate closing remarks	❏

Acromegaly: Physical Examination of the Head, Neck, and Skin

INSTRUCTIONS TO CANDIDATE: A 62-year-old man with acromegaly presents to his endocrinologist for follow-up evaluation. Examine the head, neck, and extremities for clinical signs associated with this condition. Describe your findings.

Key Points	Satisfactorily Completed
Introduces self to the patient	❏
Determines how the patient wishes to be addressed	❏
Explains nature of the examination to the patient	❏
Examines the patient in a logical manner	❏
Evaluates skin and soft tissues:	
• Thick and coarse skin	❏
• Oily, sweaty skin	❏
• Increased body hair	❏
• Acanthosis nigricans	❏
• Acne	❏
Evaluates head and neck:	
• Prognathism	❏
• Increased space between the teeth	❏
• Large nose	❏
• Prominent supraorbital ridge (frontal bossing)	❏
• Large tongue (macroglossia)	❏
• Deepened voice	❏
• Assess visual fields (bitemporal hemianopsia)	❏
Examines the thyroid gland for enlargement	❏
Evaluates the musculoskeletal system:	
• Inspects hands and feet, noting enlargement (increased shoe, glove, and ring sizes)	❏
• Inspects for thenar atrophy	❏
• Performs thumb abduction test	❏
• Performs Phalen's test	❏
• Percusses volar aspect of wrist (Tinel's sign)	❏
Drapes the patient appropriately	❏
Makes appropriate closing remarks	❏

REFERENCES

1 Siminoski K. The rational clinical examination: does this patient have a goiter? *JAMA.* 1995;273:813-817.
2 Indra R, Patil SS, Joshi R, et al. Accuracy of physical examination in the diagnosis of hypothyroidism: a cross-sectional, double-blind study. *J Postgrad Med.* 2004;50:7-11; discussion, 11.
3 Zulewski H, Müller B, Exer P, et al. Estimation of tissue hypothyroidism by a new clinical score: evaluation of patients with various grades of hypothyroidism and controls. *J Clin Endocrinol Metab.* 1997;82:771-776.

CHAPTER 10

Psychiatry

GLOSSARY OF SIGNS AND SYMPTOMS

Perception
- A **hallucination** is a subjective sensory perception in the absence of an external stimulus. Such perceptions can be visual, auditory, gustatory (taste), or olfactory in nature. **Hypnagogic** and **hypnopompic** hallucinations occur on falling asleep and waking, respectively, and are not considered pathologic.
- **Formication** is a tactile hallucination of insects crawling on or under the skin.
- An **illusion** is the misperception of an actual external stimulus (e.g., mistaking a billowing curtain for a person).
- **Depersonalization** is a state in which a person loses the sense of his or her own identity in relation to others and their environment.
- **Derealization** is a state in which a person perceives his or her environment and ordinarily familiar things as strange or unreal.

Thought Content
- A **delusion** is a fixed, false belief not shared by other individuals of the same religious or cultural background. Some common delusions are **delusions of reference** (delusional belief that insignificant comments, objects, or events have special meaning or reference to the patient), **delusions of grandeur** (delusional belief of a special talent, power, or identity), and **delusions of persecution** (delusional belief that one is being followed, monitored, or conspired against in some way by others).
- **Thought broadcasting** is the delusional belief that one's thoughts are being broadcast and can be heard by others.
- **Thought insertion** is the delusional belief that one's thoughts are not one's own, having been placed or inserted into one's mind by an external person or force.

- An **obsession** is a recurrent, intrusive thought, idea, or impulse that cannot be voluntarily suppressed.

Thought Process
- **Circumstantiality** is a disturbance in thought process evident when speech takes a circuitous route: the speaker provides excessive detail (circumstances) before finally getting to the point.
- **Tangentiality** is a disturbance in thought process evident when speech takes a tangential route: the speaker provides detail about associated thoughts as they arise, without ever reaching the point.

Affect
- **Affect** is the emotional state of an individual as observed or perceived by others, whereas **mood** is the emotional state as experienced and reported by the individual.
- **Anhedonia** is lack of pleasure in performing activities that are normally enjoyable.

Negative Symptoms
- **Avolition** is the inability to perform goal-directed activities.
- **Alogia** is poverty of speech.
- **Flat affect** is the complete lack of emotional expression, as if one is conversing with an inanimate object.

Miscellaneous
- **La belle indifference** is typically noted in conversion disorder. It is an inappropriate lack of emotion or concern about one's own disability or affliction.
- A **compulsion** is an uncontrollable impulse to perform an act, often repetitively, as a means of neutralizing anxiety caused by obsessive thoughts.

ESSENTIAL SKILLS

APPROACH TO COMPREHENSIVE PSYCHIATRIC ASSESSMENT

Starting the Interview
- Start the interview by introducing yourself to the patient and stating your role in his or her evaluation and subsequent care.
- It may be helpful to tell the patient how long you expect the interview to last.
- Confirm the identity of the patient, and determine how the patient would like to be addressed.
- Start the interview in an open-ended manner (e.g., "So tell me, what brings you in here today?"), and allow the patient to speak uninterrupted or with minimal prompting for the first 5 to 10 minutes (for a 45- to 60-minute interview).
- Be sure that there is a clear path between you and the door (means of escape as necessary) and between the patient and the door (do not be caught between a bolting patient and his or her means of escape).
- In the interest of safety, do not wear things around your neck, such as a stethoscope or identification badge.

History
- **ID:** Verify the age, sex, source, and reliability of the historian.
- **History of presenting illness:** Review the patient's current concerns and associated symptoms in detail. You may need to seek supplemental information from family members, friends, neighbors, or police.
- Ask the patient the following questions:
  - **Character:** "Can you characterize your main concern or reason for assessment, in your own words?"

- Onset: "When did the problem begin? Did it start suddenly or gradually?"
- Intensity: "How severe is the problem now? Is it getting worse or improving? Has it been constant or intermittent? How does it affect your activities of daily living (e.g., ability to work or function at home)? Have you been hospitalized for your symptoms?"
- Duration: "How long has this been going on (acute versus chronic)? If episodic, how long does it last?"
- Events associated: "Can you describe any particular events associated with the onset of symptoms?"
- Frequency: "How often does this problem occur? When was the last time this happened?"
- Palliative factors: "Does anything make the problem better? If so, what (e.g., coping strategies, medications)?"
- Provocative factors: "Does anything make the problem worse? If so, what (e.g., stressors, poor adherence to medication regimens)?"

Psychiatric Symptom Screen

- When screening for symptoms that may carry a stigma, such as delusions and hallucinations, it may be helpful to put the symptom in context and "normalize" it before asking the question. For example, "Some people tell me that when they watch television, they get special messages from God. Have you ever experienced something like that?"
  - Depression is characterized by depressed mood and the elements of the acronym **SIGE CAPS:**
    - **S**leeplessness
    - **L**oss of **i**nterest
    - **G**uilt
    - Decreased **e**nergy
    - Inability to **c**oncentrate
    - Loss of **a**ppetite
    - **P**sychomotor retardation ("Do you feel as if you are slowed down?")
    - **S**uicidal ideation
  - Mania is characterized by the elements of the acronym **ImPAIRED:**
    - **Im**pulsivity
    - **P**ressured speech
    - Increased **a**ctivity
    - **I**nsomnia
    - **R**acing thoughts
    - **E**steem inflation
    - **D**istractibility
  - Psychosis is characterized by the following behaviors or elements:
    - Hallucinations ("Do you ever see things or hear things that other people do not see or hear? Do you ever feel as if something is crawling or creeping on your skin?")
    - Delusions ("How do you get along with other people? Do you have trouble trusting others? Do you ever feel as if people are talking about you or laughing at you behind your back? Do you feel as if anyone or anything is out to get you? Do you ever get special messages while watching TV or reading the newspaper that are intended especially for you? Do you ever get the sense that other people can read your thoughts? Or that thoughts are being inserted into your mind against your will?")
    - Negative symptoms: flat affect, alogia, and avolition
    - Disorganized speech
  - Anxiety may be underlying the following conditions:
    - Panic attacks
    - Obsessions and compulsions ("Are you ever bothered by persistent thoughts that you cannot get out of your mind? What do you do about it? Do you ever

feel the need to repeat certain activities over and over again even though you do not want to?")
- ◆ Recent traumatic event (post-traumatic stress disorder)
- ▪ Suicidal thoughts
- ▪ Homicidal thoughts
- ▪ Substance abuse or dependence: Start with an open-ended question such as "Tell me about your drinking." Establish amount and frequency of alcohol consumption and other recreational drugs. Administer the **CAGE** questionnaire as a screen for alcohol abuse or dependence. Two or more affirmative answers represent a positive screening test:
  - ◆ **C**ut down: "Have you ever tried to cut down on your drinking?"
  - ◆ **A**nnoyed by criticism: "Are you annoyed by criticism about your drinking?"
  - ◆ **G**uilty about drinking: "Do you ever feel guilty about drinking?"
  - ◆ **E**ye-opener: "Do you ever need to drink first thing in the morning (eye opener)?"
- **Past psychiatric history:** Past psychiatric diagnoses and treatments (age at onset), past psychiatric admissions (quantify), most recent admission to hospital, and past suicide attempts (quantify attempts that necessitated medical evaluation and hospitalization, and ascertain the means or method)
- **Past medical history (PMH)/past surgical history (PSH):** Previous surgeries, current and past medical problems
- **Medications (MEDS):** All current medications (over-the-counter drugs, herbal or "natural" remedies, and prescription medications)
- **Allergies**
- **Social history (SH):** Smoking, use of alcohol (EtOH), use of street drugs, and sexual history
- **Family history (FH):** Psychiatric illnesses, medical illnesses (it is useful to draw a small pedigree, including grandparents, parents, siblings, and children)
- **Review of systems (ROS):** Common symptoms in each major body system

Psychosocial History
- Ask the patient the following questions:
  - ▪ "Where were you born and raised?"
  - ▪ "Were there any problems that you know of with your mother's pregnancy with you or with your delivery?"
  - ▪ "Did you reach developmental milestones (such as walking and talking) on time?"
  - ▪ "Whom did you feel close to while you were growing up?"
  - ▪ "What was your family like?"
  - ▪ "Was there any violence in your home?"
  - ▪ "When did you start school? Did you like school? Did you have any troubles in school (e.g., needing to repeat a grade)?"
  - ▪ "What were you like as a child? As a teenager?"
  - ▪ "Do you have any children of your own? How would you describe your relationship with your children?"
  - ▪ "How would you describe your relationship with your family (siblings, parents, and grandparents) now?"
  - ▪ "Do you have any close relationships right now? Tell me about that."
  - ▪ "Are you or have you been married? How would you describe your marriage?"
  - ▪ "Where do you live now? What is your home like?"
  - ▪ "Are you working right now? Tell me about your job or your trade."
  - ▪ "What kinds of jobs have you had in the past?"
  - ▪ "What kinds of things do you do for fun?"
  - ▪ "How satisfied are you with your life right now?"

Box 10-1   Outline for the Mental Status Examination

- General appearance
- Behavior
- Speech
- Affect and mood
- Thought content
- Thought process
- Perceptual disturbances
- Judgment
- Insight
- Orientation

Mental Status Examination

- The mental status examination begins as soon as you enter the room to begin the encounter with the patient. The majority of the data can be gleaned during the interview from observation alone, rather than direct questioning (Box 10-1).
- Observe the patient's **appearance,** noting hygiene, makeup, jewelry, clothing, body habitus, and any distinctive physical features.
- Characterize, the patient's **behavior,** noting body language (e.g., elaborate hand gestures), mannerisms (e.g., lip smacking), attentiveness, and psychomotor retardation or agitation. Note whether the patient appears to be responding to cues in the room (e.g., visual or auditory hallucinations).
- Observe the rate and volume of **speech.** The way the patient talks to you and responds to your questions may be equally as important as the content of his or her speech.
- Note the range and stability of the patient's **affect.** Describe the affect (an observed phenomenon) and its intensity (e.g., flat versus inflated). Elicit the patient's description of his or her **mood,** and note whether it is congruent with your observations.
- The **thought content** of the patient is inferred from the content of his or her speech. Note any delusions, obsessions, phobias, and thoughts of suicide or homicide.
- Ideas about **thought process** also are inferred from the patient's speech. Note whether the patient's speech appears to be coherent and follows a logical progression. Characterize the speech for tangentiality, circumstantiality, loose associations, and perseveration.
- Note any **hallucinations** reported by the patient or any apparent hallucinations experienced by the patient during your encounter.
- Assess **judgment** by asking the patient to respond to some questions. For example, ask the patient what he or she would do if he or she woke up in his or her home and found it to be on fire. Other such scenarios could be used instead, if preferred.
- Document whether the patient appears to have any **insight** into his or her illness or current problem.
- Assess the patient's **cognition.** At minimum, determine whether the patient is **oriented** to person, place, and time. A more detailed assessment of cognition would include administering the Folstein Mini-Mental State Examination (see pp. 368-369).

Evidence

- With a cutoff score of ≥2, the sensitivity of CAGE ranges from 43% to 100% (mean 71%), and the specificity ranges from 61% to 97% (mean 90%) across various populations.[1] The CAGE questionnaire is not useful as a screen for less severe forms of alcohol abuse. It is not adequately sensitive when used in particular populations (white women, pregnant women, and college students).[1]

SUICIDAL IDEATION: HISTORY

> **INSTRUCTIONS TO CANDIDATE: A 19-year-old woman is brought to the emergency department by the police. Her father called the police when he found that she had written a suicide note. Obtain a detailed history.**

Collateral History

- Ask the police about their interaction with the patient. Is she known to them? Did they find any pill bottles or weapons in the home? Did they bring the suicide note?
- Ask the father about the suicide note and its content. Did it state any plan? Where did he find it? Was there an argument or some type of confrontation? Has this ever happened before? Ask the father to describe stressors in the home, and ask whether he is aware of anything new.
- Establish whether any guns are in the home.

History

- Ask the patient the following questions:
  - **Character:** "Tell me what happened. Why are you here? Did you take any pills or do something else to harm yourself today? What were you planning to do? Were you planning to kill yourself?"
  - **Onset:** "When did you first start thinking about suicide? Did some particular event or stressor bring on those thoughts?"
  - **Intensity:** "How severe are your suicidal thoughts now? Have they been constant or intermittent? How do they affect your activities of daily living (e.g., ability to work, function at home)? Have you ever been hospitalized for a suicide attempt or for psychiatric evaluation?"
  - **Duration:** "How long have these thoughts been going on (acute versus chronic)?"
  - **Events associated:**
    - "How did today's events come about (planned in advance or impulsive)?"
    - "How are things at home? How are things at school? At work? How are things with your relationships?"
    - "Why did you want to kill yourself?"
    - "Are you still thinking about killing yourself? By what means?" It is important to be direct in your questioning on this manner and to determine whether the patient has a suicide plan.
  - **Frequency:** "Has this ever happened before? If so, when?"
  - **Palliative factors:** "Does anything make your state of mind better? If so, what (e.g., coping strategies, medications)?"
  - **Provocative factors:** "Does anything make your state of mind worse? If so, what (e.g., stressors, poor adherence to medication regimens)?"
- Assessment of suicidal risk with the modified **SAD PERSONS** scale, on which a score of ≥6 points to the need for emergency psychiatric evaluation or treatment, or both[2]:

Sex: male	1
Age: <19 or >45 years	1
Depression	2
Previous attempts	1
EtOH	1
Rational thinking loss	2
Separated, divorced, or widowed	1
Organized plan	2
No social support	1
Stated future intent	2

- Assessment of suicidal risk with the **Manchester Self-Harm Rule,** on which satisfaction of all criteria categorizes the patient as being at "low risk"[3]:
  - No history of self-harm
  - No prior psychiatric treatment
  - No current psychiatric treatment
  - No use of benzodiazepines in current attempt
- **Psychiatric symptom screen** (perform as outlined in the section "Approach to Comprehensive Psychiatric Assessment"; see pp. 285-286)
- **Past psychiatric history:** Past psychiatric diagnoses and treatments (age at onset), past psychiatric admissions (quantify), most recent admission to hospital, and past suicide attempts (quantify attempts that necessitated medical evaluation and hospitalization, and ascertain the means or method)
- **PMH/PSH:** Any illnesses that necessitated hospital admission or surgery; endocrine disease
- **MEDS:** Antidepressants, steroids, anxiolytics, antipsychotics, other medications
- **Allergies**
- **SH:** Smoking, use of EtOH, use of street drugs, and sexual history
- **FH:** Psychiatric illnesses, suicide, or medical illnesses
- **ROS:** Common symptoms in each major body system

Involuntary Commitment

- Suicidal patients who refuse treatment or hospitalization may need to be kept in the hospital involuntarily (certified) for their own safety. Although this is considered an acceptable intervention for acutely suicidal patients, involuntary hospitalization has not been proved to prevent future suicide.
- Laws surrounding involuntary commitment vary from province to province and from state to state; therefore, be aware of the laws in your region and the policies at your institution.
- In general, patients must have a mental illness and be deemed a danger to themselves or to others (some jurisdictions also include risk of harm to property) to be committed involuntarily.
- Patients who are certified but retain decision-making capacity (see Chapter 14, pp. 387-388) cannot be treated against their wishes.

Evidence

- Scoring systems such as the modified SAD PERSONS scale or the Manchester Self-Harm Rule are based on risk factors gleaned from population-based studies.[2,3] In practice, these "rules" are applied to individuals, but there "has not been any research which has indicated that suicide can be predicted or prevented in any individual."[4]

Pearls

- Most completed suicides are committed with guns. The presence of a gun in the household is an independent risk factor for suicide, especially among adolescents.[5,6]
- Most suicide attempts are executed with ingested toxins.[7]

MANIA: HISTORY

> **INSTRUCTIONS TO CANDIDATE:** A 39-year-old man, known to have bipolar disorder, is brought to the emergency department by his sister because he has stopped taking his medications. He has missed work for the past 3 days because he has been working fervently on projects at home. Obtain a detailed history.

DD$_X$

- Bipolar disorder
- Acute psychosis
- Cyclothymia
- Substance ingestion or withdrawal
- Schizoaffective disorder

Collateral History

- Ask the patient's sister the following questions:
  - "What about your brother's behavior worries you? What type of projects is he working on? Does he sleep?"
  - "How would you describe his mood?"
  - "How long has he been off his medications?"
  - "Have you noticed any changes in his speech?"

History

- Ask the patient the following questions:
  - **Character:** "Tell me what brings you here today. Are you here voluntarily? How are things going at home? At work?"
  - **Duration:** "Your sister is concerned about the projects you are working on. How long has this activity been going on (acute versus chronic)?"
  - **Events associated:**
    - "Have you missed work recently? Why? What have you been doing instead? Are you worried that you might lose your job?"
    - "Tell me your plans for these home projects you are working on."
    - "Have you been doing anything outside of the home?"
    - "Your sister is concerned that you have stopped taking your pills. Is this true? How long have you been off your medication? What do you normally take (include dosing schedule)?"
    - "How would you describe your mood now?"
  - **Frequency:** "Has this ever happened before? When?"
  - **Palliative factors:** "Does anything make your state of mind better? If so, what (e.g., coping strategies, medications)?"
  - **Provocative factors:** "Does anything make your state of mind worse? If so, what (e.g., stressors, poor adherence to medication regimens)?"
- Mania: Use the **ImPAIRED** acronym.
  - **Im**pulsivity ("Have you made any big decisions recently, such as a significant purchase, investment or relationship?")
  - **P**ressured speech ("Do you feel as though you are speaking fast? Do you feel the need to speak faster?")
  - Increased **a**ctivity ("Have you taken on any new projects or tasks recently? Do you find it hard to sit still?")
  - **I**nsomnia ("Do you need less sleep than usual?")
  - **R**acing thoughts ("Do you feel as if your thoughts are racing?")
  - **E**steem inflation ("Do you feel more self-confident than usual? Do you have any special talents or abilities?")
  - **D**istractibility
- **Psychiatric symptom screen** (perform as outlined in the "Approach to Comprehensive Psychiatric Assessment" section; see pp. 285-286)

- **Past psychiatric history:** Past psychiatric diagnoses and treatments (age at onset), past psychiatric admissions (quantify), most recent admission to hospital, and past suicide attempts (quantify attempts that necessitated medical evaluation and hospitalization, and ascertain the means or method)
- **PMH/PSH:** Any illnesses that necessitated hospital admission or surgery; endocrine disease
- **MEDS:** Antidepressants, mood stabilizers, steroids, anxiolytics, antipsychotics, other medications
- **Allergies**
- **SH:** Smoking, use of EtOH, use of street drugs, and sexual history
- **FH:** Bipolar disorder, other psychiatric disease, suicide, or medical illnesses
- **ROS:** Common symptoms in each major body system

Pearls
- Bipolar disorder is a lifelong illness punctuated by episodic deteriorations.
- Judgment is often impaired in acute manic episodes.

ANXIETY: HISTORY

> **INSTRUCTIONS TO CANDIDATE:** A 52-year-old woman presents to her family doctor with "anxiety." She says she just "worries about everything." She is requesting a tranquilizer to help her sleep. Obtain a detailed history.

DD$_X$
- Generalized anxiety disorder
- Panic disorder
- Agoraphobia
- Obsessive-compulsive disorder (OCD)
- Posttraumatic stress disorder (PTSD)
- Adjustment disorder
- Anxiety secondary to a general medical condition
- Anxiety secondary to substance use
- Drug seeking

History
- Ask the patient the following questions:
  - Character: "What brings you here today? What are your major worries? What kinds of things do you worry about? What is making you seek medical attention right now?"
  - Onset: "When did this trouble with anxiety start up?"
  - Intensity: "How severe is the anxiety now? Is it constant or intermittent? Is it getting better, getting worse, or staying the same? How does it affect your activities of daily living (e.g., ability to work, function at home)? Have you ever been hospitalized for it?"
  - Duration: "How long has this been going on (acute versus chronic)?"
  - Events associated:
    - "How are things going at home? At work? With your relationships?"
    - "Have you experienced any stressful events recently?"
    - "Tell me about a typical day for you. Do you go out to grocery shop? Do you go out to socialize? Do you avoid certain types of situations to get around your anxiety?"
    - "Have you ever had panic attacks?"
    - "How would you describe your mood?"
  - Frequency: "Have you ever had this trouble before? When? How often?"
  - Palliative factors: "Does anything make the anxiety better? If so, what (e.g., coping strategies, medications)?"

Box 10-2   Predictors of Anxiety with Organic Origin

- Onset of anxiety after age 35 years
- Lack of a personal or family history of anxiety disorder
- Lack of a childhood history of significant anxiety, phobia, or separation anxiety
- Absence of significant life events that would generate or exacerbate symptoms of anxiety
- Lack of avoidance behaviors
- Poor response to anxiolytics

Adapted from Marx JA, Hockberger RS, Walls RM, eds. *Rosen's Emergency Medicine: Concepts and Clinical Practice.* 5th ed. St. Louis: Mosby; 2002 [p. 1558].

Box 10-3   Some Organic Causes of Anxiety

- Myocardial infarction
- Tachyarrhythmia
- Hyperthyroidism
- Pheochromocytoma
- Pulmonary emboli
- Seizure disorders (e.g., temporal lobe epilepsy)
- Alcohol withdrawal, benzodiazepine withdrawal
- Drug intoxication

- **Provocative factors:** "Does anything make the anxiety worse? If so, what (e.g., stressors, particular situations or thoughts, poor adherence to medication regimens)?"
- **Psychiatric symptom screen** (perform as outlined in the "Approach to Comprehensive Psychiatric Assessment" section; see pp. 285-286).
- **Past psychiatric history:** Past psychiatric diagnoses and treatments (age at onset), past psychiatric admissions (quantify), most recent admission to hospital, and past suicide attempts (quantify attempts that necessitated medical evaluation and hospitalization, and ascertain the means or method)
- **PMH/PSH:** Any illnesses that necessitated hospital admission or surgery; endocrine disease
- **MEDS:** Antidepressants, mood stabilizers, steroids, anxiolytics, antipsychotics, other medications
- **Allergies**
- **SH:** Smoking, use of EtOH, use of street drugs, and sexual history
- **FH:** Anxiety disorder, other psychiatric disease, or suicide
- **ROS:** Common symptoms in each major body system

Pearl

- Anxiety disorders may manifest with symptoms of physical disease, and organic disease may manifest with symptoms of anxiety. Box 10-2 lists predictors of anxiety of organic origin, and Box 10-3 lists some items to consider in the differential diagnosis of organic anxiety.

PSYCHOSIS: HISTORY

INSTRUCTIONS TO CANDIDATE: A 49-year-old man is brought into the emergency department by a friend because he has "nowhere else to go." He has recently quit his job, sold all of his things, and given up his apartment. He was going to travel to another city to stay with family but could not get on the bus because it was "infested with bugs." He wanted to leave town to get away from the infestation. Obtain a detailed history.

DD$_X$
- Brief psychotic disorder
- Schizophrenia
- Bipolar disorder
- Psychosis secondary to a medical condition
- Substance ingestion or withdrawal
- Schizoaffective disorder
- Organic brain syndrome

Collateral History
- Ask the patient's friend the following questions:
  - "Tell me what has been going on with your friend. How long have you known him?"
  - "When did you first notice this change in his behavior? How long has he been concerned about bugs? Has he had any other strange concerns?"
  - "Has this ever happened before?"
  - "Are you aware of whether he has any psychiatric or medical problems?"
  - "Does he drink alcohol or use recreational drugs?"

History
- Ask the patient the following questions:
  - **Character:** "What brings you here today? Are you here voluntarily? How are things going at home? At work?"
  - **Onset:** "When did you first start noticing the bug infestation? How did you come to notice it?"
  - **Duration:** "How long have you been concerned about this infestation (acute versus chronic)?"
  - **Events associated:**
    - "Did you quit your job? Why? Were there any bugs in your workplace?"
    - "What happened with your apartment? Why were you leaving town?"
    - "Were there bugs in your apartment? What did you do to get rid of them?"
    - "How would you describe your mood now?"
    - "Have you been sleeping? How much?"
    - "Do you ever see or hear things that other people do not see or hear?"
    - "Do you ever feel like there is something crawling or creeping on your skin?"
    - "Do you ever get special messages while watching TV or reading the newspaper that are intended especially for you?"
    - "Do you feel as if anyone or anything is out to get you?"
    - "Do you ever get the sense that other people can read your thoughts? Or that thoughts are being inserted into your mind against your will?"
  - **Frequency:** "Has this ever happened before? When?"
  - **Palliative factors:** "Does anything alleviate your concerns about the bugs? If so, what (e.g., coping strategies, medications)?"
  - **Provocative factors:** "Does anything make you more concerned? If so, what (e.g., stressors, poor adherence to medication regimens)?"

- **Orientation** to person, place, and time (assess)
- **Psychiatric symptom screen** (perform as outlined in the "Approach to Comprehensive Psychiatric Assessment" section; see pp. 285-286).
- **Past psychiatric history:** Past psychiatric diagnoses and treatments (age at onset), past psychiatric admissions (quantify), most recent admission to hospital, and past suicide attempts (quantify attempts that necessitated medical evaluation and hospitalization, and ascertain the means or method)
- **PMH/PSH:** Any illnesses that necessitated hospital admission or surgery; endocrine disease
- **MEDS:** Antidepressants, mood stabilizers, steroids, anxiolytics, antipsychotics, other medications
- **Allergies**
- **SH:** Smoking, use of EtOH, use of street drugs, and sexual history
- **FH:** Schizophrenia, bipolar disorder, other psychiatric disease, or suicide
- **ROS:** Common symptoms in each major body system

Pearl

- Psychosis can be caused by organic brain syndrome (Table 10-1). The organic causes of psychosis include (but are not limited to) central nervous system tumor or infection, electrolyte disturbances, toxic ingestion, and drug withdrawal.

Table 10-1 Differentiating Organic from Functional Psychosis

"MAD FOCS" Mnemonic	Organic	Functional
Memory deficits	Recent impairment	Remote impairment
Activity	Psychomotor retardation	Repetitive activity
	Tremor	Posturing
	Ataxia	Rocking
Distortions	Visual hallucinations	Auditory hallucinations
Feelings	Emotional lability	Flat affect
Orientation	Disoriented	Oriented
Cognition	Islands of lucidity	Continuous scattered thoughts
	Attends occasionally	Unable to attend (focus)
		Unfiltered perceptions
Some other findings	Age >40 years	Age <40 years
	Sudden onset	Gradual onset
	Abnormal physical examination	Normal physical examination
	Abnormal vital signs	Normal vital signs
	Social immodesty	Social modesty
	Aphasia	Intelligible speech
	Impaired consciousness	Awake and alert

Adapted from Marx JA, Hockberger RS, Walls RM, eds. *Rosen's Emergency Medicine: Concepts and Clinical Practice.* 5th ed. St. Louis: Mosby; 2002 [p. 1544].

SAMPLE CHECKLISTS

Depression: History

> **INSTRUCTIONS TO CANDIDATE: A 33-year-old man presents for evaluation of depression. Obtain a focused history.**

Key Points	Satisfactorily Completed
Introduces self to the patient	❏
Determines how the patient wishes to be addressed	❏
Washes hands	❏
Explains the purpose of the encounter	❏
Develops good patient rapport	❏
Asks about depressed mood:	❏
• Inquires about sleep patterns (**s**leeplessness or hypersomnia)	❏
• Asks about normal daily activities (loss of **i**nterest)	❏
• Asks about feelings of **g**uilt or worthlessness	❏
• Inquires about level of energy (decreased **e**nergy)	❏
• Asks about inability to **c**oncentrate	❏
• Asks about changes in **a**ppetite and weight	❏
• Observes for **p**sychomotor retardation or agitation	❏
Asks about suicidal ideation:	
• "Do you feel like life is not worth living?"	❏
• "Have you thought about killing yourself?"	❏
• "Do you have any suicide plan?"	❏
Asks about duration of symptoms	❏
Asks about effect of symptoms on daily activities (severity)	❏
Asks about recent events and stressors	❏
Asks about social supports	❏
Asks about past psychiatric problems	❏
Asks about history of medical or surgical problems	❏
Prescription medications:	
• Asks about adherence to prescribed therapies	❏
Asks about use of alcohol and recreational drugs	❏
Makes appropriate closing remarks	❏

Evidence

- Depression is more likely to be present in patients who have chronic medical illness, chronic pain, recent life changes or stressors, self-ratings of fair or poor health, and unexplained physical symptoms.[8,9]
- Physicians who ask questions about feelings or psychosocial issues such as stress are more likely to recognize depression.[10]

Mania: History

> **INSTRUCTIONS TO CANDIDATE:** A 39-year-old man, known to have bipolar disorder, is brought to the emergency department by his sister because he has stopped taking his medications. He has missed work for the past 3 days because he has been working fervently on projects at home. Obtain a focused history.

Key Points	Satisfactorily Completed
Introduces self to the patient	❏
Determines how the patient wishes to be addressed	❏
Washes hands	❏
Explains the purpose of the encounter	❏
Develops good patient rapport	❏
Asks about elevated, expansive, or irritable mood:	❏
• Asks about **im**pulsive decisions and involvement in pleasurable but risky activities (e.g., gambling, sexual encounters)	❏
• Asks about (and observes) **p**ressured speech	❏
• Asks about increased involvement in goal-directed **a**ctivity (socially, at work, at school)	❏
• Inquires about sleep patterns (**i**nsomnia)	❏
• Asks about **r**acing thoughts or ideas	❏
• Asks about **e**steem inflation or grandiosity	❏
• Asks about (and observes) **d**istractibility	❏
Asks about duration of symptoms	❏
Asks about effect of symptoms on daily activities (severity)	❏
Asks about social supports	❏
Asks about past psychiatric problems	❏
Asks about history of medical or surgical problems	❏
Prescription medications:	
• Asks about adherence to prescribed therapies	❏
Asks about use of alcohol and recreational drugs	❏
Makes appropriate closing remarks	❏

Obsessive-Compulsive Disorder: History

> **INSTRUCTIONS TO CANDIDATE:** A 21-year-old woman is visiting her family doctor because of increased preoccupation with cleaning and germs. She knows her level of cleanliness is "over the top" but she "can't help it." Obtain a focused history.

Key Points	Satisfactorily Completed
Introduces self to the patient	❏
Determines how the patient wishes to be addressed	❏
Washes hands	❏
Explains the purpose of the encounter	❏
Develops good patient rapport	❏
Asks about recurrent and persistent thoughts about cleanliness	❏
Clarifies the nature of these recurrent thoughts	❏
Asks about where these thoughts come from	❏
Asks about how she copes with these thoughts	❏
Asks whether these repetitive thoughts are distressing	❏
Asks about repetitive behaviors or mental acts she must perform	❏
Asks whether these repetitive activities serve a purpose (i.e., whether they decrease anxiety or distress)	❏
Clarifies how much time is spent engaging in these repetitive activities	❏
Asks about effect of symptoms on daily activities (severity)	❏
Asks about duration of symptoms	❏
Asks whether the patient sees her recurrent thoughts and repetitive behaviors as excessive	❏
Asks about social supports	❏
Asks about past psychiatric problems	❏
Asks about history of medical or surgical problems	❏
Prescription medications:	
• Asks about adherence to prescribed therapies	❏
Asks about use of alcohol and recreational drugs	❏
Makes appropriate closing remarks	❏

Suicide: Risk Assessment

> **INSTRUCTIONS TO CANDIDATE: A 69-year-old man is visiting his family doctor at the insistence of his daughter. She has been concerned about him since her mother died 6 months ago because he "just isn't himself anymore." Obtain a focused history to assess risk for suicide in this man.**

Key Points	Satisfactorily Completed
Introduces self to the patient	❏
Determines how the patient wishes to be addressed	❏
Washes hands	❏
Explains the purpose of the encounter	❏
Develops good patient rapport	❏
Asks the patient about his future plans	❏
Asks whether he feels hopeless	❏
Asks whether he feels as if life is not worth carrying on	❏
Asks whether the patient is considering self-harm	❏
Asks whether the patient has considered specific methods of self-harm	❏
Asks whether the patient has a specific suicide plan at this time:	❏
• Asks how recently the patient has considered suicide	❏
• Asks the patient to describe his plan	❏
• Inquires about the patient's rationale for suicide at this time	❏
Asks about duration of symptoms	❏
Asks about suicidal ideation in the past	❏
Asks about previous suicide attempts	
• Clarifies the means by which suicide was attempted	❏
• Asks whether the patient required medical or psychiatric evaluation or admission	❏
Asks about the presence of a gun in the home	❏
Asks about history of depression	❏
Quantifies the patient's daily intake of alcohol	❏
Asks about social supports in his family and community	❏
Assesses orientation to person, place, and time	❏
Asks about past psychiatric problems	❏
Asks about history of medical or surgical problems	❏
Prescription medications:	
• Asks about adherence to prescribed therapies	❏
Makes appropriate closing remarks	❏

REFERENCES

1. Dhalla S, Kopec JA. The CAGE questionnaire for alcohol misuse: a review of reliability and validity studies. *Clin Invest Med.* 2007;30:33-41.
2. Hockberger RS, Rothstein RJ. Assessment of suicide potential by nonpsychiatrists using the SAD PERSONS score. *J Emerg Med.* 1988;6(2):99-107.
3. Cooper J, Kapur N, Dunning J, et al. A clinical tool for assessing risk after self-harm. *Ann Emerg Med.* 2006;48:459-466.
4. Paris J. Predicting and preventing suicide: do we know enough to do either? *Harv Rev Psychiatry.* 2006;14:233-240.
5. Wiebe DJ. Homicide and suicide risks associated with firearms in the home: a national case-control study. *Ann Emerg Med.* 2003;41:771.
6. Killias M. International correlations between gun ownership and rates of homicide and suicide. *CMAJ.* 1993;148:1721.
7. Birkhead GS, Galvin VG, Meehan PJ, et al. The emergency department in surveillance of attempted suicide: findings and methodologic considerations. *Public Health Rep.* 1993;108:323.
8. Kroenke K, Jackson JL, Chamberlin J. Depressive and anxiety disorders in patients presenting with physical complaints: clinical predictors and outcome. *Am J Med.* 1997;103:339-347.
9. Kroenke K, Spitzer RL, Williams JB, et al. Physical symptoms in primary care: predictors of psychiatric disorders and functional impairment. *Arch Fam Med.* 1994;3:774-779.
10. Carney PA, Eliassen MS, Wolford GL, et al. How physician communication influences recognition of depression in primary care. *J Fam Pract.* 1999;48:958-964.

Women's Health

ANATOMY

Vulva

- The external female genitalia, known as the **vulva,** consist of the mons veneris, labia majora, labia minora, clitoris, urethral meatus, vaginal introitus, Bartholin's gland, and posterior fourchette (Figure 11-1).
- The female urethra is four to five times shorter than the male urethra. The **urethral meatus** is directly inferior to the clitoris and is the opening through which urine passes externally.

Internal Genitalia

- The internal female genitalia consist of the vagina, cervix, uterus, fallopian tubes, and ovaries (Figure 11-2).
- The **uterus** is a pear-shaped, hollow muscular organ. The uterus can be palpated in bimanual pelvic examination and its position described using standard terminology (Figure 11-3).

Breasts

- Accessory breast tissue may be present along the embryonic milk lines (Figure 11-4).
- Each breast has lobules of glandular tissue that produce milk. These lobules are drained by **lactiferous ducts,** which drain into **lactiferous sinuses** behind the areola (Figure 11-5). The ducts open onto the **nipple,** the prominence at the center of the pigmented **areola.**

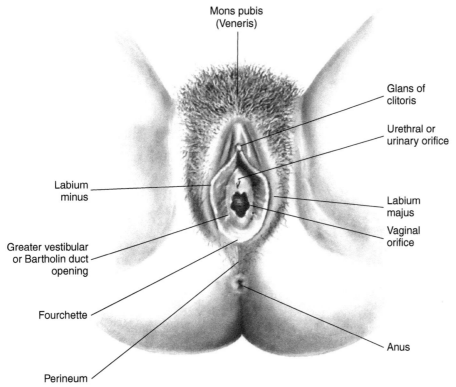

Figure 11-1 External female genitalia. (Adapted from Seidel HM, Dains JE, Ball JW, et al. *Mosby's Guide to Physical Examination.* 5th ed. St. Louis: Mosby; 2003 [p. 585].)

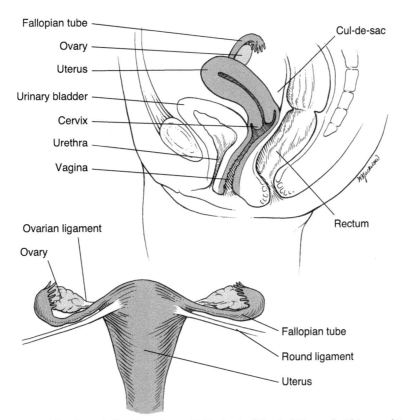

Figure 11-2 Internal female genitalia. (From Swartz M. *Textbook of Physical Diagnosis: History and Examination.* 6th ed. Philadelphia: Elsevier; 2010 [p. 552].)

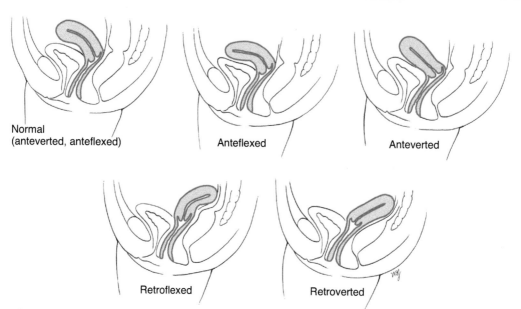

Normal
(anteverted, anteflexed)

Anteflexed

Anteverted

Retroflexed

Retroverted

Figure 11-3 Describing uterine position. (From Swartz M. *Textbook of Physical Diagnosis: History and Examination.* 6th ed. Philadelphia: Elsevier; 2010 [p. 579].)

Figure 11-4 Embryonic milk line. (From Powell DE, Stelling CB. *The Diagnosis and Detection of Breast Tissue.* St. Louis: Mosby; 1994 [Figure 1-1, *A*].)

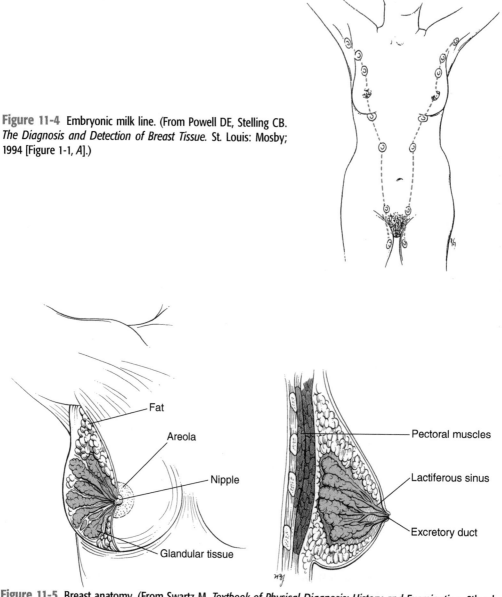

Fat

Areola

Nipple

Glandular tissue

Pectoral muscles

Lactiferous sinus

Excretory duct

Figure 11-5 Breast anatomy. (From Swartz M. *Textbook of Physical Diagnosis: History and Examination.* 6th ed. Philadelphia: Elsevier; 2010 [p. 456].)

ESSENTIAL SKILLS

APPROACH TO OBSTETRIC/GYNECOLOGIC HISTORY

- Ask the patient's age, occupation, relationship with partner, gravida, and parity.
- Use the mnemonic **ChLORIDE FPP** to structure your approach to the presenting concern.

Menstrual History
- Age at menarche
- Duration of menstrual cycle
- Duration and character of menses: Amount of flow (number of sanitary pads or tampons used per day), presence of clots, and dysmenorrhea
- Premenstrual syndrome (PMS): Bloating, breast tenderness, mood changes, decreased concentration and motivation, food cravings
- Age at menopause and associated symptoms: Fatigue, hot flashes, nervousness or irritability, headache, insomnia, depression, aches or pains, vaginal itch or dryness
- Postmenopausal bleeding
- Hormone replacement therapy

Sexual History
- Age at first sexual intercourse
- Number of sexual partners
- Previous sexually transmitted infections (STIs)
- Use of precautions, such as condoms (STI prevention), and use of other contraceptive devices

Obstetric History
- Blood type: Rh positive versus Rh negative
- Date of last menstrual period (LMP)
- Infertility: Lack of conception after attempts to conceive for 1 year
- **Nägele's rule** for estimated date of confinement (EDC):
  - EDC = date of LMP − 3 months + 7 days + 1 year
- Contraceptive use (e.g., oral contraceptive pill may change the reliability of the LMP)
- Pregnancy history: Bleeding, discharge, premature rupture of membranes, nausea or vomiting, STIs, other infections, gestational diabetes mellitus, anemia, gastroesophageal reflux (GER)
- Gravida, parity, and abortions (written $G_{number}P_{number}A_{number}$). Specifically ascertain whether deliveries were full-term or preterm or stillbirth.
- Date and gestation at delivery
- Onset of labor: Spontaneous versus induced
- Duration of labor: Use of augmentation
- Type of anesthetic: Oral or intravenous pain medications, nitrous oxide, epidural anesthetic, or no anesthetic at all
- Type of delivery: Normal spontaneous vaginal delivery, lower segment cesarean section, use of forceps or vacuum
- Episiotomy: Midline versus mediolateral or none
- Maternal complications: Tears (first to fourth degree), postpartum hemorrhage, infection
- Newborn: Sex, weight, fed breast milk versus formula, complications, and general health

Pap Smear History
- Date of last Pap smear
- History of abnormal Pap smears and type of follow-up evaluation and investigations
- History of human papillomavirus (HPV)

- **Past medical history (PMH)/past surgical history (PSH):** Bleeding diathesis, diabetes mellitus, hypertension, cardiovascular disease, thyroid problems, renal problems, anemia, epilepsy, asthma, STIs, psychiatric problems, anesthetic problems, or malignancy; previous surgery (including cryotherapy and loop electrocautery excision procedure [LEEP]), complications, or trauma
- **Medications (MEDS):** It is important to document all medications (prescription and over-the-counter [OTC] drugs) and consider all effects on pregnancy.
- **Allergies**
- **Immunizations:** Routine immunizations and immune status or exposure to infectious diseases such as rubella, human immunodeficiency virus (HIV), hepatitis B virus (HBV), and syphilis
- **Social history (SH):** Nutrition, folic acid intake, smoking history, present smoking status, exposure to second-hand smoke, use of alcohol (EtOH), use of street drugs, family support, and occupational and financial situation
- **Family history (FH):** Malformations, developmental delay, known hereditary disorders, or diabetes mellitus

BREAST: EXAMINATION

Inspection

- Inspect both breasts. Ask the patient to sit with arms at her side, with arms overhead, and with hands resting on the knees (Figure 11-6). Finally, ask the patient to lie supine, and inspect the breast with the ipsilateral arm resting under the head (Figure 11-7). Using these different positions helps to accentuate dimpling, skin retraction, or asymmetry between the breasts.
- Inspect for breast symmetry, and note the direction to which each nipple points (the two directions should be similar). Note dimpling, skin retraction, peau d'orange (like the skin of an orange), eczema or rash, local swelling, or discoloration. Assess the color, quantity, consistency, and odor of any breast or nipple discharge.

Palpation

- With the patient supine, ask her to place her ipsilateral hand behind her head (see Figure 11-7).
- Wear gloves if open lesions are present or if discharge is observed.
- Begin by palpating at the junction of the clavicle and sternum. Follow a grid pattern, palpating each quadrant, medially to laterally and back (Figure 11-8). Be sure to palpate breast tissue in the axillary area and below the breast. Use the pads of your second, third, and fourth fingers in a rotatory motion, applying light, moderate, and deeper pressure.

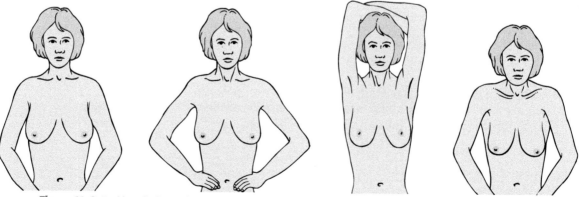

Figure 11-6 Positions for breast inspection. (From Munro JF, Campbell IW, editors. *Macleod's Clinical Examination.* 10th ed. Edinburgh: Churchill Livingstone; 2000 [p. 66].)

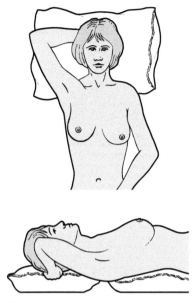

Figure 11-7 Position for breast palpation. (From Munro JF, Campbell IW, editors. *Macleod's Clinical Examination.* 10th ed. Edinburgh: Churchill Livingstone; 2000 [p. 66].)

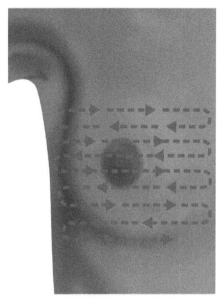

Figure 11-8 Direction of breast palpation. (Modified from Seidel HM, Ball JW, Dains JE, et al. *Mosby's Guide to Physical Examination.* 5th ed. St. Louis: Mosby; 2003 [p. 510].)

- Palpate around the areola, noting the presence of discharge.
- Palpate supraclavicular, infraclavicular, and axillary lymph nodes. For a woman with large breasts, it may be easier to examine axillary nodes when the patient is in a sitting position.
- Describe the size, shape, location (Figure 11-9), consistency, and contour of any lesions (Box 11-1). Note tenderness, pulsatility, warmth, and color.
- You may be asked to simulate a breast examination by using a synthetic **breast model.** The following assessments, however, cannot be performed adequately with a breast model:
  - Assessment of skin changes: color, dimpling, skin retraction, eczema or rash, and peau d'orange
  - Assessment of nipple discharge
  - Assessment of warmth and tenderness
  - Palpation of breast tissue in axillae and axillary lymph nodes
  - Needle aspiration or core biopsy

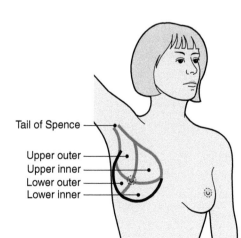

Tail of Spence

Upper outer
Upper inner
Lower outer
Lower inner

Figure 11-9 Terms to describe location of a breast lesion. (From Munro JF, Campbell IW, editors. *Macleod's Clinical Examination.* 10th ed. Edinburgh: Churchill Livingstone; 2000 [p. 65].)

> **Box 11-1   Findings Associated with Breast Malignancy**
>
> • Hard, fixed lump with irregular borders
> • Asymmetry, fixation of lesion to chest wall
> • Skin changes: Retraction, dimpling, peau d'orange, and ulceration
> • Nipple retraction or inversion and bloody discharge
> • Lymphadenopathy: Axillary, infraclavicular, and supraclavicular
> • Edema of ipsilateral arm (lymphedema or venous obstruction)
> • Metastasis: Hepatomegaly, lung nodules, pleural effusion, bone pain, and seizure (central nervous system metastases)

BREAST LUMP: HISTORY

> **INSTRUCTIONS TO CANDIDATE: A 61-year-old woman presents to her family doctor after finding a lump in her right breast. Obtain a detailed history, focusing on risk factors for malignancy.**

DD$_X$: VITAMINS C
- **Traumatic:** Fat necrosis
- **Idiopathic/iatrogenic:** Fibrocystic changes, cystic lesion (e.g., galactocele, abscess)
- **Neoplastic:** Breast malignancy (Box 11-2), mammary duct ectasia, intraductal papilloma, and fibroadenoma

History
- Ask the patient the following questions:
  - **Character:** "What does the lump feel like? What is its shape? What is its consistency: hard versus soft, nodular versus uniform, and mobile versus fixed? What is its contour: well-defined regular margins versus ill-defined irregular margins? Does it feel tender? Have you noted redness or warmth?"
  - **Location:** "In which breast did you find the lump (e.g., right breast)? Where is it located?"
  - **Onset:** "When and how did you first notice the lump? Do you perform monthly self-examinations? What was the lump like when you first noticed it? Has there been any change in the size or consistency of the lump or in any other feature? Does the lump change in relation to your menstrual cycle?"

> **Box 11-2   Historical Risk Factors for Breast Malignancy**
>
> • Age: >40 years, female sex
> • Age at menarche: <13 years
> • Age at menopause: >50 years
> • Parity: Nulliparity or late first pregnancy (at age >30 years)
> • History of breast malignancy, dysplasia, or atypia
> • Paget disease of the breast
> • Lynch II syndrome: Endometrial, ovarian, and colon
> • Radiation therapy or exposure
> • Obesity, diet high in fats, and excessive alcohol (EtOH) consumption
> • Family history: Breast cancer in first-degree relatives, Lynch II syndrome

- Intensity: "How large is the lump? Is it a single lump or multiple lumps?"
- Duration: "How long have you had this lump?"
- Events associated:
  - "Have you noticed any retraction of skin or nipple? Have you noticed any dimpling?"
  - Skin changes: "Do you have eczema, rash, ulceration, or skin breakdown on the breast?"
  - Nipple discharge: "Have you noticed bloody, milky, clear, or purulent discharge (green or straw-colored fluid is less worrisome)?"
  - "Have you had a breast injury recently (fat necrosis)?"
  - Constitutional symptoms: "Have you had fever, chills, night sweats, weight loss, anorexia, or asthenia?"
- Frequency: "Have you had any breast lumps before this one? If so, when? How frequently do you notice lumps?"
- Palliative factors: "Does anything make the lump better? If so, what?"
- Provocative factors: "Does anything make the lump worse? If so, what (e.g., menses)?"

- **Previous investigations:** Breast biopsy, mammography, and cytologic study (cyst aspiration, nipple discharge)
- **PMH/PSH:** Previous breast malignancy or dysplasia, breast lumps, fibrocystic changes, other medical problems, previous surgery, trauma, or radiation therapy
- **MEDS:** Immunosuppressive medications (increase the risk of malignancy)
- **SH:** Nutrition, smoking history, use of EtOH, use of street drugs, and family or social support network
- **FH:** Breast cancer in first-degree relatives, Lynch II syndrome (breast, endometrial, ovarian, colon)

AMENORRHEA: HISTORY

> **INSTRUCTIONS TO CANDIDATE: A 21-year-old woman presents to her family doctor with a history of several "missed" periods. Until last year, she had regular menses. Obtain a detailed history, exploring possible causes.**

DD$_X$: VITAMINS C
- Traumatic: Asherman syndrome
- Metabolic: Lactation, premature ovarian failure, polycystic ovarian syndrome, Cushing syndrome, hyperthyroidism, acromegaly, Sheehan syndrome, and malnutrition
- Idiopathic/iatrogenic: Intense athletic training, systemic disease
- Neoplastic: Prolactinoma
- Substance abuse and psychiatric: Pseudocyesis

DD$_X$: Other
- Pregnancy

History
- Ask the patient the following questions:
  - **Character:** "Can you describe your usual menstrual cycle (amount of flow [number of pads/tampons per day] and presence of clots)? What was your last period like? Was it normal for you?"
  - **Onset:** "When did you start menstruating (menarche)?"
  - **Intensity:** "How many periods have you missed? What is the date of your LMP? Any bleeding or spotting since then?"
  - **Duration:** "How long does your menses usually last?"

- Events associated:
  - "Have you experienced dysmenorrhea?"
  - "Are you pregnant? Have you recently had a baby? Are you breastfeeding?"
  - "Have you sustained recent trauma, illness, or surgery (especially pelvic)?"
  - Symptoms of PMS: "Have you experienced bloating, breast tenderness, mood changes, decreased concentration and motivation, or food cravings?"
  - Symptoms of estrogen deficiency: "Have you experienced hot flashes, nervousness or irritability, insomnia, or vaginal itch or dryness?"
  - Symptoms of virilization: "Have you had acne, increased hair growth, temporal balding, deepening voice, or decreased breast size?"
  - Lifestyle: "Have you experienced obesity, malnutrition (anorexia, bulimia), intense exercise, and stress?"
  - Hyperthyroidism: "Have you noticed heat intolerance, weight loss despite increased appetite, or palpitations?"
  - Prolactinoma: "Have you had milk leaking from your breasts or visual changes (bitemporal hemianopsia)?"
  - Cushing syndrome: "Have you had truncal obesity, round face (moon facies), stretch marks (striae), and increased hair growth (hirsuitism)?"
  - Acromegaly: "Have you noticed acne; increased space between the teeth; or increased shoe, hat, glove, and ring sizes?"
- Frequency: "How frequently do you usually menstruate? Have you ever missed periods before? How often?"
- Palliative factors: "Does anything make this problem better? If so, what?"
- Provocative factors: "Does anything make this problem worse? If so, what?"

Sexual History
- Recent sexual activity
- Current or past STIs
- Dyspareunia
- Signs of pregnancy
- Use of hormonal contraception, other contraception

Obstetric/Gynecologic History
- Previous pregnancies or abortions
- Uterine instrumentation
- Most recent Pap smear
- **PMH/PSH:** Oophorectomy, hysterectomy, or pelvic surgery; radiation therapy or chemotherapy; endocrinopathy, polycystic ovarian syndrome, or hepatic or renal disease
- **MEDS:** Hormonal contraception, steroids
- **SH:** Smoking, use of EtOH, and use of street drugs
- **FH:** Amenorrhea, age at onset of menopause in mother and sisters (premature ovarian failure), or endocrinopathies

PELVIC INFLAMMATORY DISEASE: HISTORY AND PHYSICAL EXAMINATION

> **INSTRUCTIONS TO CANDIDATE:** A 32-year-old woman presents with fever and lower abdominal pain that have lasted 12 hours. She also has noted some foul-smelling vaginal discharge. Obtain a focused history, and perform a focused physical examination.

DD$_X$: VITAMINS C
- Infectious: Pelvic inflammatory disease (PID)/tubo-ovarian abscess, cystitis, pyelonephritis, and psoas abscess
- Traumatic: Musculoskeletal injury
- Idiopathic/iatrogenic: Ruptured ectopic pregnancy, ovarian torsion, renal colic, appendicitis, mesenteric adenitis, diverticulitis, incarcerated hernia, and inflammatory bowel disease

History
- Ask the patient the following questions:
  - **Character:** "What is the pain like: sharp? Crampy? Dull? What is the vaginal discharge like (color, consistency, odor)?"
  - **Location:** "Where does the pain originate?"
  - **Onset:** "When did the pain start? How did it come on (sudden versus gradual)? When did the vaginal discharge start? What is the temporal relationship to your menstrual cycle?"
  - **Radiation:** "Does the pain move anywhere?"
  - **Intensity:** "How severe is the pain on a scale of 1 to 10, with 1 being mild pain and 10 being the worst? How much discharge are you having (number of sanitary pads or tampons)? Are the symptoms getting better, getting worse, or staying the same?"
  - **Duration:** "How long has the pain been there (12 hours)? How long have you had the discharge (acute versus chronic)?"
  - **Events associated:**
    - PID: "Have you had intermenstrual bleeding, vaginal discharge, fever, and pain?"
    - Pregnancy: "What is the date of your LMP? Have you had vaginal bleeding?"
    - Appendicitis: "Have you had fever, nausea or vomiting, decreased appetite, or initial dull central abdominal pain that later localizes to the right lower quadrant (RLQ)?"
    - Cystitis: "Have you noticed urinary frequency, pain with urination, blood in the urine, urinary retention, urgency, or incontinence?"
    - Inflammatory bowel disease: "Have you had chronic diarrhea, weight loss, and extraintestinal manifestations (e.g., uveitis, erythema nodosum, peripheral arthritis)?"
  - **Frequency:** "Have you ever had this pain before? How often does the pain come (intermittent versus constant)? Have you ever had this discharge before? If so, when? How often do you notice it?"
  - **Palliative factors:** "Does anything make the pain better? If so, what? Lying in one position?
  - **Provocative factors:** "Does anything make the pain worse? If so, what? Movement?
- **PMH/PSH:** STIs, PID, ectopic pregnancy, diverticular disease, previous surgery, malignancy, inflammatory bowel disease, or renal colic
- **MEDS:** Analgesics, antibiotics
- **SH:** Smoking, use of EtOH, use of street drugs, and sexual history

Physical Examination

- **Vital signs (Vitals):** Evaluate heart rate (HR), respiratory rate (RR), blood pressure (BP), and temperature.
  - Note fever and any tachycardia or hypotension.
- **General:** Check capillary refill. Note the patient's position on the stretcher and whether she is moving about or lying still.
- **Respiratory (Resp):** Check chest expansion (symmetry), and auscultate the lungs (breath sounds, adventitious sounds).
- **Cardiovascular system (CVS):** Measure the jugular venous pressure (JVP). Palpate peripheral pulses. Note pulse volume, contour, and rhythm. Auscultate the heart, listening for extra heart sounds or flow murmurs associated with hyperdynamic circulation.
- **Abdomen:** Inspect the abdomen. Auscultate for bowel sounds (may be decreased in peritonitis). Percuss lightly in all four quadrants. Percussion produces pain in a patient with peritonitis. Before palpation, ask the patient to cough and to point to the most tender area with one finger. Palpate the most tender area last. Perform light and deep palpation, and identify any masses or areas of tenderness. Check for rebound tenderness. Examine the liver and spleen. Perform a digital rectal examination. A retrocecal appendix may produce tenderness on palpation of the rectal walls.
- **Genitourinary (GU):** It is important to perform a pelvic examination (Figure 11-10). Inspect the cervical os, and note any discharge, inflammation, or lesions (Figure 11-11). In PID, the cervix may appear inflamed and friable. If the speculum examination yields unremarkable findings, proceed with a bimanual pelvic examination. Note any discharge, cervical motion tenderness, adnexal tenderness, or pelvic masses.

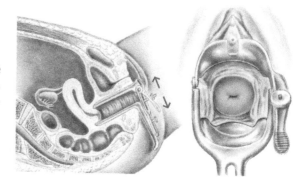

Figure 11-10 Speculum examination of the pelvis. (From Seidel HM, Ball JW, Dains JE, et al. *Mosby's Guide to Physical Examination.* 6th ed. St. Louis: Mosby; 2006 [p. 600].)

Figure 11-11 Cervical descriptors. (From Wilson SF, Giddens JF. *Health Assessment for Nursing Practice.* 2nd ed. St. Louis: Mosby; 2001 [p. 540].)

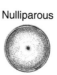

Nulliparous   Parous (after childbirth)   Cervical eversion   Nabothian cysts

SAMPLE CHECKLISTS

Breast Lump: History

> **INSTRUCTIONS TO CANDIDATE:** A 48-year-old woman presents to your office after finding a lump during routine breast self-examination. Obtain a detailed history, focusing on risk factors for malignancy.

Key Points	Satisfactorily Completed
Introduces self to the patient	❏
Determines how the patient wishes to be addressed	❏
Washes hands	❏
Explains purpose of the encounter	❏
Asks about the qualities of the lump:	
• Location	❏
• Size and shape	❏
• Consistency	❏
Asks about associated breast pain	❏
Asks about performance of monthly examinations	❏
Asks when this lump was first noted and whether it has changed	❏
Asks about changes in the lump throughout the menstrual cycle	❏
Asks about a history of injury to the area (fat necrosis)	❏
Notes skin changes:	
• Skin retraction or dimpling	❏
• Eczema or rash on the breast	❏
• Ulceration	❏
• Peau d'orange	❏
• Redness	❏
Notes any nipple discharge	❏
Notes constitutional symptoms:	
• Fever, chills, night sweats, weight loss, anorexia, or asthenia	❏
Asks age at menarche (increased risk if age <13 years)	❏
Asks age at menopause	❏
Notes parity (nulliparity or late first pregnancy [at age >30 years])	❏
Asks about past exposure to radiation	❏
Asks about previous mammographic results	❏
Asks about previous breast lumps:	
• Malignancy	❏
• Dysplasia	❏
Asks about eczema on the breast (Paget disease of the breast)	❏
Asks about family history:	
• Breast cancer in first-degree relatives	❏
• Lynch II syndrome: cancers in breast, endometrium, ovary, and colon	❏
Asks about social history: smoking, use of EtOH, use of street drugs, obesity, and high-fat diet	❏
Makes appropriate closing remarks	❏

Intimate Partner Violence: Screen and Counsel

> **INSTRUCTIONS TO CANDIDATE:** A 32-year-old woman presents to the emergency department with a fractured wrist and some facial contusions. Perform a screen for intimate partner violence and counsel.

Key Points	Satisfactorily Completed
Introduces self to the patient	❑
Determines how the patient wishes to be addressed	❑
Washes hands	❑
Explains purpose of the encounter	❑
Asks persons other than the patient to leave the room, to ensure privacy	❑
Assures the patient that this encounter is confidential, although information will be recorded on her medical record	❑
Asks about her relationship with her partner	❑
Prefaces screening questions with a framing statement such as "Domestic violence is a very common problem" or "I have met a lot of patients who have experienced domestic violence"	❑
Asks whether her partner (or someone else close to her) has ever hit, pushed, shoved, punched, or kicked her	❑
Asks whether she is ever threatened	❑
Asks whether she feels safe at home, and clarifies any areas of concern identified by the patient	❑
Asks whether she has been involved in any abusive relationships in the past	❑
Asks about the presence of weapons in the home and asks specifically about guns	❑
Asks about hospitalizations or previous visits to the emergency department for abuse-related problems	❑
Asks whether she has ever tried to leave the relationship, and acknowledges the difficulty of leaving	❑
States that domestic assault is illegal	❑
Expresses concern for her safety (violence tends to escalate)	❑
Asks whether she has any children	❑
Informs her that you are obligated to report any suspicion of child abuse to the authorities (e.g., Child Protective Services)	❑
Asks whether the children have been abused or have witnessed any abuse	❑
Asks about support systems such as family and friends (abusers often isolate their partners)	❑
Provides contacts for community resources such as legal aid, safe houses, and counseling services	❑

Key Points	Satisfactorily Completed
Asks the patient what avenues she would like to pursue, and provides support (the patient must be empowered to make these decisions herself and should also be supported even if she chooses to stay in the abusive relationship)	❏
Encourages the patient to develop and follow a safety plan:	
• Have a plan of escape from the home	❏
• If possible, tell a neighbor to call the police in the event of a disturbance	❏
• Hide money, identification, credit cards, important documents, and important sentimental objects to take in the event of a quick departure	❏
• Have emergency telephone numbers nearby	❏
• Choose a safe place to go in the event of an emergency, such as a women's shelter or with family or friends	❏
Sets up a follow-up encounter	❏
Makes appropriate closing remarks	❏

First Trimester Pain and Bleeding: History

INSTRUCTIONS TO CANDIDATE: A 26-year-old G_1P_0 woman who is 9 weeks' pregnant presents to the emergency department with severe pelvic pain and vaginal bleeding. Obtain a focused history.

Key Points	Satisfactorily Completed
Introduces self to the patient	❏
Determines how the patient wishes to be addressed	❏
Washes hands	❏
Explains purpose of the encounter	❏
Asks about the character of the pain:	
• Specific descriptors (sharp, cramping, dull)	❏
Asks about the character of the bleeding:	
• Volume or quantity of blood (number of sanitary napkins or pads soaked per hour)	❏
• Color, presence of clots, or presence of tissue	❏
• Heavier than normal menstrual period	❏
Establishes location of pain	❏
Asks about onset:	
• Specific time of onset	❏
• Activity at onset	❏
• Order of symptoms	❏
Asks about radiation of pain	❏
Establishes intensity of pain, using pain scale	❏
Asks about duration of symptoms:	
• Whether pain is getting worse, getting better, or staying the same	❏
• Whether bleeding is getting worse, getting better, or staying the same	❏

Continued

Key Points	Satisfactorily Completed
Asks about events associated with pain and bleeding:	
• Vaginal intercourse or penetration (local trauma)	❏
• Presyncope, shortness of breath, palpitations, syncope (hemorrhagic shock)	❏
• Fever, chills, rigors (sepsis)	❏
• Other sites of bleeding (bleeding disorder)	❏
Asks about frequency of symptoms:	
• Previous episodes of pain during the pregnancy	❏
• Previous episodes of bleeding during the pregnancy	❏
Asks about palliative factors	❏
Asks about provocative factors:	
• Position, walking, any slight movement (peritonitis)	❏
• Palpation	❏
Asks about past medical history:	
• Ectopic pregnancy risk factors:	❏
• Pelvic inflammatory disease (chlamydia, gonorrhea)	❏
• Previous ectopic pregnancy	❏
• Intrauterine device in place at the time of conception	❏
• Fertility treatment	❏
• Smoking	❏
• Previous uterine or tubal instrumentation	❏
• Bleeding disorders	❏
• Pregnancy or miscarriage	❏
• Ovarian cysts or tumors, endometriosis (risk for ovarian torsion)	❏
Asks about medications:	
• Anticoagulants (warfarin)	❏
• Antiplatelet agents (aspirin, clopidogrel)	❏
Asks about allergies	❏
Asks about social history:	
• Use of alcohol	❏
• Smoking	❏
• Use of street drugs	❏
• Living situation and social supports	❏
Makes appropriate closing remarks	❏

ADVANCED SKILLS

PREGNANCY: HISTORY AND DETERMINATION OF GESTATIONAL AGE AND PRESENTING PART

> **INSTRUCTIONS TO CANDIDATE: An 18-year-old woman, G_1P_0, presents to the labor and delivery unit with "contractions." She concealed her pregnancy until recently. Obtain a detailed history. Determine the gestational age and presenting part by using the Leopold maneuvers (see Figure 11-12).**

History
- Ask the patient the following questions:
  - Character: "Tell me about the contractions. What are they like: sharp? Crampy? Dull?"
  - Location: "Where does the pain originate?"
  - Onset: "When did it start? How did it come on (sudden versus gradual)?"
  - Radiation: "Does the pain move anywhere?"
  - Intensity: "How severe is the pain on a scale of 1 to 10, with 1 being mild pain and 10 being the worst? Is it getting better, getting worse, or staying the same?"
  - Duration: "How long does each contraction last (seconds or minutes)?"
  - Events associated:
    - "Have you had vaginal bleeding?"
    - "Have you noticed leakage of fluid (rupture of membranes)?"
    - "Have you felt fetal movements?"
  - Frequency: "Have you ever had this sensation before? How often does the pain come (in minutes)? Does it come regularly?"
  - Palliative factors: "Does anything make the pain better? If so, what?"
  - Provocative factors: "Does anything make the pain worse? If so, what?"

Pregnancy History
- This aspect of the history, especially determination of the gestational age, is pivotal. Because of the concealment of the pregnancy, the patient has probably not received prenatal care.
- Nägele's rule: EDC = date of LMP − 3 months + 7 days + 1 year
  - Nägele's rule depends on menstrual cycles that span 28 to 30 days and are regular.
  - Determine duration of the patient's menstrual cycle, whether her cycles are regular, and the date of her LMP.
  - Determine whether she has used hormonal contraceptives (e.g., the oral contraceptive pill may change the reliability of the LMP).
- Date of first positive pregnancy test
- Date when patient first noted fetal movement (quickening; the date of quickening is usually 18 to 20 weeks in a primigravida patient)
- Blood type: Rh positive versus Rh negative
- Pregnancy history: Bleeding, discharge, nausea or vomiting, gestational diabetes mellitus, anemia, or GER
- STIs: Previous and current infections, especially gonococcal and herpes infections (may preclude vaginal delivery)
- Type of anesthetic the patient desires for labor and delivery: Oral/intravenous pain medications, nitrous oxide, epidural anesthetic, or no medications at all
- **PMH/PSH:** Bleeding diathesis, diabetes mellitus, hypertension, cardiovascular disease, thyroid problems, renal problems, anemia, epilepsy, asthma, STIs, psychiatric problems, anesthetic problems, previous surgery (including cryotherapy and LEEP), complications, or trauma
- **MEDS:** *All* medications (prescription and OTC drugs) taken during pregnancy
- **Allergies**

- **Immunizations:** Routine immunizations and immune status or exposure to infectious diseases such as rubella, HIV, HBV, and syphilis
- **SH:** Nutrition, intake of folic acid, smoking, use of EtOH, and use of street drugs during pregnancy; family support; occupational/financial situation; and relationship with the infant's father
- **FH:** Malformations, developmental delay, or known hereditary disorders

Leopold Maneuvers

- The **Leopold maneuvers** are used to determine fetal lie, presentation, and position. These maneuvers are not useful before 28 weeks of gestation.
  - The fetal **lie** refers to the relationship of the fetal long axis to the maternal long axis:
    - Oblique
    - Transverse
    - Longitudinal
  - The fetal **presentation** refers to the part of the fetus that first passes through the birthing canal:
    - Cephalic
    - Breech
  - The **position** of the fetus refers to the relationship of the fetus to the maternal pelvis. In cephalic presentations, the position is defined in relation to the occiput, whereas breech presentations are defined with regard to the fetal sacrum.
- **First maneuver** (Figure 11-12, *A*): Facing the patient's head, palpate the fundus of the uterus to determine which part of the fetus occupies the fundus (head versus bottom). The head feels firm, round, and smooth.
- **Second maneuver** (see Figure 11-12, *B*): Place your hands on either side of the patient's abdomen to determine on which side the fetal back lies. The back is linear and firm, whereas the extremities are lumpy. Use one hand to steady the uterus and the other to palpate the fetus.
- **Third maneuver** (see Figure 11-12, *C*): Place one hand just above the patient's symphysis pubis to determine the presenting part. Grasp the presenting part between the thumb and forefinger. The head will feel round, firm, and ballottable, whereas in the breech position, the specific body part will feel irregular.

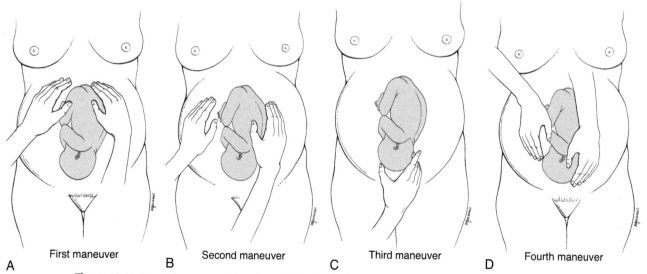

A First maneuver   B Second maneuver   C Third maneuver   D Fourth maneuver

Figure 11-12 Leopold maneuvers. (From Swartz M. *Textbook of Physical Diagnosis: History and Examination.* 6th ed. Philadelphia: Elsevier; 2010 [pp. 725-727].)

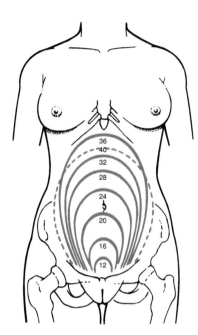

Figure 11-13 Measuring fundal height. (From Seidel HM, Ball JW, Dains JE, et al. *Mosby's Guide to Physical Examination.* 6th ed. St. Louis: Mosby; 2006 [p. 617].)

- **Fourth maneuver** (see Figure 11-12, *D*): Face the patient's feet. Place your hands on the patient's lower abdomen just above the pelvic inlet to determine the side of cephalic prominence. Exert pressure toward the inlet. One hand usually descends further than the other, which is stopped by the cephalic prominence. If the cephalic prominence is on the same side as the fetal parts, the fetal head is flexed. Alternatively, if the prominence is on the same side as the fetal back, the head is extended.

Fundal Height

- Estimate **gestational age** by measuring **fundal height** from the pubis symphysis to the superior border of the fundus (Figure 11-13). In the third trimester, this measurement in centimeters is equivalent to the gestational age in weeks.

PAINLESS THIRD TRIMESTER BLEEDING: HISTORY AND PHYSICAL EXAMINATION

> **INSTRUCTIONS TO CANDIDATE: A 32-year-old woman, G_2P_1, presents to the labor and delivery unit with painless bleeding. She is 37 weeks pregnant, according to the date of her LMP. Obtain a focused history, and perform a focused physical examination.**

DD_X: VITAMINS C

- **Vascular:** Placenta previa, vasa previa, and (although the bleeding is painless) placental abruption
- **Traumatic:** Trauma or lesion on the external genitalia
- **Idiopathic/iatrogenic:** Cervicitis
- **Neoplastic:** Cervical polyp, cervical malignancy

History

- Ask the patient the following questions:
  - **Character:** "What color is the blood (bright red versus dark red versus brown)? Have you seen any clots? Are you still bleeding?"
  - **Location:** "Where is the blood coming from (vaginal, vulvar, bowel, bladder)?"
  - **Onset:** "How did the bleeding start (sudden versus gradual)?"
  - **Intensity:** "How much blood have you passed (number of sanitary pads or tampons)?"

Table 11-1 Risk Factors for Placenta Previa and Placental Abruption

Condition	Risk Factors
Placenta previa	Previous placenta previa Grand multiparity Multiple gestation Increased maternal age Uterine scar (previous lower segment cesarean section, therapeutic abortion, or myomectomy)
Placental abruption	Previous placental abruption Hypertension, preeclampsia Trauma Premature rupture of membranes Cigarette smoking, cocaine use Folate deficiency

- **Duration:** "How long have you been bleeding?"
- **Events associated:**
  - "Have you felt fetal movements?"
  - "What is your blood type (Rh positive versus Rh negative)?"
  - "Have you had an ultrasound examination during this pregnancy? When?"
  - Placenta previa (Table 11-1): "Have you had previous bleeding that stopped spontaneously, with no abdominal pain or tenderness?"
  - Vasa previa: "How much blood have you passed?" (Because it is fetal blood, even a small amount can be catastrophic.)
  - Pregnancy history: "Have you had bleeding along with discharge, premature rupture of membranes, nausea or vomiting, infections or STIs, gestational diabetes mellitus, anemia, or GER?"
  - Placental abruption (see Table 11-1): "Have you had abdominal pain and tenderness along with dark blood?"
  - Labor: "Have you felt uterine contractions?"
  - Were you injured recently? "Did you recently have sexual intercourse (localized trauma)?"
- **Frequency:** "Has this ever happened to you before? If so, when? How often do you bleed?"
- **Palliative factors:** "Does anything seem to slow the bleeding? If so, what?"
- **Provocative factors:** "Does anything seem to make the bleeding worse? If so, what?"
- **Past obstetric history:** Previous placenta previa, previous placental abruption, preterm cesarean section, gestation at delivery, type of delivery, maternal complications (tears, postpartum hemorrhage, infection), or complications and general health of the newborn
- **PMH/PSH:** Bleeding diathesis, liver disease, urogenital malignancy, abnormal results of Pap smears, or urogenital surgery
- **MEDS:** Anticoagulants
- **Allergies**
- **SH:** Smoking, use of EtOH, use of street drugs (e.g., cocaine), and physical abuse

Physical Examination
- **Vitals:** Evaluate HR, RR, BP, and temperature.
  - Obstetric vitals also include the fetal HR and its trends (beat-to-beat variability, accelerations).
- **General:** Assess whether the patient is apprehensive or in apparent distress. Check capillary refill.

- **Resp:** Check chest expansion (symmetry), and auscultate the lungs (breath sounds, adventitious sounds).
- **CVS:** Measure the JVP. Palpate peripheral pulses. Note pulse volume, contour, and rhythm. Auscultate the heart, listening for extra heart sounds or flow murmurs associated with hyperdynamic circulation.
- **Abdomen:** Inspect the abdomen. Auscultate for bowel sounds. Percuss lightly. Perform light and deep palpation, and identify any masses or areas of tenderness. At 37 weeks, the uterus occupies nearly all of the palpable abdomen. In placental abruption, the uterus is exquisitely tender.
- **Obstetric/gynecologic (Obs/Gyne):** Measure the fundal height from the pubis symphysis (in the third trimester, height in centimeters is correlated with gestational age in weeks). Use the Leopold maneuvers to determine the position, presentation, and lie of the infant (see Figure 11-12). In placenta previa, the presenting part is high riding and not engaged in the pelvis. It is important to perform a speculum examination of the cervix (see Figure 11-10). Inspect the cervical os, and note any discharge, inflammation, or lesions (see Figure 11-11). If the speculum examination yields unremarkable results, proceed with a manual vaginal examination. Do not perform a blind vaginal examination because this may incite catastrophic bleeding if placenta previa or vasa previa is present. Note whether the os is open or closed.

PRETERM LABOR: HISTORY AND PHYSICAL EXAMINATION

INSTRUCTIONS TO CANDIDATE: A 25-year-old woman, G_1P_0, presents to the labor and delivery unit with intermittent abdominal and back pain. She is 27 weeks pregnant, according to ultrasound findings. Obtain a focused history, and perform a focused physical examination.

- **Preterm labor** is the onset of labor before 37 weeks of gestation. It is diagnosed on the basis of documented, regular uterine contractions (four per 20 minutes) and cervical effacement of 80% or cervical dilation of >2 cm. The onset of spontaneous preterm labor is usually idiopathic. Prematurity (20 to 37 weeks of gestation) is the leading cause of perinatal morbidity and mortality.
- **Maternal risk factors** include previous preterm delivery, uterine abnormalities, incompetent cervix, vaginal bleeding, bacterial vaginosis, smoking, maternal age <18 or >40 years, low socioeconomic status, drug addiction, and poor nutrition.

DD_X: VITAMINS C
- **I**nfectious: Pyelonephritis
- **T**raumatic: Musculoskeletal injury
- **I**diopathic/**i**atrogenic: Braxton-Hicks contractions, preterm labor, and renal colic
- **S**ubstance abuse and **p**sychiatric: Use of cocaine

History
- Ask the patient the following questions:
  - **Character:** "Tell me about the pain. What is it like: sharp? Crampy? Dull?"
  - **Location:** "Where does the pain originate?"
  - **Onset:** "When did it start? How did it come on (sudden versus gradual)?"
  - **Radiation:** "Does the pain move anywhere?"
  - **Intensity:** "How severe is the pain on a scale of 1 to 10, with 1 being mild pain and 10 being the worst? Is it getting better, getting worse, or staying the same?"
  - **Duration:** "How long does the pain last (seconds or minutes)?"
  - **Events associated:**
    - "Have you had vaginal bleeding?"
    - "Have you noticed leakage of fluid (rupture of membranes)?"
    - "Have you felt fetal movements?"

- **Frequency:** "Have you ever had this pain before? How often does the pain come (quantify in minutes)? Does it come regularly?"
- **Palliative factors:** "Does anything make the pain better? If so, what?"
- **Provocative factors:** "Does anything make the pain worse? If so, what?"

Pregnancy History

- This aspect of the history, especially confirmation of the gestational age, is pivotal.
- Nägele's rule: EDC = date of LMP − 3 months + 7 days + 1 year
  - Nägele's rule depends on menstrual cycles that span 28 to 30 days and are regular.
  - Determine duration of the patient's menstrual cycle, whether her cycles are regular, and the date of her LMP.
  - Determine whether she has used hormonal contraceptives (e.g., the oral contraceptive pill may change the reliability of the LMP).
- Date of first positive pregnancy test
- Date when patient first noted fetal movement (quickening; the date of quickening is usually 18 to 20 weeks in a primigravida patient)
- Results of the ultrasound examination
- Blood type: Rh positive versus Rh negative
- Pregnancy history: Bleeding, discharge, nausea or vomiting, gestational diabetes mellitus, anemia, or GER
- STIs: Previous and current infections, especially gonococcal and herpes infections (may preclude vaginal delivery)
- **PMH/PSH:** Bleeding diathesis, diabetes mellitus, hypertension, cardiovascular disease, thyroid problems, renal problems, anemia, epilepsy, asthma, STIs, psychiatric problems, anesthetic problems, previous surgery (including cryotherapy and LEEP), complications, or trauma
- **MEDS**
- **Allergies**
- **Immunizations:** Routine immunizations and immune status or exposure to infectious diseases such as rubella, HIV, HBV, and syphilis
- **SH:** Nutrition, intake of folic acid, smoking, use of EtOH, and use of street drugs during pregnancy; family support; occupational/financial situation; and relationship with the infant's father
- **FH:** Malformations, developmental delay, or known hereditary disorders

Physical Examination

- **Vitals:** Evaluate HR, RR, BP, and temperature.
  - Obstetric vitals also include the fetal HR and its trends (beat-to-beat variability, accelerations).
- **General:** Assess whether the patient is apprehensive or in apparent distress. Check capillary refill.
- **Resp:** Check chest expansion (symmetry), and auscultate the lungs (breath sounds, adventitious sounds).
- **CVS:** Measure the JVP. Palpate peripheral pulses. Note pulse volume, contour, and rhythm. Auscultate the heart, listening for extra heart sounds or flow murmurs associated with hyperdynamic circulation.
- **Abdomen:** Inspect the abdomen. Auscultate for bowel sounds. Percuss lightly. Perform light and deep palpation, and identify any masses or areas of tenderness.
- **Obs/Gyne:** Measure the fundal height from the pubis symphysis (in the third trimester, height in centimeters is correlated with gestational age in weeks). Use the Leopold maneuvers to determine the position, presentation, and lie of the infant (see Figure 11-12). If there is any bleeding, perform a speculum examination of the cervix (see Figure 11-10). Inspect the cervical os, and note any discharge, inflammation, or lesions. If the speculum examination yields unremarkable findings, proceed with a manual vaginal examination. Note whether the os is open or closed. Document effacement and dilation of the cervix.

BREASTFEEDING DIFFICULTIES: HISTORY

> **INSTRUCTIONS TO CANDIDATE: A 29-year-old woman with a 1-week-old infant presents to her family doctor with difficulty breastfeeding. She is concerned that the baby is not getting enough milk. Obtain an appropriate history.**

DD$_X$
- Improper latch
- Perceived lack of milk
- Baby-related problem (e.g., thrush, neurologic disorder, heart failure)
- Mastitis

History
- Ask the patient the following questions:
  - **Character:** "What kind of difficulty are you having with the breastfeeding? Does the baby latch well? The baby should latch on to nearly the whole areola rather than only the nipple. Is breastfeeding painful for you? Are your nipples sore (with proper latch, it should not be painful)?"
  - **Location:** "Where do you breastfeed: at home? In public places? Is your breastfeeding position comfortable for you?"
  - **Onset:** "When did you start to have difficulty? From the start?"
  - **Intensity:** "What was the baby's birth weight? What is his or her weight now?" (It is normal for infants to lose 10% of birth weight in the first week.)
  - **Events associated:**
    - "Is this your first child? Have you ever breastfed before?"
    - "How do you know whether the baby is getting milk? Does he or she swallow?" (The baby's mouth should open, pause, and close. The baby swallows during the pause.)
    - "Is your milk in? Do you feel your breasts filling up? Do they feel softer after each feed?"
    - "Do your breasts leak milk? Do you feel contractions in your uterus when you breastfeed?"
    - "How many bowel movements is the baby having each day? What color are they?" (The baby should have at least one bowel movement per day, usually a loose-consistency [seedy], mustard yellow stool [after meconium]. The stool may appear green if the milk is not yet in.)
    - "How many wet diapers does the baby have each day?" (He or she should have at least five to six wet diapers per day.)
    - "Does your baby wake for feedings? Is the baby easily roused from sleep?"
    - "Are you sleeping when you can, and are you eating a healthy diet? Are you drinking enough?"
  - **Frequency:** "How often do you breastfeed?" It is normal to breastfeed 8 to 12 times per 24 hours.)
  - **Palliative factors:** "Does anything make the breastfeeding easier? If so, what?"
  - **Provocative factors:** "Does anything make it more difficult? If so, what?"

Pregnancy History
- Date and gestational age at delivery
- Onset of labor: Spontaneous versus induced
- Duration of labor: Use of augmentation
- Type of delivery: Normal, spontaneous vaginal delivery; lower segment cesarean section; use of forceps or vacuum
- Maternal complications: Tears (first- to fourth-degree), postpartum hemorrhage, infection, and so on
- **PMH/PSH:** Endocrinopathies, psychiatric problems

- **MEDS:** *All* medications (prescription and OTC drugs) taken during pregnancy and since delivery and their effects on lactation
- **SH:** Nutrition, smoking, use of EtOH, use of street drugs, family support, and occupational/financial situation
- **FH:** Malformations, developmental delay, or known hereditary disorders

When to Return for Assessment
- If the baby sleeps for long periods or is difficult to arouse
- If the baby has <5 to 6 wet diapers per day
- If the mother has fever or chills and a red, painful area in the breast
- If the mother has sore nipples with no improvement
- See Dr. Jack Newman's Website for excellent resource information for breastfeeding moms (it provides printable handouts for patients, one of which is "Is my baby getting enough milk?"): http://www.breastfeedingonline.com/newman.shtml

CHAPTER 12

Pediatrics

ANATOMY

- Children are not merely "small adults"; there are many anatomic differences between children and adults, and just a few key differences are outlined below.

General

- Children have a large head-to-body ratio in comparison with adults, which raises their center of gravity and makes them more prone to head trauma in falls and motor vehicle collisions.
- Children also have a larger body surface area-to-mass ratio, which predisposes them to hypothermia. It is important to bear this in mind when children are disrobed for

Table 12-1   Normal Ranges for Vital Signs by Age

Age	Heart Rate (Beats/Minute)	Systolic Blood Pressure (mm Hg)	Respiratory Rate (Breaths/Minute)
Infant	120–160	>60	30–50
6 months to 1 year	120–140	70–80	30–40
2–4 years	100–110	80–95	20–30
5–8 years	90–100	90–100	14–20
8–12 years	80–100	100–110	12–20
>12 years	60–90	100–120	12–16

Adapted from Marx JA, Hockberger RS, Walls RM, editors. *Rosen's Emergency Medicine: Concepts and Clinical Practice.* 5th ed. St. Louis: Mosby; 2002 [p. 2221].

examination in a chilly emergency department, especially in trauma or resuscitation situations.
- Heart rate (HR), blood pressure (BP), and respiratory rates (RR) vary with age (Table 12-1).

Airway
- In comparison with adults, children have a larger tongue in relation to the size of the oral cavity (a common cause of upper airway obstruction).
- The epiglottis is larger and floppier, and the larynx is more anterior and cephalad than that of an adult.
- The cricoid ring is the narrowest part of the pediatric airway, which allows for the use of an uncuffed endotracheal tube in children aged <8 years (in adults, the larynx is the narrowest part of the airway).

Breathing
- The chest wall of a child is very compliant. Rib fractures are thus uncommon in children, but the underlying organs are susceptible to injury nonetheless.

Circulation
- Pediatric blood volume is approximately 8% of total body weight, in contrast to 6% of body weight in adults.
- Because the absolute blood volume in a child is less than that of an adult, the hemodynamic consequences of a given volume of blood loss are more severe in a child.

Abdomen
- Solid abdominal organs are more susceptible to injury because of the more anterior location and larger relative size of these organs and the laxity of the abdominal wall (less musculature and subcutaneous tissue).

Musculoskeletal System
- The presence of growth plates in children sometimes makes the interpretation of radiographs challenging. It may be helpful to take a comparative radiograph of the contralateral joint to identify the normal anatomy.
- The growth plate is the weakest part of the bone. Children are more likely to sustain a growth plate injury than a sprain (the ligamentous connective tissue is stronger relative to the cartilaginous growth plate).
- The bony pelvis in children is more shallow, frequently allowing the urinary bladder to become an abdominal rather than a pelvic organ.

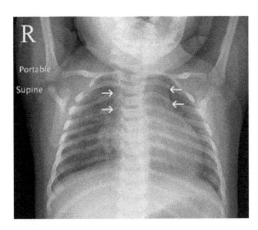

Figure 12-1 Portable anteroposterior chest radiograph in a neonate. *Arrows* point out left and right margins of the thymus.

Thymus
* In relation to the body, the thymus is largest at birth. This is evident on infant chest radiographs as a "mediastinal mass" (Figure 12-1).
* It reaches its largest absolute mass during puberty and begins to involute thereafter.

ESSENTIAL SKILLS

APPROACH TO PEDIATRIC PATIENTS

Communication
* Children are often accompanied by one or both parents or another family member. Although it is important to get information from the caregiver about the reasons for the visit, do not ignore the importance of communicating directly with the child, because he or she is a valuable source of clinical data.
* Address the caregivers' concerns. It may be helpful to ask a question such as "What is your biggest worry or concern today?" This helps identify expectations for the visit and perceptions about the child's illness.
* Avoid using technical jargon. Establishing a good rapport with the caregiver is important in your encounter with the child, who is likely to pick up on the discomfort of his or her caregiver.
* Follow the lead of the caregiver to ensure that you communicate with the child at an appropriate level. When you address a child, ensure that your eyes are on the same horizontal plane by sitting, kneeling, or crouching as necessary. Engage the child by talking about things he or she likes, such as a favorite toy or activity, friends, or school.
* An older child or adolescent should be addressed primarily in the interview; garner supplemental information from the caregiver afterwards.
* For children, the prenatal, natal, and neonatal history may be relevant for evaluating their current presentation. This type of history should definitely be sought in children aged <2 years.

Initial Assessment
* The initial pediatric assessment should take into account the general appearance of the child, the work of breathing, and circulation to the skin (Table 12-2). This simple assessment will help identify cardiorespiratory compromise (Table 12-3).

Physical Examination
* A great deal can be learned from simply observing the pediatric patient. By watching the parent-child interaction and watching the child play, socialize, and interact with his or her environment, you can obtain valuable data about development. Furthermore, through observation, you can identify respiratory distress, cry, physical limitations

Table 12-2   Initial Assessment of the Pediatric Patient

Appearance	Work of Breathing	Circulation to the Skin

Tone
Irritable, interactive
Consolable
Look/gaze
Speech/cry
	Abnormal sounds: stridor, grunting,
	  snoring, wheezing
	Abnormal positioning: sniffing,
	  tripoding, refusal to lie down
	Retractions
	Head bobbing
	Nasal flaring
		Pallor
		Mottling
		Cyanosis
		Petechiae

Adapted from Dieckmann R, Brownstein D, Gausche-Hill M, eds. *Pediatric Education for Prehospital Professionals.* Sudbury, MA: Jones & Bartlett/American Academy of Pediatrics; 2000 [p. 36-40].

Table 12-3   Correlation of the Initial Assessment Findings with Underlying Physiologic State

Physiologic State	Appearance	Work of Breathing	Circulation to the Skin
Respiratory distress	Normal	Abnormal	Normal
Respiratory failure	Abnormal	Abnormal	Normal/abnormal
Compensated shock	Normal	Normal	Abnormal
Decompensated shock	Abnormal	Normal/abnormal	Abnormal
Brain injury/dysfunction	Abnormal	Normal	Normal
Cardiopulmonary failure	Abnormal	Abnormal	Abnormal

Adapted from Dieckmann R, Brownstein D, Gausche-Hill M, eds. *Pediatric Education for Prehospital Professionals.* Sudbury, MA: Jones & Bartlett/American Academy of Pediatrics; 2000 [p. 30-57].

such as a limp, or handedness. Overall, a great deal of the neuromuscular examination and developmental assessment can be documented without laying hands on the child.
- The remainder of the physical examination is largely opportunistic in nature. The order of the examination is not important, and you should routinely leave the most invasive or uncomfortable parts for last. For example, if the child is quiet, take the opportunity to auscultate the heart and lungs.
- To improve the comfort level of the child and increase cooperation, it is helpful to examine the child on the parent's lap or with the parent close by.

Pearl
- Always consider the possibility of abuse. The majority of children are well cared for, but failure to consider the possibilities may cause you to overlook red flags.

EARS AND THROAT: EXAMINATION

Inspection
- Are both ears present and normally formed, and are they positioned normally (Figure 12-2)?
  - The appearance of small, malformed, and low-set ears may be associated with genetic syndromes.
- Inspect the pinnae and tragi (Figure 12-3). Note signs of trauma, eczema, redness, swelling, or tenderness.
- Inspect the palate and pharynx (Figure 12-4). Look at the size of the tonsils. "Kissing" tonsils may be large enough to cause airway obstruction. Note any petechiae, erythema, exudate, or vesicles.
  - Petechiae and exudate may be present in streptococcal pharyngitis.

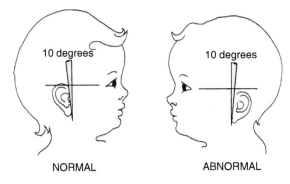

NORMAL   ABNORMAL

Figure 12-2 Ear alignment. (From Barkauskas VH, Baumann LC, Darling-Fisher CS. *Health and Physical Assessment.* 3rd ed. St Louis: Mosby; 2002 [p. 656].)

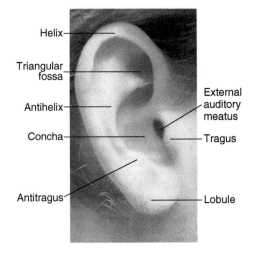

Helix
Triangular fossa
Antihelix
Concha
Antitragus
External auditory meatus
Tragus
Lobule

Figure 12-3 External ear. (From Seidel HM, Ball JW, Dains JE, et al. *Mosby's Guide to Physical Examination.* 6th ed. St. Louis: Mosby; 2006 [p. 318].)

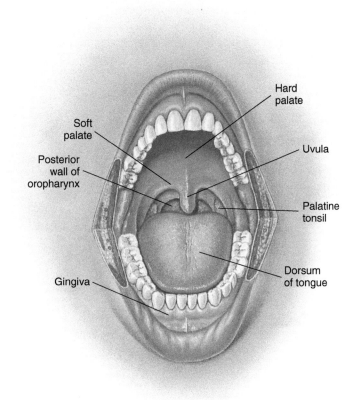

Soft palate
Posterior wall of oropharynx
Gingiva
Hard palate
Uvula
Palatine tonsil
Dorsum of tongue

Figure 12-4 Oropharynx. (From Seidel HM, Ball JW, Dains JE, et al. *Mosby's Guide to Physical Examination.* 6th ed. St. Louis: Mosby; 2006 [p. 323].)

- Vesicles or ulcerations may be suggestive of herpangina, hand-foot-mouth disease, or herpetic gingivostomatitis.
- "Cobblestoning" of the posterior pharynx may be seen in postnasal drip.

Palpation
- Palpate the external ear. In acute otitis externa, movement of the pinna and tragus is painful.
- Palpate the mastoid. Tenderness may be suggestive of mastoiditis.
- Examine the lymph nodes of the head and neck (see pp. 244-246).

Otoscopic Examination
- Explain the examination to the parent and child. You may allay anxiety in the child by seating him or her on the parent or caregiver's lap. If the child needs to be restrained, ask the parent or caregiver to turn the child's head to one side, holding the head against the parent's body. Protect the ear by bracing your hand between the child's head and the otoscope.
- Grasp the auricle, and pull it upward, backward, and slightly away from the head to straighten the external auditory canal. Hold the otoscope between your thumb and fingers. Gently insert the speculum of the otoscope into the ear canal. Describe any abnormalities such as discharge, erythema, or swelling. Inspect for any obstructions in the external auditory canal, such as cerumen or a foreign body.
- Examine the tympanic membrane, and identify landmarks (Figure 12-5). The normal tympanic membrane has a translucent appearance. Opacification is usually caused by thickening or effusion. Note the color, contour, and any bulging or retraction. Note any perforation, scars, or the presence of myringotomy "tubes."
- Acute otitis media usually manifests with a hyperemic, opaque, bulging tympanic membrane and loss of normal landmarks. A middle ear effusion may produce a bluish (serous) or yellow (pus) appearance to the tympanic membrane.
- **Pneumootoscopy:** Using a bulb attached to the otoscope, apply positive and negative pressure in the ear canal. Decreased compliance with positive pressure is suggestive of a bulging tympanic membrane, whereas decreased compliance with negative pressure is suggestive of a retracted tympanic membrane.

Auditory Acuity
- If a parent believes his or her child cannot hear, this belief should be assumed correct until proved otherwise.
- Occlude one ear with a finger and whisper softly into the other ear, using words or numbers of equally accented syllables.
- **Acoustic blink test:** To test an infant's hearing, observe blinking in response to a sudden sharp sound produced approximately 12 inches from the ear (e.g., snapping fingers, clapping).

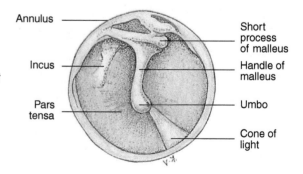

Figure 12-5 Tympanic membrane. (From Wilson SF, Gidden JF. *Health Assessment for Nursing Practice.* 2nd ed. St. Louis: Mosby; 2001 [p. 289].)

- If acuity is decreased, use Weber's and Rinne's tests to distinguish sensorineural from conductive hearing loss. These tests, however, are not useful in young children.
  - **Weber's test:** Place a vibrating tuning fork (512 Hz or 1024 Hz) firmly on top of the patient's head. Ask the patient whether he or she hears it in one or both ears. Normally, the sound is heard midline. In conductive hearing loss, sound is heard laterally in the impaired ear. In sensorineural hearing loss, the sound is heard laterally in the normal ear.
  - **Rinne's test:** Place a vibrating tuning fork (512 Hz or 1024 Hz) on the mastoid bone, behind the ear and level with the external auditory canal. When the patient can no longer hear the sound, place the tuning fork close to the ear canal (the "U" of the fork facing forward), and ask whether the sound is now audible. In conductive hearing loss, sound is best transmitted by bone conduction.

EYES: EXAMINATION

Inspection
- **Alignment:** Check the eyes for position and alignment with each other, noting any deviation or protrusion.
- **Lids:** Inspect the lids, noting their position in relation to the eye itself. Document any swelling or redness in the area of the lacrimal glands.
  - **Ptosis** is the drooping of the upper lid and may be related to myasthenia gravis, Horner's syndrome, or cranial nerve III palsy (congenital and acquired).
  - **Retracted lid** is present when a rim of sclera can be seen between the upper lid and the iris. When the lids are retracted, also look for lid lag. Ask the child to follow an object with his or her eyes from midline, up to down. The lid normally overlaps the iris slightly throughout this movement. In lid lag, a rim of sclera is seen between the upper lid and iris when the patient gazes downward. The presence of retracted lids and lid lag may be suggestive of hyperthyroidism.
- **Eyes:** Note any excessive tearing or dryness. Inspect the sclerae, noting any icterus or redness. If the conjunctiva is injected, qualify this finding by noting the pattern (e.g., peripheral versus ciliary). Look at the iris; its margins should be clearly defined.
- **Pupils:** Inspect size, shape, and symmetry of the pupils. If the pupils are large (>5 mm), small (<3 mm), or unequal, measure them. Use the swinging flashlight test to assess the direct and consensual response to light. Pupillary constriction can also be observed during accommodation; ask the child to look at your finger or an object, and bring it progressively closer until the child's eyes cross.
  - **Miosis** is constriction of the pupil.
  - **Mydriasis** is dilation of the pupil.
  - **Anisocoria** is pupillary inequality (up to 1 mm of asymmetry is considered within normal limits).

Visual Acuity
- Test visual acuity with the Snellen eye chart. For young children, use a Snellen E chart, and ask them to identify which way the letter is facing. It is difficult to quantify visual acuity in children aged <3 years. Patients who have prescription glasses should wear them. Position the child 20 feet from the chart. Cover one eye, and ask the child to read the smallest print possible. Visual acuity is expressed as two numbers (e.g., 20/20), in which the first number indicates the distance of the patient from the chart, and the second number is the distance at which the average person can read the line of letters. Normal visual acuity at age 3 is 20/40 and usually reaches 20/20 by age 6. A discrepancy in visual acuity between the eyes is abnormal and

may lead to amblyopia. Refractive errors improve when the patient looks through a pinhole.

- **Myopia** is impaired far vision (i.e., near-sighted).
- **Hyperopia** is impaired near vision (i.e., far-sighted).
- **Amblyopia** is unilateral decreased visual acuity without any detectable cause. It is related most commonly to suppression of vision in patients with strabismus.

Visual Fields

- Seat the child on the parent's lap. Hold the child's head in midline position, and bring a brightly colored object into the child's field of vision from behind (upper and lower temporal fields). Eye deviation toward the object indicates that the child has seen it. The blind spot is 15 degrees temporal.

Extraocular Movements

- Using a light or an object, assess the extraocular eye movements (Figure 12-6). Note any dysconjugate movement or nystagmus at the extremes of gaze. Dysconjugate movements may be caused by a cranial nerve palsy (cranial nerves III, IV, and VI) or by a muscular problem (strabismus). Brief nystagmus (<3 beats) on extreme lateral gaze is normal.

Strabismus Screening

- Shine a light on the patient's eyes, and ask the patient to look at it. Observe the reflection of the light on the corneas. Normally, the reflection is visible slightly nasally with regard to the center of the pupil and is symmetric (Figure 12-7).

Funduscopic Examination

- Darken the room. Tell the child you are going to shine a light in his or her eyes. Have the child pick which eye he or she would like you to look in first. Use your left eye to examine the patient's left eye. Approach the patient from the temporal side at a 15-degree angle to elicit the red reflex. Absence of the red reflex is suggestive of corneal opacity (e.g., cataracts) or retinoblastoma. Inspect the cornea, lens, and vitreous for opacities.

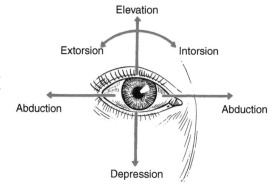

Figure 12-6 Extraocular movements. (From Swartz M. *Textbook of Physical Diagnosis: History and Examination.* 6th ed. Philadelphia: Elsevier; 2010 [p. 215].)

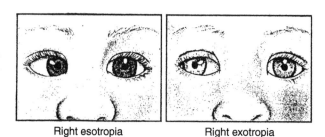

Figure 12-7 Asymmetric corneal light reflex. (Adapted from Jarvis CJ. *Physical Examination and Health Assessment.* 2nd ed. Philadelphia: Saunders; 1996 [p. 340].)

Right esotropia   Right exotropia

- Inspect each optic disc. Compare the discs for symmetry, and note the following:
  - Clarity of the disc margins and color. Papilledema is rarely seen in children aged <3 years because the sutures can open to accommodate increased intracranial pressure (ICP).
  - Inspect the retina. Follow the course of the vessels to each of four quadrants. Note exudates, hemorrhages, or other lesions. Inspect the macula and fovea.

DEVELOPMENTAL DYSPLASIA OF THE HIP IN A NEWBORN: EXAMINATION

Anatomy
- The hip is a ball-and-socket joint (the femoral head is the ball, and the acetabulum is the socket). The components of the joint are interdependent for normal growth and development. The cause of developmental dysplasia of the hip (DDH) is multifactorial.

Definition
- **Developmental dysplasia of the hip** is congenital dislocation of the hips. The cause is multifactorial, and the condition is progressive unless corrected; thus, every newborn should be examined for DDH. Beyond 2 months of age, DDH becomes more difficult to detect clinically because of increases in muscle strength and in soft tissue.

Inspection
- Inspect the contour of the legs while the infant is lying supine. **Count the skin folds** on the medial aspect of the thigh (Figure 12-8). Asymmetry is suggestive of dislocation of the femoral head (skin folds are increased ipsilaterally).
- **Visualization of the perineum** in this position is suggestive of bilateral hip dislocations. The normal position of the thighs should cover most of the perineum.
- Flex the infant's knees and hips. Place the infant's feet side by side with the plantar aspects of the feet against the examination table. Observe the relative heights of the knees. If the knees are symmetric, either both hips are normal or both are dislocated. If the knee height is asymmetric, suspect either dislocation of the femoral head on the side of the shorter knee **(Galeazzi's sign)** or a congenitally short femur.

Range of Motion
- Test the passive range of motion of the hip: flexion, extension, abduction, adduction, and internal and external rotation. Limitation of abduction is abnormal and may be indicative of DDH. The neonatal joints are agile; in normal infants, the hips should readily abduct to nearly 90 degrees.

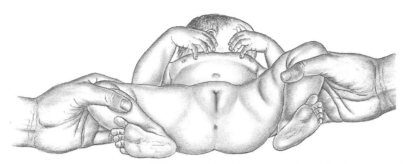

Figure 12-8 Asymmetric gluteal folds. (From Seidel HM, Ball JW, Dains JE, et al. *Mosby's Guide to Physical Examination.* 6th ed. St. Louis: Mosby; 2006 [p. 737].)

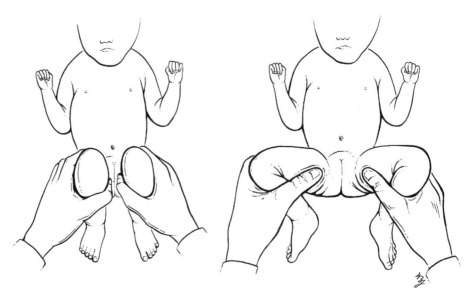

Figure 12-9 Ortolani's test. (From Swartz M. *Textbook of Physical Diagnosis: History and Examination.* 4th ed. Philadelphia: Saunders; 2002 [Figure 23-14].)

Special Tests
- Perform these tests with the infant supine, legs pointing toward you.
- **Ortolani's test** (Figure 12-9): Flex the infant's knees and hips to 90 degrees. Place your index finger over the greater trochanter and your thumb over the lesser trochanter. Simultaneously abduct both hips until the lateral aspect of each knee touches the examination table. When DDH is present, you will feel and sometimes hear a "clunk" as the dislocated femoral head reenters the acetabulum.
- **Barlow's test:** Place your index finger over the greater trochanter and your thumb over the lesser trochanter. Using the opposite hand to stabilize the pelvis, push your thumb posterolaterally and feel for movement of the femoral head as it slips out onto the posterior lip of the acetabulum. Then, with your index finger, press the greater trochanter anteromedially. Feel for movement of the femoral head as it reenters the acetabulum. Normally, no movement is felt. Movement felt in both directions constitutes a positive result of Barlow's test indicating hip instability.

DENVER DEVELOPMENTAL SCREENING TEST

- The **Denver Development Screening Test (DDST)** assesses development of children from birth to 6 years of age in four categories:
  - Personal-social
  - Fine motor–adaptive
  - Language
  - Gross motor
- The DDST is not a test of intelligence. The criteria for passing the DDST are set low to minimize labeling normal children as abnormal, which makes the test more specific than sensitive. Children with "borderline" or "questionable" scores should be monitored closely.
- **To use the DDST** (Figure 12-10): Draw a line from top to bottom according to the age of the child. Test each of the milestones crossed by this line. Failure to perform an item passed by 90% of children is significant. Two failures in any of the four categories are indicative of a developmental delay in that domain.

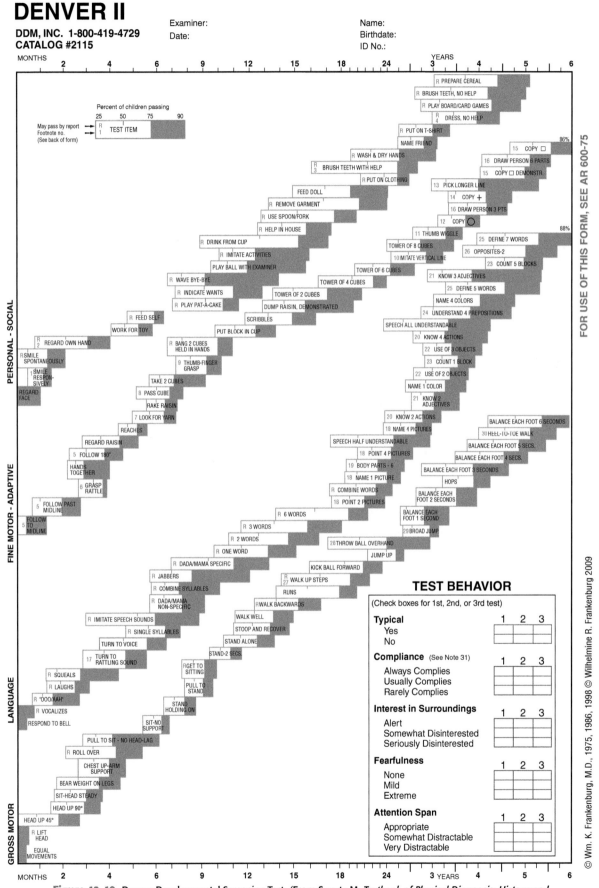

Figure 12-10 Denver Developmental Screening Test. (From Swartz M. *Textbook of Physical Diagnosis: History and Examination.* 6th ed. Philadelphia: Elsevier; 2010 [p. 738-739].)

Continued

DIRECTIONS FOR ADMINISTRATION

1. Try to get child to smile by smiling, talking, or waving. Do not touch him/her.
2. Child must stare at hand several seconds.
3. Parent may help guide toothbrush and put toothpaste on brush.
4. Child does not have to be able to tie shoes or button/zip in the back.
5. Move yarn slowly in an arc from one side to the other, about 8" above child's face.
6. Pass if child grasps rattle when it is touched to the backs or tips of fingers.
7. Pass if child tries to see where yarn went. Yarn should be dropped quickly from sight from tester's hand without arm movement.
8. Child must transfer cube from hand to hand without help of body, mouth, or table.
9. Pass if child picks up raisin with any part of thumb and finger.
10. Line can vary only 30 degrees or less from tester's line.
11. Make a fist with thumb pointing upward and wiggle only the thumb. Pass if child imitates and does not move any fingers other than the thumb.

         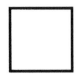

| 12. Pass any enclosed form. Fail continuous round motions. | 13. Which line is longer? (Not bigger.) Turn paper upside down and repeat. (pass 3 of 3 or 5 of 6) | 14. Pass any lines crossing near midpoint. | 15. Have child copy first. If failed, demonstrate. |

When giving items 12, 14, and 15, do not name the forms. Do not demonstrate 12 and 14.

16. When scoring, each pair (2 arms, 2 legs, etc.) counts as one part.
17. Place one cube in cup and shake gently near child's ear, but out of sight. Repeat for other ear.
18. Point to picture and have child name it. (No credit is given for sounds only.)
    If less than 4 pictures are named correctly, have child point to picture as each is named by tester.

   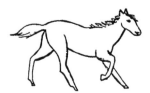   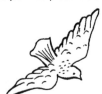   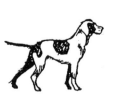   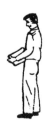

19. Using doll, tell child: Show me the nose, eyes, ears, mouth, hands, feet, tummy, hair. Pass 6 of 8.
20. Using pictures, ask child: Which one flies?... says meow?... talks?... barks?... gallops? Pass 2 of 5, 4 of 5.
21. Ask child: What do you do when you are cold?... tired?... hungry?   Pass 2 of 3, 3 of 3.
22. Ask child: What do you do with a cup? What is a chair used for? What is a pencil used for?
    Action words must be included in answers.
23. Pass if child correctly places <u>and</u> says how many blocks are on paper. (1, 5).
24. Tell child: Put block **on** table; **under** table; **in front of** me, **behind** me. Pass 4 of 4.
    (Do not help child by pointing, moving head or eyes.)
25. Ask child: What is a ball?... lake?... desk?... house?... banana?... curtain?... fence?... ceiling? Pass if defined in terms of use, shape, what it is made of, or general category (such as banana is fruit, not just yellow). Pass 5 of 8, 7 of 8.
26. Ask child: If a horse is big, a mouse is __? If fire is hot, ice is __? If the sun shines during the day, the moon shines during the __? Pass 2 of 3.
27. Child may use wall or rail only, not person. May not crawl.
28. Child must throw ball overhand 3 feet to within arm's reach of tester.
29. Child must perform standing broad jump over width of test sheet (8 1/2 inches).
30. Tell child to walk forward, ⚬⚬⚬⚬⚬⚬➤ heel within 1 inch of toe. Tester may demonstrate.
    Child must walk 4 consecutive steps.
31. In the second year, half of normal children are non-compliant.

OBSERVATIONS:

Figure 12-10, cont'd Denver Developmental Screening Test. (From Swartz M. *Textbook of Physical Diagnosis: History and Examination.* 6th ed. Philadelphia: Elsevier; 2010 [p. 738-739].)

IMMUNIZATION HISTORY

INSTRUCTIONS TO CANDIDATE: A 28-month-old girl is brought to her family physician by her mother for the first time. They have recently immigrated to this country. Obtain an immunization history.

Immunization History
- Ask the mother the following questions:
  - "From where did you emigrate?" (Specific immunization schedules vary from country to country and within jurisdictions.)
  - "Has your child had any vaccinations?" (If so, determine the age at immunization and type of immunizations received.)
  - "Do you have an immunization record or a copy of your daughter's health records?"
  - "Can you describe any adverse reactions to past vaccinations?"
    - Local reactions: Induration, tenderness, redness, and, on occasion, edema and abscess formation at the injection site.
    - Systemic reactions: Fever, exanthem, joint or muscle pains, fainting, seizures, and other central nervous system (CNS) symptoms; irritability is common
    - Allergic reactions (rare): Urticaria, rhinitis, bronchospasm, anaphylaxis
- Persons lacking written documentation of immunization should be started on an age-appropriate immunization schedule (Table 12-4).

Prenatal, Natal, and Neonatal History
- Ask the mother the following questions:
  - "Did you have prenatal care? Any difficulties during the pregnancy?"
  - "Did you use alcohol or recreational drugs during the pregnancy? Did you smoke during the pregnancy?"
  - "Was this a singleton or multiple gestation?"
  - "What was the child's gestational age at delivery?"
  - "When did labor begin? How long did labor last? What type of delivery did you have (normal spontaneous vaginal delivery [NSVD], lower segment cesarean section [LSCS], forceps, vacuum)?"
  - "What was your daughter's birth weight? Was she fed breast milk or formula?"
  - "What were her Apgar scores at 1 and 5 minutes?"
  - "Did your daughter have any health problems as a baby? Any hospital admissions? Any surgeries?"
  - "Did your daughter have any delay in speech, language, or motor development?"

Pearls
- There are few *true* contraindications to vaccination: Allergy to vaccine component, pregnancy (live vaccines contraindicated), and severe immunocompromise (live vaccines contraindicated). Minor illnesses such as the common cold are not contraindications to immunization. Infections do not increase the risk of adverse effects from immunization and do not interfere with immune responses to vaccines.
- Immunization schedules in Canada can be accessed through the Public Health Agency of Canada online (http://www.phac-aspc.gc.ca/im/iyc-vve/is-cv-eng.php).

Table 12-4   Routine Immunization Schedule for Children <7 Years Not Immunized in Infancy

Time of Immunization	DTaP IPV*	Hib†	MMR‡	Hep B§	Pneum¶	Men¶¶	HPV**	Td††	Comments
First visit	✓	✓	✓	✓	✓	✓			
2 months later	✓	(✓)	✓	✓	(✓)				
2 months later	✓				(✓)				
6–12 months later	✓	(✓)		✓					Hib not needed if child's age >5 years
4–6 years	(✓)								DTaP-IPV may be omitted if the fourth dose is given after the fourth birthday.
12 years						✓			Girls aged 9–13 years (three doses)
14–16 years								✓	Td booster should be given every 10 years after this vaccination.

Adapted from National Advisory Committee on Immunization. *Canadian Immunization Guide,* 7th ed. Ottawa: Public Health Agency of Canada; 2006, [Table 2].
*Diphtheria, tetanus, acellular pertussis, and inactivated polio virus vaccine.
†*Haemophilus influenzae* type b conjugate vaccine.
‡Measles, mumps, and rubella vaccine.
§Hepatitis B vaccine.
¶Pneumococcal conjugate vaccine–7-valent vaccine.
¶¶Meningococcal C conjugate vaccine.
**Human papillomavirus vaccine.
††Diphtheria and tetanus vaccine.
Parentheses around a check mark mean that the dose may not be required, depending on the age of the child.

MALAISE AND LYMPHADENOPATHY: PHYSICAL EXAMINATION

INSTRUCTIONS TO CANDIDATE: A 15-year-old girl presents to her family physician with malaise and "swollen glands." Perform a focused physical examination.

DD$_X$: VITAMINS C
- Infectious: Mononucleosis, other viral illness, tuberculosis, and human immunodeficiency virus (HIV) infection
- Neoplastic: Lymphoma (Hodgkin's and non-Hodgkin's types), leukemia, and other malignancies

Physical Examination

- **Vital signs (Vitals):** Evaluate HR, BP, RR, and temperature (low-grade fever may be present).
- **General:** Assess the patient's general appearance, noting signs of cachexia.
- **Skin:** Inspect the skin and nails, noting any diaphoresis, jaundice, pallor (lips, buccal mucosa, conjunctiva, palmar creases), petechiae, or ecchymosis.
- **Lymphatic system:** Note size, shape, mobility, consistency, tenderness, warmth, and number of enlarged nodes. Seat the patient in a chair, and stand behind him or her. Flex the neck slightly. Using the pads of your fingers, palpate in a rotatory motion (moving the skin over the underlying tissues):
  - Occipital: Base of skull posteriorly
  - Postauricular: Superficial to mastoid process
  - Preauricular: Anterior to ear
  - Tonsillar: Angle of mandible
  - Submandibular: Midway between the angle and the tip of the mandible
  - Submental: Midline behind the tip of the mandible (helpful to palpate with one hand while bracing the top of the head with the other hand)
  - Anterior cervical: Along the anterior border of the sternocleidomastoid muscle
  - Posterior cervical: Along the anterior edge of the trapezius muscle
  - Deep cervical: Deep to the sternocleidomastoid muscle (the lymph nodes here are often inaccessible; hook your thumb and fingers around the sternocleidomastoid muscle, and roll the muscle between your fingers)
  - Supraclavicular: Deep in the angle between the clavicle and sternocleidomastoid muscle
  - Infraclavicular: Inferior to the clavicle
  - Axillary
  - Epitrochlear
  - Inguinal
- **Respiratory system (Resp):** Inspect for thoracic deformity. Assess chest expansion for symmetry. Evaluate the position of the trachea. Auscultate the lungs, noting breath sounds and adventitious sounds. Note any signs of infection, pleural effusion, or tracheobronchial compression.
- **Cardiovascular system (CVS):** Check capillary refill. Palpate peripheral pulses, noting contour, volume, and rhythm. Auscultate the heart, listening for extra heart sounds or murmurs. Look for signs of anemia such as hyperdynamic precordium and aortic flow murmur.
- **Abdomen:** Inspect the abdomen. Auscultate for bowel sounds. Percuss lightly in all four quadrants. Perform light and deep palpation, and identify any masses or areas of tenderness. Check for rebound tenderness. Examine the liver and spleen (looking for organomegaly).
- Note any signs or sources of infection.

DIARRHEA: HISTORY AND PHYSICAL EXAMINATION

> **INSTRUCTIONS TO CANDIDATE: A 14-month-old girl is brought to the emergency department by her parents because of diarrhea. Obtain a focused history, and perform a focused physical examination.**

DD$_X$: VITAMINS C
- **Infectious:** Bacterial/parasitic/viral infection, pseudomembranous colitis
- **Autoimmune/allergic:** Celiac disease
- **Metabolic:** Drugs (e.g., antibiotics)
- **Idiopathic/iatrogenic:** Toddler's diarrhea, inflammatory bowel disease (IBD), irritable bowel syndrome
- **Congenital/genetic:** Cystic fibrosis, lactose intolerance

History

- Ask the parents the following questions:
  - **Character:** "Can you describe the bowel movements (BMs)?"
    - "Are the stools frequent, voluminous, and poorly formed (diarrhea)? Are any food particles visible?"
    - "Are the stools large, oily, and malodorous, but somewhat formed (steatorrhea)?"
    - "Are the stools frequent and formed but small?"
    - "Any blood, pus, or mucus in the stool? What color is the stool?"
    - "Does diarrhea persist despite fasting?"
    - "Does your child experience diarrhea at night?"
    - "Describe her usual BMs."
  - **Location:** "Where was she when this started? Have you traveled recently?"
  - **Onset:** "When did the diarrhea start (sudden versus insidious)?"
  - **Intensity:** "How severe is the diarrhea (number of stools per day and approximate volume of stool)? Has it gotten worse?"
  - **Duration:** "How long has the diarrhea been going on (acute versus chronic)?"
  - **Events associated:**
    - "Has your child had nausea or vomiting? Fever or chills? Abdominal pain? How is her appetite?"
    - "Did your child eat meat or seafood products in the 72 hours before the diarrhea started (undercooked hamburger or chicken, shellfish)? Has she eaten excessive amounts of cereal, prunes, or other roughage? Has she consumed artificial sweeteners?"
    - "Has your child had periods of constipation (possibility of stool overflow)?"
    - "Has your child traveled to tropical or subtropical regions or gone camping? Has she been in contact with persons with infections? Has she drunk contaminated water?"
    - IBD: "Has she had chronic diarrhea, abdominal pain, weight loss, perianal disease, and extraintestinal manifestations?"
    - Constitutional symptoms: "Has she had fever, chills, night sweats, weight loss, anorexia, or asthenia?"
  - **Frequency:** "Has this ever happened before? Is every BM like diarrhea (intermittent versus constant)?"
  - **Palliative factors:** "Does anything make it better? If so, what? Fasting?"
  - **Provocative factors:** "Does anything make it worse? If so, what? Dairy products? Solid foods?"
- **Previous investigations:** Stool analysis
- **Past medical history (PMH)/past surgical history (PSH):** IBD, celiac disease, hyperthyroidism, previous gastrointestinal (GI) surgery, cystic fibrosis, HIV infection or acquired immune deficiency syndrome (AIDS), or malignancy
- **Medications (MEDS):** Laxatives, antidiarrheal agents, recent antibiotics, or corticosteroids
- **Allergies:** Medications, food allergies or intolerances
- **Social history (SH):** Diet
- **Family history (FH):** IBD, cystic fibrosis, GI malignancy, celiac disease, or HIV infection or AIDS

Prenatal, Natal, and Neonatal History

- Ask the mother the following questions:
  - "Did you have prenatal care? Any difficulties during the pregnancy?"
  - "Did you use alcohol or recreational drugs during the pregnancy? Did you smoke during the pregnancy?"
  - "Was this a singleton or multiple gestation?"

- "What was the child's gestational age at delivery?"
- "Did labor begin spontaneously, or was it induced? How long did labor last? Was any type of augmentation used in the delivery? What type of delivery did you have (NSVD, LSCS, forceps, or vacuum)?"
- "What was your daughter's birth weight? Was she fed breast milk or formula?"
- "What were her Apgar scores at 1 and 5 minutes?"
- "Has your daughter had any delay in speech, language, or motor development?"

Examination

- **Vitals:** Evaluate HR, BP (lying and standing), RR, and temperature
- **General:** Assess the patient's general appearance, work of breathing, and circulation to the skin. Correlate the findings of the initial assessment with the underlying physiologic state (see Table 12-3). Note signs of dehydration (sunken eyes, dry buccal mucosa, loss of skin turgor, delayed capillary refill, lethargy).
- **Skin:** Inspect the skin and nails, noting any diaphoresis, jaundice, or pallor.
- **Head, eyes, ears, nose, and throat (HEENT):** Inspect the sclerae. Note any aphthous oral ulcers (extraintestinal manifestation of IBD), glossitis, or cheilosis (signs of anemia).
- **Resp:** Inspect for thoracic deformity. Assess chest expansion for symmetry. Auscultate the lungs, noting breath sounds and adventitious sounds.
- **CVS:** Check capillary refill. Palpate peripheral pulses, noting contour, volume, and rhythm. Auscultate the heart, listening for extra heart sounds or murmurs.
- **Abdomen:** Inspect the abdomen. Hyperperistalsis may be evident. Auscultate for bowel sounds, noting borborygmus. Percuss lightly in all four quadrants. Perform light and deep palpation, and identify any masses or areas of tenderness. Check for rebound tenderness. Examine the liver and spleen. Inspect the perianal area for fissures, fistulas, skin tags, or other lesions.
- **Examine the stool:** Note the proportion of water to solids and the presence of pus, mucus, fat globules, and food particles. Note any fresh blood, and test for the presence of occult blood.

Evidence

- The reliability of the clinical examination for diagnosing dehydration in children (Table 12-5) is only fair to moderate. Combinations of the clinical examination yield more reliable results than do single signs in the evaluation of dehydration.[1]

Table 12-5	Usefulness of Clinical Examination for Diagnosing Dehydration in Children	
Clinical Feature	**+LR (95% CI)**	**−LR (95% CI)**
Poor overall appearance	1.9 (0.97–3.8)	0.46 (0.34–0.61)
Delayed capillary refill	4.1 (1.7–9.8)	0.57 (0.39–0.82)
Abnormal respiratory pattern	2.0 (1.5–2.7)	0.76 (0.62–0.88)
Sunken eyes	1.7 (1.1–2.5)	0.49 (0.38–0.63)
Sunken fontanelle	0.9 (0.6–1.3)	1.12 (0.82–1.54)
Dry mucous membranes	1.7 (1.1–2.6)	0.41 (0.21–0.79)
Absence of tears	2.3 (0.9–5.8)	0.54 (0.26–1.13)
Loss of skin turgor	2.5 (1.5–4.2)	0.66 (0.57–0.75)

Modified from Steiner MJ, DeWalt DA, Byerley JS. Is this child dehydrated? *JAMA.* 2004;291: 2746-2754.

CI, Confidence interval; −LR, negative likelihood ratio; +LR, positive likelihood ratio.

ASTHMA: HISTORY AND PHYSICAL EXAMINATION

> **INSTRUCTIONS TO CANDIDATE: A 10-year-old girl with a history of asthma is brought to the emergency department from gym class. At the triage desk, she is tachypneic and has an audible wheeze. Obtain a focused history, and perform a focused physical examination.**

DD$_X$: VITAMINS C

- "All that wheezes is not asthma," although it is a common cause of wheeze in children.
- **V**ascular: Cardiac wheeze
- **T**raumatic: Foreign body aspiration
- **A**utoimmune/**a**llergic: Angioedema
- **I**diopathic/**i**atrogenic: Asthma, gastroesophageal reflux (GER)
- **C**ongenital/genetic: Cystic fibrosis
- First evaluate **appearance, work of breathing,** and **circulation to the skin** (see Table 12-2). If no immediate interventions are required, proceed to obtain an appropriate history and perform a physical examination.

History

- Ask the patient the following questions:
  - **Character:** "Can you describe the wheeze? What time of day is the wheeze at its worst?"
    - "Is the wheeze high-pitched or low-pitched? Can you hear it on inspiration or expiration?"
    - "Do you feel short of breath? Describe the nature of your breathing difficulty."
  - **Location:** "Where were you when this started? What were you doing?"
  - **Onset:** "How did the wheeze begin (sudden versus insidious onset)? How did the shortness of breath start?"
  - **Intensity:** "How severe is the wheeze right now on a scale of 1 to 10, with 10 being the most severe? How severe has the wheeze been in the past? How is it affecting your daily activities? How severe is the shortness of breath?"
  - **Duration:** "How long have you had this wheeze (acute versus chronic)? How long have you been short of breath?"
  - **Events associated:**
    - Asthma: "Do you have nocturnal cough, decreased exercise tolerance, eczema, sensitivity to acetylsalicylic acid (ASA) or nonsteroidal anti-inflammatory drugs (NSAIDs), and nasal polyps?"
    - Foreign body aspiration: "Have you aspirated a foreign body (often followed by a choking spell, cyanosis, cough, and wheeze localized to one area of the chest)?"
    - GER: "Have you had heartburn, nonspecific chest pain, trouble swallowing, and symptoms aggravated by lying or bending and specific foods (e.g., peppermint, fatty foods)?"
    - Anaphylaxis: "Have you been exposed to a known allergen (exposure may be accompanied by anxiety and apprehension; urticaria and edema; choking sensation/cough/bronchospasm or laryngeal edema; abdominal pain; nausea or vomiting; and hypotension)?"
  - **Frequency:** "Have you had this wheeze before? Have you been short of breath before? If so, when? How frequently does it occur (continuous versus intermittent)?"
  - **Palliative factors:** "Does anything make the wheeze or shortness of breath better? If so, what?"
    - Inhalers
    - Steroids

- ■ Provocative factors: "Does anything make the wheeze or shortness of breath worse? If so, what?"
  - ◆ Exposure to known allergens: Animal dander, dust mites, pollen, and feathers
  - ◆ Pets or stuffed animals, carpets, pillow
  - ◆ Environment: Exposure to cold air, type of heating system in the home, industrialized area, air pollution or smog, and scented products
  - ◆ Smoking, smokers in the home (second-hand smoke)
  - ◆ Infections: Upper respiratory tract infection (URTI), pneumonia, and influenza
  - ◆ Exercise: Change in exercise habits, exposure to cold air
  - ◆ Emotional stress: Crying, screaming, or hard laughing
- **PMH/PSH:** Asthma, atopy, GER, or congenital anomalies
- **MEDS:** Respiratory medications (including method of delivery and use of a holding chamber, if applicable)
  - ■ Check for any increase or decrease in medication dosage and more frequent use of inhalers.
  - ■ Consider adherence to regimen of prescribed medications.
  - ■ Check for prescriptions of new medications.
- **FH:** Asthma, allergic rhinitis, atopy, or eczema

Physical Examination
- **Vitals:** Evaluate HR and heart rhythm, BP, RR (depth, effort, and pattern), pulsus paradoxus, and temperature.
- **General:** Assess the patient's general appearance, work of breathing, and circulation to the skin. Correlate the findings of the initial assessment with the underlying physiologic state (see Table 12-3).
  - ■ Respiratory distress: tachypnea, pursed lips, nasal flare, tripod positioning, tracheal tug, accessory muscle use, intercostal or subcostal retractions, and thoracoabdominal dissociation
- **Skin:** Inspect the skin and nails, noting any diaphoresis, cyanosis, clubbing, or eczema.
- **HEENT:** Inspect the nose and oropharynx, noting any polyps or evidence of URTI. Examine the lymph nodes in the head and neck.
- **Resp** (Table 12-6): Inspect for thoracic deformity. Assess chest expansion for symmetry. Evaluate tracheal position (tug may be noted). Assess tactile fremitus and percussion. Auscultate the lungs, noting breath sounds and adventitious sounds.
- **CVS:** Measure the jugular venous pressure, and assess for hepatojugular reflux (signs of venous congestion may herald a pneumothorax). Palpate peripheral pulses, noting contour, volume, and rhythm. Inspect and palpate the apical impulse. Auscultate the heart, listening for extra heart sounds or murmurs.

Table 12-6 Expected Findings in an Acute Exacerbation of Asthma

Examination	Expected Findings
Thoracic deformity	Barrel chest: hyperinflation
Chest movement	May be asymmetric in case of associated pneumothorax
Trachea	Midline; tracheal tug may be noted
Tactile fremitus	Decreased
Percussion	Hyperresonant, flattened diaphragms
Breath sounds	Prolonged expiratory phase; localized disappearance of breath sounds can occur temporarily as a result of bronchial plugging
Adventitious sounds	High-pitched wheezes

Evidence

- One study[2] revealed at least moderate reliability for aspects of the clinical assessment in asthma, including rated work of breathing, wheeze, decreased air entry, prolonged expiration, breathlessness, respiratory rate, mental status, and overall severity.

Pearls

- **Asthma** is a pulmonary disease characterized by reversible airway obstruction, airway inflammation, and increased airway responsiveness to a variety of stimuli. Airway obstruction in asthma is caused by spasm of airway smooth muscle, edema of airway mucosa, increased mucus secretion, cellular infiltration of airway walls, and injury and desquamation of the airway epithelium.
- **Asthma triad** consists of atopy, ASA sensitivity, and nasal polyps.
- A quiet-sounding chest in a patient having an asthma attack may be a *warning* of patient fatigue or obstruction of small airways. It can quickly become *life-threatening*.
- The most reliable signs of a severe attack are dyspnea at rest, inability to speak, accessory muscle use, cyanosis, and pulsus paradoxus. An asthma attack may begin with cough and wheezing and rapidly progress to dyspnea. Confusion and lethargy may indicate respiratory failure and CO_2 narcosis. A normal or increased partial pressure of arterial CO_2 ($Paco_2$) may be indicative of respiratory failure (hyperventilation should result in a decreased $Paco_2$).

SORE THROAT AND FEVER: HISTORY AND PHYSICAL EXAMINATION

> **INSTRUCTIONS TO CANDIDATE: A 7-year-old boy is brought to his family doctor by his father. The boy has had a sore throat and fever for 2 days. Obtain a focused history, and perform a physical examination.**

DD_X: VITAMINS C

- Infectious: Viral infection (e.g., adenovirus, herpangina), bacterial infection (e.g., "Strep throat"), pharyngeal abscess, and epiglottitis
- Traumatic: Ingestion of a caustic substance

History

- Ask the patient the following questions:
  - Character: "What is your sore throat like? Does it hurt when you swallow? Does your neck hurt?"
  - Location: "Can you point to where it hurts?"
  - Onset: "How did it come on (sudden versus insidious)?"
  - Intensity: "Can you rate the discomfort on a pain scale (Figure 12-11)? Are the symptoms preventing you from sleeping? From attending school? From playing?"
  - Events associated (ask the patient's father):
    - Strep throat: "Has the fever been >38.3° C, with rash (macular exanthem), swollen glands (adenopathy), and infectious contacts?"

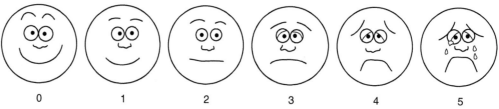

0	1	2	3	4	5

Figure 12-11 Adapted version of Wong-Baker FACES Pain Rating Scale. (From Wong DL, Hockenberry-Eaton M, Wilson D, et al. *Wong's Essentials of Pediatric Nursing.* 6th ed. St. Louis: Mosby; 2001 [p. 1301].)

♦ URTI: "Has your son had clear rhinorrhea, cough, myalgia, headache with or without fever, decreased appetite, and infectious contacts?"

♦ Adenovirus: "Has your son had rhinorrhea, conjunctivitis, and GI symptoms (e.g., diarrhea)?"

♦ Infectious contacts: "Is anyone else at home sick? Any known sick contacts at school?

▪ Frequency: "Has your child ever had this before? If so, when? How frequently does it occur?"

▪ Palliative factors: "Does anything make him feel better? If so, what?"

▪ Provocative factors: "Does anything make him feel worse? If so, what?"

- **PMH/PSH:** URTIs, atopy, and tonsillectomy
- **MEDS:** Antibiotics, decongestants
- **SH:** Smokers in the home

Physical Examination

- **Vitals:** Evaluate HR and heart rhythm, BP, RR (depth, effort, and pattern), and temperature.
- **General:** Assess the patient's general appearance, work of breathing, and circulation to the skin. Correlate the findings of the initial assessment with the underlying physiologic state (see Table 12-3). Note the posture of the head and neck and any drooling.
- **Skin:** Inspect the skin and nails, noting any eruptions (particularly a macular exanthem).
- **HEENT:** Ensure that the neck is supple. Inspect the conjunctiva, noting any injected appearance. Inspect the nasal mucosa for inflammation or polyps, noting any discharge (e.g., clear versus purulent). Ask the patient to open his mouth. Inspect the oropharynx, noting any erythema, petechiae, or vesicles on the palate and any trismus. Note the size of the tonsils and the presence of any exudate (Figure 12-12). Examine for cervical lymphadenopathy.
- **Resp:** Inspect for thoracic deformity. Assess chest expansion for symmetry. Auscultate the lungs, noting breath sounds and adventitious sounds.
- **CVS:** Check capillary refill. Palpate peripheral pulses, noting contour, volume, and rhythm. Auscultate the heart, listening for extra heart sounds or murmurs.
- **Abdomen:** Inspect the abdomen. Auscultate for bowel sounds. Percuss lightly in all four quadrants. Identify any masses or areas of tenderness. Examine the liver and spleen.

Evidence (Table 12-7)

- No *one* clinical feature is sufficient to make a diagnosis of strep throat.[3] Combinations of clinical features, such as the McIsaac modification of the Centor Strep Score, are quite useful. A score of −1 or 0 has a likelihood ratio (LR) of 0.05, whereas a score of 4 or 5 has a LR of 4.9. The score is calculated as follows: history of fever or measured temperature of >38.3° C (1 point); absence of cough (1 point); tender anterior cervical lymphadenopathy (1 point); tonsillar swelling or exudates (1 point); age <15 years (1 point); and, age ≥45 years (−1 point).[4]

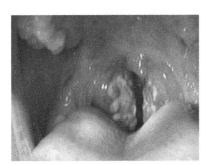

Figure 12-12 Enlarged tonsils with exudate. (Courtesy Dr. Brett Taylor, Dalhousie University, Halifax, Nova Scotia.)

Table 12-7 Usefulness of Clinical Examination for Strep Throat

Clinical Feature	+LR Range or +LR (95% CI)	−LR Range or −LR (95% CI)
Temperature >38.3° C	0.68–3.9	0.54–1.3
Absence of cough	1.1–1.7	0.53–0.89
Pharyngeal exudate	2.1 (1.4–3.1)	0.9 (0.75–1.1)
Tonsillar exudate	3.4 (1.8–6)	0.72 (0.6–0.88)
Enlarged tonsils	1.4–3.1	0.63 (0.56–0.72)
Enlarged cervical nodes	0.47–2.9	0.58–0.92
Tender cervical nodes	1.2–1.9	0.6 (0.49–0.71)
Exposure to *Streptococcus* organisms in past 2 weeks	1.9 (1.3–2.8)	0.92 (0.86–0.99)

Modified from Ebell MH, Smith MA, Barry HC, et al. The rational clinical examination: does this patient have strep throat? *JAMA.* 2000;284:2912-2918.
CI, Confidence interval; −LR, negative likelihood ratio; +LR, positive likelihood ratio.

RESPIRATORY DISTRESS: HISTORY AND PHYSICAL EXAMINATION

INSTRUCTIONS TO CANDIDATE: A 2½-month-old boy is brought to the emergency department by his parents because of cough, fever, and rapid breathing. Obtain a focused history, and perform a focused physical examination.

DD$_X$: VITAMINS C
- **Vascular:** Congestive heart failure (pulmonary edema)
- **Infectious:** Pneumonia, bronchiolitis, URTI, croup, tracheitis, pertussis, urinary tract infection (UTI), meningitis, acute otitis media
- **Idiopathic/iatrogenic:** GER
- **Neoplastic:** Tracheobronchial tree neoplasm or neoplasm compressing the tracheobronchial tree (e.g., lymphoma, thymoma)
- First evaluate **appearance, work of breathing,** and **circulation to the skin** (see Table 12-2). If no immediate interventions are required, proceed to obtain an appropriate history and perform a physical examination.

History
- Ask the parents the following questions:
  - **Character:** "What is the cough like? Is your son producing any sputum? If so, what color and how much (mucus, blood, pus)? Has he had any post-tussive vomiting?"
    - Clearing of the throat: GER and postnasal drip
    - Barking cough (like a seal): Croup
    - Hacking cough: Pharyngitis, tracheobronchitis, and early pneumonia
    - Whooping cough: Pertussis
  - **Onset:** "How did this illness start (sudden versus gradual)? Was the onset of cough sudden and paroxysmal (possible foreign body aspiration)?"
  - **Intensity:** "How severe is the cough? At what time of day (if any) is the cough most severe? Have you taken the child's temperature? By what means (tympanic, axillary, oral, rectal or forehead)? How high has the temperature been?"
  - **Duration:** "How long has the illness been going on (acute versus chronic versus paroxysmal versus seasonal versus perennial)? Is it getting better, getting worse, or staying the same?"
  - **Events associated:**
    - "Is your son having difficulty breathing? Is his breathing noisy?"
    - "Has he had difficulty feeding (fatigue, color change, difficulty breathing)?"

- ◆ "How many diapers has he wet in the past 24 hours? Any change in quality or quantity of stool?"
- ◆ "Has he been irritable?"
- ◆ "Has he been lethargic? Have you noticed a change in his sleep patterns? Have you had difficulty rousing him for feedings?"
- ◆ "Has he had rhinorrhea?"
- ◆ "Has he been exposed to infectious contacts (e.g., family, day care)?"
- ◆ "Has he been exposed to irritants?"
  - ▪ Frequency: "Has your child ever had this cough before? When? How often?"
  - ▪ Palliative factors: "Does anything make the cough better? If so, what?"
  - ▪ Provocative factors: "What brings on the cough? What makes the cough worse?"
- **PMH/PSH:** Congenital heart disease, cystic fibrosis, bronchopulmonary dysplasia, tracheomalacia, or HIV infection or AIDS
- **MEDS:** Antipyretics, antibiotics, other medications
- **Allergies:** Medications, foods
- **SH:** Smokers in the home
- **Immunizations**
- **FH:** Cystic fibrosis or α_1-antitrypsin deficiency

Prenatal, Natal, and Neonatal History

- Ask the parents the following questions:
  - ▪ "Did you have prenatal care? Any difficulties during the pregnancy?"
  - ▪ "Did you use of alcohol or recreational drugs during the pregnancy? Did you smoke during the pregnancy?"
  - ▪ "Was this a singleton or multiple gestation?"
  - ▪ "What were the date and the child's gestational age at delivery?"
  - ▪ "Did labor begin spontaneously, or was it induced? How long did labor last? Was any type of augmentation used in the delivery? What type of delivery did you have (NSVD, LSCS, forceps, or vacuum)?"
  - ▪ "What was your son's birth weight? Is he fed breast milk or formula?"
  - ▪ "What were his Apgar scores at 1 and 5 minutes?"

Physical Examination

- **Vitals:** Evaluate HR and heart rhythm, BP, RR (depth, effort, and pattern), pulsus paradoxus, and temperature.
- **General:** Assess the patient's general appearance, work of breathing, and circulation to the skin. Correlate the findings of the initial assessment with the underlying physiologic state (see Table 12-3). Characterize any cough observed during the encounter.
- **HEENT:** Inspect the oropharynx, noting any erythema, petechiae, or vesicles on the palate. Note the size of the tonsils and the presence of any exudate. Inspect the tympanic membranes. Ensure that the neck is supple, and palpate the anterior fontanelle. Examine for cervical lymphadenopathy.
- **Resp:** Inspect for thoracic deformity. Assess chest expansion for symmetry. Auscultate the lungs, noting breath sounds and adventitious sounds.
- **CVS:** Check capillary refill. Palpate peripheral pulses, noting contour, volume, and rhythm. Auscultate the heart, listening for extra heart sounds or murmurs.
- **Abdomen:** Inspect the abdomen. Auscultate for bowel sounds. Percuss lightly in all four quadrants. Identify any masses or areas of tenderness. Examine the liver and spleen.

Evidence

- In infants, the respiratory assessment, with regard to work of breathing, has moderate reliability, whereas agreement on auscultatory findings is poorer. The measurement of the RR is more reproducible if it is counted over 1 minute or if it is calculated as the average of two 30-second counts. Determining the

Table 12-8	Usefulness of Clinical Examination for Diagnosing Pneumonia in Infants	
Clinical Feature	**+LR Range**	**−LR Range**
Fever	1.2–1.5	0.17–0.95
Tachypnea	1.6–8	0.32–0.75
Intercostal indrawing	1.3–26	0.53–0.78
Nasal flaring	1.2–6.6	0.71–0.83
Grunting	1.2–3.2	0.86–0.89
Crackles	1.8–15	0.36–0.86
Wheezes	0.19–4	0.97–1.3

Modified from Margolis P, Gadomski A. The rational clinical examination. Does this infant have pneumonia? *JAMA.* 1998;279:308-313.
−LR, Negative likelihood ratio; +LR, positive likelihood ratio.

RR on the basis of a single 30-second count appears to yield an overestimate. In general, normal findings on the clinical examination mean that pneumonia is unlikely, but individual clinical findings are not accurate enough to be considered diagnostic[5] (Table 12-8).

Pearl

• The **Rochester criteria** can be used to help identify febrile infants at low risk for serious bacterial infections (Box 12-1). To be considered at low risk, all criteria must be met.

Box 12-1   Rochester Criteria

Infant appears well (no signs of toxicity)
No skin, soft tissue, bone, joint, or ear infection
Previously healthy infant
• Term birth
• No perinatal antibiotic therapy
• No history of unexplained hyperbilirubinemia
• No previous or current antibiotic therapy
• Not previously hospitalized except for birth (not hospitalized for longer than the mother
• No chronic or underlying illness
Laboratory values
• Peripheral WBC count of 5000–15,000/mm³
• Total band count of <1500/mm³
• ≤10 WBCs per high-power field (×40) on microscopic examination of spun urine sediment
• ≤5 WBCs per high-power field (×40) on microscopic examination of a stool smear (in infants with diarrhea)

Adapted from Lopez JA, McMillin KJ, Tobias-Merrill EA, et al. Managing fever in infants and toddlers, *Postgrad Med.* 1997;101:242.
WBC, White blood cell.

FEBRILE SEIZURE: HISTORY AND PHYSICAL EXAMINATION

INSTRUCTIONS TO CANDIDATE: A 31-month-old boy is brought to the emergency department via ambulance because of a seizure. His parents say that he was "shaking all over" and his eyes rolled back in his head. The triage nurse notes that he has a temperature of 39.3° C. Obtain a focused history, and perform a focused physical examination.

DD$_X$: VITAMINS C
- **V**ascular: Intracranial hemorrhage (e.g., arteriovenous malformation)
- **I**nfectious: CNS infection (meningitis, encephalitis, abscess)
- **T**raumatic: Head injury
- **M**etabolic: Disturbance in sodium, calcium, magnesium, or glucose level; disturbance in renal function
- **I**diopathic/**i**atrogenic: Febrile seizure, epilepsy
- **N**eoplastic: Intracranial malignancy
- **S**ubstance abuse and psychiatric: Toxic ingestion, pseudoseizure
- **C**ongenital/genetic: Congenital structural defects

History
- Ask the parents the following questions:
  - **Character:** "What happened? What did you see? Did he fall? Was there any trauma? Was he well before this episode? What was happening at the time of this episode? Were there any movements (e.g., automatisms, tonic-clonic activity)? Was he able to talk to you? What was he like afterward? How long did it take for him to get back to normal (postictal period)?"
  - **Location:** "Where did this happen?"
  - **Onset:** "Was there any warning? Has this ever happened before? If so, what was your son's age at onset? How did it start?"
  - **Duration:** "How long did this episode last? How long did it take to get back to normal?"
  - **Events associated:**
    - Fever: "Has your son had a cold, headache, or urinary tract infection?"
    - "Did you notice salivation, color change, tongue biting, or incontinence during this episode?"
    - Postictal symptoms: "Has your son mentioned having muscle aches, tongue soreness, or headache? Did you find him drowsy or confused after this episode?"
  - **Frequency:** "Has this ever happened before? When? How often?"
  - **Palliative factors:** "Did anything seem to help? If so, what (e.g., medications)?"
  - **Provocative factors:** "Does anything seem to have brought on the 'seizure'? If so, what?"
    - "Did he have fever or other illness? How high was the fever? How quickly did it come on?"
    - "Has he had a head injury?"
- **PMH/PSH:** Birth injury, head trauma, stroke, CNS infection, previous seizures, or developmental delay
- **MEDS:** Antipyretics, antibiotics, or anticonvulsants
- **FH:** Seizures (febrile, epilepsy)

Physical Examination
- **Vitals:** Evaluate HR and heart rhythm, BP, RR (depth, effort, and pattern), and temperature.
- **General:** Assess the patient's general appearance, work of breathing, and circulation to the skin. Correlate the findings of the initial assessment with the underlying physiologic state (see Table 12-3).

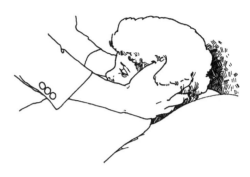

Figure 12-13 Gently move the patient's neck through the range of motion, assessing for stiffness in flexion. (From Gill D, O'Brien N. *Paediatric Clinical Examination Made Easy.* 4th ed. London: Churchill Livingstone; 2002 [p. 146].)

- **Skin:** Inspect the skin and nails, noting any diaphoresis, flushing, or eruption (petechiae, purpura).
- **HEENT:** Ensure that the neck is supple (Figure 12-13). Inspect the conjunctiva, noting any injected appearance. Inspect the nasal mucosa, noting any discharge (e.g., clear versus purulent). Inspect the oropharynx, noting any erythema, petechiae, or vesicles on the palate. Note the size of the tonsils and the presence of any exudate. Examine for cervical lymphadenopathy. Perform funduscopy, looking for papilledema (increased ICP) or hemorrhage.
- **Resp:** Inspect for thoracic deformity. Assess chest expansion for symmetry. Auscultate the lungs, noting breath sounds and adventitious sounds.
- **CVS:** Check capillary refill. Palpate peripheral pulses, noting contour, volume, and rhythm. Auscultate the heart, listening for extra heart sounds or murmurs.
- **Abdomen:** Inspect the abdomen. Auscultate for bowel sounds. Percuss lightly in all four quadrants. Identify any masses or areas of tenderness. Examine the liver and spleen.
- **Neuro:** Look for focal neurologic deficits that are suggestive of a space-occupying lesion. Most of the neurologic examination can be performed by simply observing the child play (motor function, cranial nerves).

Pearls
- Febrile seizures are common in children.
- Criteria for **febrile seizures:**
  - Age: 3 months to 5 years
  - Temperature >38.8° C
  - Non-CNS source of infection
- Features that increase the risk of recurrent seizures include the following:
  - >1 seizure in 24 hours
  - Seizure duration >15 minutes
  - Focal seizure (most febrile seizures are generalized tonic-clonic type)
  - Age <1 year
  - Family history of seizure disorder

HEADACHE AND FEVER: HISTORY AND PHYSICAL EXAMINATION

INSTRUCTIONS TO CANDIDATE: A 13-year-old boy presents to the emergency department with a headache and fever. He recently returned from army cadet camp. Obtain a focused history, and perform a focused physical examination.

DD$_X$: VITAMINS C
- **V**ascular: Cavernous sinus thrombosis, vasculitis
- **I**nfectious: CNS infection (meningitis, encephalitis, intracranial abscess)
- **I**diopathic/iatrogenic: Collagen vascular disease

DD$_X$: Other

- Consider the differential diagnosis of headache in the presence of a coincidental fever: migraine, tension headache, intracranial hemorrhage, increased ICP, and trauma.

History

- Ask the patient the following questions:
  - **Character:** "Can you describe the headache? Is it bandlike? Pulsatile? Nonspecific? Did you take your temperature at home? By what means (e.g., axillary, oral, tympanic, rectal, forehead)?"
  - **Location:** "Where is the headache? Bilateral? Unilateral? Occipital? Does it involve your neck?"
  - **Onset:** "How did it start (sudden maximal intensity versus gradual buildup)?"
  - **Radiation:** "Does the pain move anywhere (e.g., neck)?"
  - **Intensity:** "What is the severity of the pain on a scale of 1 to 10, with 1 being mild and 10 being the worst? How high is your temperature?"
  - **Duration:** "How long have you had the headache and fever (acute versus chronic)? Which came on first?"
  - **Events associated:**
    - "Have you felt malaise? Lethargy? Loss of appetite?"
    - "Have you had nausea or vomiting? Skin lesions (e.g., petechiae)?"
    - "Have you had a head injury? Have you had previous neurosurgery? Do you have a shunt?"
    - "Have you had a facial infection (venous drainage to cavernous sinus), sinusitis, or retropharyngeal abscess (extension into CNS)?"
    - "Have you been exposed to infectious contacts (family, cadet camp)?"
  - **Frequency:** "Have you ever had a headache like this before? When? How frequently (intermittent versus constant)?"
  - **Palliative factors:** "Does anything make the headache better? If so, what?"
    - NSAIDs
    - Acetaminophen
  - **Provocative factors:** "Does anything make the headache worse? If so, what?"
    - Movement
    - Bright light (photophobia)
    - Loud noises (phonophobia)
- **PMH/PSH:** Head trauma, CNS infection, HIV infection or other immunosuppression, asplenia, migraines, previous neurosurgery, or presence of a shunt
- **MEDS:** Antibiotics, antipyretics, or immunosuppressants
- **FH:** Seizures, cerebral aneurysms, migraine

Physical Examination

- **Vitals:** Evaluate HR and heart rhythm, BP, RR (depth, effort, and pattern), and temperature
- **General:** Assess the patient's general appearance, work of breathing, and circulation to the skin. Correlate the findings of the initial assessment with the underlying physiologic state (see Table 12-3).
- **Skin:** Inspect the skin and nails, noting any diaphoresis, flushing, or acute eruption (petechiae, purpura).
- **HEENT:** Ensure that the neck is supple (see Figure 12-13). Inspect the conjunctiva, noting any injected appearance. Inspect the nasal mucosa, noting any discharge. Inspect the oropharynx, noting any erythema, petechiae, or vesicles on the palate. Note the size of the tonsils and the presence of any exudate. Examine for cervical lymphadenopathy. Perform funduscopy, looking for papilledema (indicative of increased ICP).
- **Resp:** Inspect for thoracic deformity. Assess chest expansion for symmetry. Auscultate the lungs, noting breath sounds and adventitious sounds.

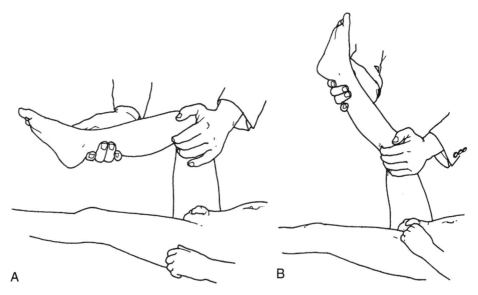

A   B

Figure 12-14 Examination for Kernig's sign. (From Gill D, O'Brien N. *Paediatric Clinical Examination Made Easy.* 4th ed. London: Churchill Livingstone; 2002 [p. 148].)

- **CVS:** Check capillary refill. Palpate peripheral pulses, noting contour, volume, and rhythm. Auscultate the heart, listening for extra heart sounds or murmurs.
- **Abdomen:** Inspect the abdomen. Auscultate for bowel sounds. Percuss lightly in all four quadrants. Identify any masses or areas of tenderness. Examine the liver and spleen.
- **Neuro:** Look for focal neurologic deficits that are suggestive of a space-occupying lesion.
  - **Kernig's sign** (Figure 12-14): With the patient supine, flex the hip and knee to 90 degrees. Attempt to extend the knee. In patients with meningeal irritation, full extension may be impossible (Kernig's sign) because of resistance and pain (extension increases meningeal stretch).
  - **Brudzinski's sign:** With the patient supine, gently attempt to flex the neck. Brudzinski's sign is said to be present when this produces neck pain and simultaneous flexion of the knees (to decrease meningeal stretch).

Pearl
- In patients with true meningism, the neck is stiff (board-like rigidity); you could actually lift the patient's upper body, as well as the head, off the bed.

ADVANCED SKILLS

ROUTINE NEONATAL EXAMINATION

> **INSTRUCTIONS TO CANDIDATE: You are a senior medical student on your neonatology rotation. The nurse in charge asks you to measure the height, weight, and head circumference of a newborn boy and plot them on the growth charts provided (Figure 12-15). Perform a routine neonatal examination.**

- Height, weight, and head circumference should be plotted on standardized **growth charts** at routine health encounters. Serial measurements are much more valuable than single measurements because they reflect changes in the child's growth pattern.

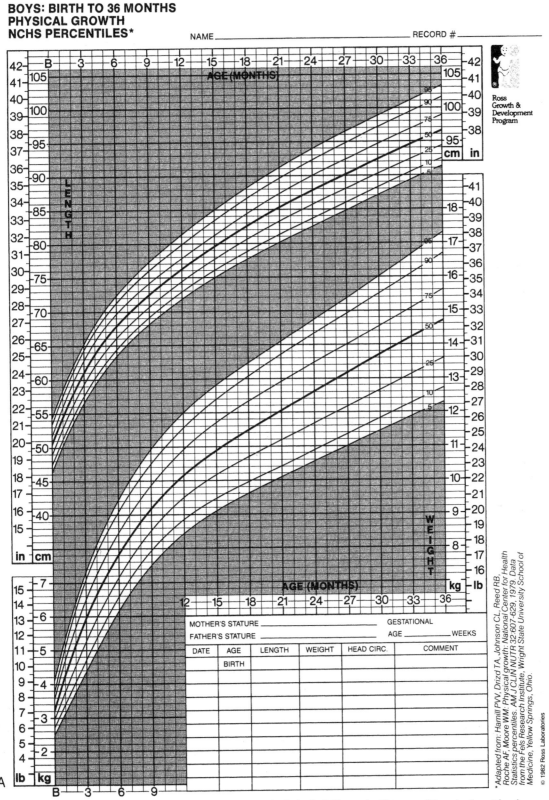

Figure 12-15 Growth chart. (From Swartz M. *Textbook of Physical Diagnosis: History and Examination.* 4th ed. Philadelphia: Saunders; 2002 [Figure 23-16, *A*].)

The most common reason for deviation from the growth curve is measuring error. Take every measurement at least twice, and take a third measurement if the first two have any discrepancy.

Head Circumference
- Use a nonstretchable measuring tape to measure the head circumference. Place the tape over the occipital, parietal, and frontal prominences to maximize the measured circumference of the head.

DD$_X$: VITAMINS C
Decreased Head Circumference
- **Idiopathic/iatrogenic:** Premature closure of the sutures
- **Congenital/genetic:** Familial microcephaly

Increased Head Circumference
- **Idiopathic/iatrogenic:** Hydrocephalus (obstructive and nonobstructive)
- **Neoplastic:** Space-occupying lesion in CNS
- **Congenital/genetic:** Familial megalocephaly

Height
- Use a measuring board to quantify the height. (Use of a measuring tape yields inaccurate results.) Hold the infant's head against the upper board, and adjust the lower board. Ensure that both the infant's feet are flat against the base.

Weight
- Use an infant scale to measure the weight. Remove all clothing, including the diaper, and ensure that the infant is not touching the wall.
- When caloric intake is inadequate, the weight percentile decreases first, followed by height and finally head circumference. The World Health Organization (WHO)[6] recommends that **weight for height** be used as an index of acute malnutrition (wasting) and **height for age** be used as an index of chronic malnutrition (stunting).

Newborn Examination
- **Vitals:** Observe the baby undressed for 1 to 2 minutes. A normal RR in a newborn is 30 to 50 breaths per minute. Note any signs of respiratory distress, such as grunting, nasal flare, intercostal or subcostal retractions, tracheal tug, and thoracoabdominal dissociation. Use a well-lubricated rectal thermometer to determine temperature. Determine the HR by auscultation. The average HR in a newborn is 120 to 140 beats per minute (<90 beats per minute is abnormal).
- **General:** The limbs should be moving in a random and asymmetric manner. Jerky or symmetric movements are abnormal.
- **Skin:** Inspect the skin, noting the color and any lesions. Note any signs of birth trauma, especially if instrumentation was used in the delivery.
  - **Acrocyanosis** is the presence of cyanosis in the extremities while the trunk is pink and warm.
  - **Pallor** may be associated with anemia, vasoconstriction, or edema.
  - The yellow discoloration of **jaundice** is common in newborns and most noticeable on the brow and face. Jaundice occurring in the first 24 hours after birth is considered abnormal.
  - **Milia** are sebaceous retention cysts, appearing as small white papules on the face.
- **HEENT:** Examine the fontanelles, and assess the shape and symmetry of the head. Inspect the face for symmetry, noting the presence of epicanthal folds or low-set ears. Ensure that the nares are patent. Inspect the palate. Use your gloved finger

to palpate it, noting any clefts. Inspect the gums for neonatal teeth (these probably need to be removed to prevent aspiration). Inspect the eyes, and perform a funduscopic examination. Absence of the red reflex may indicate congenital cataracts or retinoblastoma.

- **Caput succedaneum** is edema of the soft tissues of the vertex related to the birth.
- **Esophageal atresia** may be detected by the presence of excessive saliva in the mouth; saliva production is normally limited in the neonate.
- **Coloboma** is any defect of ocular tissue (e.g., coloboma iridis).
- **Resp:** Inspect for thoracic deformity and symmetry of chest expansion. Percuss the chest bilaterally. The chest should be hyperresonant and symmetric (dullness can indicate diaphragmatic hernia). Auscultate the lungs (breath sounds and adventitia).
- **CVS:** Palpate the radial and femoral pulses, noting any radial-femoral delay that may be related to coarctation of the aorta. Auscultate the heart, listening for any extra heart sounds or murmurs.
- **Abdomen:** In normal newborns, the abdomen is protuberant. Inspect for umbilical herniation (associated with congenital hypothyroidism). Auscultate for bowel sounds. Palpate the abdomen, noting any masses or apparent tenderness. Attempt to palpate the liver and spleen.
- **Genitalia:** Inspect the genitalia for ambiguity. Look at the urethral meatus, and identify any hypospadias.
- **Musculoskeletal system:** Inspect the feet. Forefoot adduction is usually a result of intrauterine positioning and resolves spontaneously. Clubfoot deformity is more extensive and serious and includes forefoot adduction, hindfoot inversion, and internal tibial torsion. Note the position of the head and neck. Tilting toward one side may indicate torticollis.
- **Neuro:** The following reflexes should be present:
    - **Rooting reflex:** Touch the corner of the infant's mouth. A normal response is opening of the mouth and turning the head toward the stimulus.
    - **Palmar grasp:** Place your finger or an object in the palm of the infant's hand. A normal response is a complete grasp.
    - **Moro's reflex (startle reflex):** Supporting the infant's head, allow the infant to drop suddenly. A normal response is abduction of the arms and extension of the fingers, followed by arm adduction.
    - **Plantar reflexes** are usually upgoing (positive **Babinski** sign).
    - **Plantar grasp:** With the infant's knee and hip flexed, press your thumb into the sole of the foot. Normally the toes flex, as if to grasp the thumb.

NEONATAL JAUNDICE: HISTORY

INSTRUCTIONS TO CANDIDATE: The next day, the nurse in charge asks you to reassess the boy because he appears jaundiced. Obtain a detailed history from his mother, exploring possible causes.

DD$_X$: VITAMINS C
- Infectious: Toxoplasmosis, **o**ther agents, **r**ubella, **c**ytomegalovirus, and **h**erpes simplex (**TORCH**); sepsis
- Traumatic: Hematoma resorption (birth trauma)
- **A**utoimmune/**a**llergic: blood group incompatibility
- Metabolic: Gilbert syndrome, Crigler-Najjar syndrome
- **I**diopathic/**i**atrogenic: Physiologic jaundice, breast milk–related jaundice, and meconium ileus
- Congenital/genetic: Hereditary hemolytic anemia (e.g., spherocytosis), sickle cell anemia, thalassemia, biliary atresia, and Hirschsprung disease
- Many more diagnoses are associated with neonatal jaundice!

Prenatal History
- Ask the mother the following questions:
  - "Did you have prenatal care? Any difficulties during the pregnancy?"
  - "Did you have any bleeding? Premature rupture of the membranes? Gestational diabetes mellitus?"
  - "Have you had sexually transmitted infections? TORCH infections?"
  - "Did you use alcohol or recreational drugs during the pregnancy?"
  - "Did you smoke during the pregnancy?"
  - "Was this a singleton or multiple gestation?"
  - "What was your Rh status? Do you have any history of isoimmunization?"

Birth History
- Ask the parents the following questions:
  - "What were the date and the child's gestational age at delivery?"
  - "Did labor begin spontaneously, or was it induced?"
  - "How long did labor last? Was any type of augmentation used in the delivery?"
  - "What type of delivery did you have (NSVD, LSCS, forceps, or vacuum)?"
  - "Did the baby experience birth trauma (e.g., cephalohematoma)?"

Neonatal History
- Obtain the following information from the hospital's records:
  - Birth weight
  - Apgar scores at 1 and 5 minutes
  - Breastfed versus formula-fed
  - The color of the baby now, the part of the baby where this color change is noted (e.g., trunk, face), and when the change in color was first noted
  - Whether the baby has passed any stools yet (meconium)
  - Any systemic symptoms:
    - Fever, lethargy
    - Vomiting
    - Poor feeding
- **Maternal PMH:** Hepatitis, hemolytic disorders, or metabolic disorders (e.g., Gilbert syndrome)
- **Maternal MEDS:** Hepatotoxic drugs (ASA, anticonvulsants, antipsychotics, herbal supplements)
- **FH:** Jaundice, metabolic disorders, or unexplained infant deaths

Pearls
- Jaundice appearing in the first 24 hours of life is usually pathologic.
- Direct hyperbilirubinemia in a neonate is always pathologic.
- Several online tools are available to help evaluate the need for phototherapy, such as http://BiliTool.org.

VOMITING INFANT: HISTORY

> **INSTRUCTIONS TO CANDIDATE: A 1-month-old boy is brought to the emergency department because of a 1-day history of vomiting. His mother is concerned that he is becoming dehydrated because he is not feeding well. Obtain a detailed history, exploring possible causes.**

DD$_X$: VITAMINS C
- **Infectious:** Sepsis, gastroenteritis, UTI, pneumonia
- **Traumatic:** Head injury (nonaccidental trauma)
- **Autoimmune/allergic:** Food allergy (milk protein intolerance)
- **Idiopathic/iatrogenic:** GER, GI obstruction (e.g., malrotation and volvulus), necrotizing enterocolitis, systemic illness, and increased ICP

- Congenital/genetic: Inborn errors of metabolism, pyloric stenosis
- Other: Overfeeding

History
- Ask the mother the following questions:
  - Character: "What is the vomiting like: projectile? Spitting up? What is the temporal relationship to feeds? Did the child retch before vomiting or retch without vomiting at all?"
    - Color (clear, bilious, bloody, feculent), quantity, and smell
    - Bilious vomiting: suggestive of obstruction distal to the ampulla of Vater
    - Hematemesis: bright red blood versus coffee grounds
  - Location: "Where were you when this started? Has the family been traveling?"
  - Onset: "How did the vomiting begin (sudden versus gradual)? Does it come on after a meal (postprandial)? Is it post-tussive? What time of day does it occur (morning vomiting may be related to increased ICP)?"
  - Intensity: "How severe is the vomiting? How many episodes of vomiting occur per day? Are the volumes of vomitus small or large?"
  - Duration: "When did the vomiting begin? Is it getting better, getting worse, or staying the same?"
  - Events associated:
    - "Has your child had a fever? Lethargy?"
    - "How is his appetite? Does he eat readily? Have you noticed any change in volume of feeding?"
    - "Does he appear to have any pain? Jaundice?"
    - "Have you noticed any change in BMs (diarrhea, constipation, melena, hematochezia, steatorrhea)?"
    - "Have you noticed any change in the size of the baby's head (hydrocephalus, space-occupying lesion)?
    - Diet: "Is your son fed breast milk or formula? Any other foods?"
    - "Has he been exposed to infectious contacts (day care, recent parties, school, and babysitter)?"
  - Frequency: "Has this ever happened to your child before? When? How frequently (intermittent versus constant)?"
  - Palliative factors: "Does anything lessen the vomiting? If so, what?"
  - Provocative factors: "Does anything make the vomiting worse? If so, what?"
- **PMH/PSH:** IBD, cystic fibrosis, or gastric obstruction
- **MEDS:** Antibiotics, antipyretics
- **SH:** Other children at home, stressors (e.g., financial, relationships)
- **FH:** IBD, cystic fibrosis

Prenatal, Natal, and Neonatal History
- Ask the mother the following questions:
  - "Did you have prenatal care? Any difficulties during the pregnancy?"
  - "Did you use alcohol or recreational drugs during the pregnancy? Did you smoke during the pregnancy?"
  - "Was this a singleton or multiple gestation?"
  - "What were the date and the child's gestational age at delivery?" (Prematurity is a risk factor for necrotizing enterocolitis.)
  - "When did labor begin? How long did labor last? What type of delivery did you have (NSVD, LSCS, forceps, vacuum)?"
  - "What was your son's birth weight? "
  - "What were his Apgar scores at 1 and 5 minutes?"

Pearl
- **Vomiting** is the forceful ejection of gastric contents. **Regurgitation** is different from vomiting and is generally nonforceful reflux.
- **Bilious vomit** in a neonate is always abnormal—in fact, it is a *surgical emergency.*

NOCTURNAL ENURESIS: HISTORY

> **INSTRUCTIONS TO CANDIDATE: A 5-year-old girl is brought to her family doctor by her mother because of ongoing bedwetting. Obtain a detailed history, exploring possible causes.**

DD$_X$: VITAMINS C

Primary Enuresis
- **I**diopathic/iatrogenic: Idiopathic enuresis, delayed maturation of the urethral sphincter
- **C**ongenital/genetic: Congenital anomalies

Secondary Enuresis
- **I**nfectious: UTI
- **T**raumatic: Chemical distal urethritis (e.g., caused by bubble bath)
- **M**etabolic: Diabetes mellitus
- **I**diopathic/iatrogenic: Polydipsia, fecal impaction
- **S**ubstance abuse and psychiatric: Psychologic stress

History
- Ask the mother the following questions:
  - **Character:** "Can you tell me about the bedwetting? Is your daughter at all incontinent during the daytime?"
  - **Location:** "Does the bedwetting happen at home? Does it happen at sleepovers?"
  - **Onset:** "When did the bedwetting begin? Has your daughter ever been continent at night?"
  - **Intensity:** "How frequently does this occur? Every night? More than once a night? Is it getting better, getting worse, or staying the same? Does it interfere with any of her activities?"
  - **Duration:** "How long has the bedwetting been going on?"
  - **Events associated:**
    - UTI: "Have you noticed urinary frequency, painful urination, blood in the urine, urinary retention, or urgency?"
    - Chemical urethritis: "Has she used bubble bath or perfumed soaps?"
    - "Does she need to strain to urinate? Any dribbling or small-caliber stream?"
    - "Does she have stress incontinence? Continuous dampness?"
    - "Does she drink a lot?"
    - "Have you noticed any difficulty with walking or balance? Change in behavior?"
    - "Does she have any encopresis? Constipation?"
    - "What do you do when she wets the bed? Is she punished? Have you tried any reward systems?"
  - **Frequency:** "How often does the bedwetting occur (times per night, times per week)?"
  - **Palliative factors:** "Does anything make the bedwetting better? If so, what?"
    - Behavior modification, such as emptying the bladder before sleep
    - Limiting fluid intake before bed
  - **Provocative factors:** "Does anything make the bedwetting worse? If so, what?"
    - Drinking before bed
    - Caffeine
    - Soft drinks
    - Use of bubble bath or perfumed soaps
    - Constipation
- **PMH/PSH:** Diabetes, spina bifida, fecal impaction, or genitourinary (GU) malformations
- **MEDS:** Imipramine, desmopressin (DDAVP)
- **SH:** Psychologically stressful situations in the home
- **FH:** Bedwetting

Table 12-9	Usefulness of Clinical Examination for Diagnosing Urinary Tract Infection in Verbal Children	

Clinical Feature	+LR (95% CI)	−LR (95% CI)
Abdominal pain in patients with temperature >38° C	6.3 (2.5–16.0)*	0.80 (0.65–0.99)
Back pain	3.6 (2.1–6.1)	0.84 (0.75–0.95)
Dysuria	2.4 (1.8–3.1)	0.65 (0.51–0.81)
Urinary frequency	2.8 (2.0–4.0)	0.72 (0.60–0.86)
New-onset urinary incontinence	4.6 (2.8–7.6)	0.79 (0.69–0.90)
Foul-smelling urine	Range: 0.82–0.93	Range: 1.01–1.2

From Shaikh N, Morone NE, Lopez J, et al. Does this child have a urinary tract infection? *JAMA.* 2007;298:2895-2904.
CI, Confidence interval; −LR, negative likelihood ratio; +LR, positive likelihood ratio.
*LR > 5 means that this feature is more useful.

Pearl
- **Nocturnal enuresis** is nighttime urinary incontinence. It is **primary** when the child has never been continent for a prolonged period and **secondary** when incontinence recurs after a 6- to 12-month period of continence.

Evidence
- Table 12-9 lists features that are informative in the examination for UTI.

SPEECH DELAY: HISTORY

> **INSTRUCTIONS TO CANDIDATE: A 30-month-old boy is brought to his pediatrician by his mother, who is concerned about his small vocabulary. Obtain a detailed history, exploring possible causes.**

DD$_X$: Language Delay
- Global developmental delay
- Isolated language delay
- Hearing impairment
- Social deprivation
- Autism
- Oral-motor abnormalities

History
- Ask the mother the following questions:
  - **Character:** "Tell me about your concern about your son's language. What have you noticed? What is your biggest concern? Does he understand you? Does he follow instructions? Does he have trouble expressing his wants? Does he get frustrated?"
  - **Onset:** "When did you notice his trouble with words? Has his speech taken any steps backward? Is he continuing to gain words? Has he stopped progressing?"
  - **Intensity:** "How many words does he use? How many words does he know?"
  - **Duration:** "How long has this been going on (acute versus chronic)?"
  - **Events associated:** "Does he have any social or motor troubles (gross and fine)?"

- Frequency: "Is his language difficulty constant, or does it fluctuate?"
- Palliative factors: "Does anything improve his language skills? If so, what?"
- Provocative factors: "Does anything worsen his language skills? If so, what?"
  - Unfamiliar situations or people
- **PMH/PSH:** Meningitis, prematurity, or birth defects
- **MEDS:** Aminoglycosides, loop diuretics
- **Immunizations**
- **SH:** Other children in the home, day care, and stress or tension in the home
- **FH:** Speech/language delay, hearing deficit, autism, or Tourette syndrome

Prenatal and Natal History
- Ask the mother the following questions:
  - "Did you have prenatal care? Any difficulties during the pregnancy?"
  - "Did you have bleeding, discharge, premature rupture of membranes, or abdominal trauma during the pregnancy?"
  - "Did you have nausea or vomiting, malnutrition, gestational diabetes mellitus, anemia, or GER?"
  - Infections: "Do you have any sexually transmitted infections, UTI, or TORCH infections?"
  - "Did you use alcohol or recreational drugs during the pregnancy? Did you use over-the-counter and prescription drugs? Did you smoke?"
  - "Was this a singleton or multiple gestation?"
  - "What was the child's gestational age at delivery?"
  - "Did labor begin spontaneously, or was it induced?"
  - "How long did labor last? Was any type of augmentation used in the delivery?"
  - "What type of delivery did you have (NSVD, LSCS, forceps, or vacuum)?"
  - "Were there complications at delivery?"

Neonatal History
- Ask the mother the following questions:
  - "What was your son's birth weight? Was he fed breast milk or formula?"
  - "What were his Apgar scores at 1 and 5 minutes?"

Growth and Development
- Ask whether the child has reached normal developmental milestones.
- Use the DDST to screen for language items.

Hearing
- Ask the mother whether she has any concerns about her child's hearing and whether his hearing has ever been tested.
- Risk factors for hearing loss include congenital hearing loss in a family member; high bilirubin level (neonatal); congenital rubella; congenital defects in the ears, nose, or throat; very low birth weight (<1500 g); meningitis; and ototoxic medications.

Environmental Stimulation
- Ask the mother the following questions:
  - "Does your child play with other children?"
  - "Do you read or talk/interact with your child?"
  - "Has your child ever been abused (physical, verbal, sexual), or has he witnessed and/or experienced a traumatic event?"

LIMP: HISTORY

INSTRUCTIONS TO CANDIDATE: A 4-year-old boy is brought in by his mother because she has noticed him limping for the past 2 days. Obtain a focused history, exploring possible causes.

DD$_X$: VITAMINS C

- **V**ascular: Avascular necrosis of the femoral head (Legg-Calvé-Perthes disease), hemarthrosis (e.g., hemophilia)
- **I**nfectious: Septic arthritis, osteomyelitis
- **T**raumatic: Injury to bone or soft tissue (known traumatic history or occult trauma, as in abuse)
- **A**utoimmune/allergic: Inflammatory arthritis (e.g., juvenile rheumatoid arthritis)
- **I**diopathic/iatrogenic: Transient synovitis
- **N**eoplastic: CNS malignancy (ataxia), localized malignancy (e.g., osteosarcoma)
- **C**ongenital/genetic: DDH, sickle cell crisis

History

- Ask the child the following questions:
  - **Character:** "Can you describe the limp. Is it painful? What is the pain like?"
  - **Location:** "Where does the pain originate?"
  - **Onset:** "When did the limp start? When did the pain start (before or after the limp)? How did it come on (sudden versus gradual)?"
  - **Radiation:** "Does the pain move anywhere?"
  - **Intensity:** "How severe is the pain, if present?" (See Figure 12-11.)
    - "How does the limp affect activities (getting dressed, going to the bathroom, participating in sports, playing with friends)?"
    - "Is the limp getting better, getting worse, or staying the same?"
  - **Duration:** "How long has the limp or pain been present (2 days)?"
  - **Events associated** (ask the mother):
    - "Has he experienced trauma? Describe the mechanism of injury."
    - "Does he play sports? Has he started new activities?"
    - "Has he had fever or chills? Has he lost weight? Does he have nighttime pain?"
    - "Has he had a recent illness? Has he recently taken antibiotics?"
    - "Does he have a rash on his lower extremities (purpura as in Henoch-Schönlein purpura)?
    - "Have you noticed limitation of movement?"
    - "Does he have morning stiffness (as in inflammatory arthritides)? Swelling? Redness?"
    - "Does he have muscle pain (thigh, calf)? Wasting? Weakness?"
  - **Frequency:** "Has this ever happened before? How often (intermittent versus constant)?"
  - **Palliative factors:** "Does anything make the pain better? If so, what?"
    - "Does rest help? What is the position of comfort?"
    - "Does certain activity help?"
    - "Do NSAIDs or acetaminophen help?"
  - **Provocative factors:** "Does anything make the pain worse? If so, what: rest? Activity? Particular movements?"
  - **PMH/PSH:** DDH, hemophilia, sickle cell anemia, arthritis, connective tissue disease, past injuries, and previous surgery
  - **MEDS:** NSAIDs, acetaminophen, narcotics, ASA, steroids, or immunosuppressants
  - **Allergies:** Cefaclor hypersensitivity (associated with serum sickness and migratory arthritis)
  - **SH:** Living arrangements, family dynamics
  - **FH:** Arthritis, connective tissue disease

Motor Development
- Sitting unsupported at age 6 months
- Crawling and pulling to standing position at age 9 months
- Walking unaided at ages 12 to 15 months
- Running at age 18 months

Pearls
- A child with a hip effusion may prefer to lie with the hip flexed, abducted, and externally rotated to minimize intra-articular pressure.
- Be sure to differentiate a painless "limp" from ataxia, which may be caused by a posterior fossa tumor.
- Beware of the painful limp that is worsening, limits activity, and is unrelieved by NSAIDs; it may herald a serious pathologic process.

EYE SWELLING: HISTORY AND PHYSICAL EXAMINATION

> **INSTRUCTIONS TO CANDIDATE: A 3-year-old boy is brought in by his parents because of a very swollen right eye (Figure 12-16), which he can no longer open voluntarily. Obtain a focused history, and perform a focused physical examination.**

DD$_X$: VITAMINS C
- Infectious: Orbital cellulitis, periorbital cellulitis
- Trauma
- Allergic reaction
- Idiopathic/iatrogenic: Localized reaction to an insect bite

History
- Ask the parents the following questions:
  - Character: "Can you describe the swelling? Is it painful? Is he otherwise well?"
  - Location: "What part of the eye is swollen (e.g., upper lid, lower lid, or both)? Any troubles with the other eye?"
  - Onset: "How did the swelling start: Did it come about suddenly, or has it been worsening over several hours or days?"
  - Intensity: "How severe is the pain, if present (see Figure 12-11)? Is the pain worse with eye movement?"
  - Duration: "How long has this swelling been going on?"
  - Events associated:
    - "Has your son had malaise? Lethargy? Loss of appetite? Nausea or vomiting?"
    - "Has he had a head or face injury? Recent infection? Sinusitis? Dental surgery?"
    - "Has he had a change in vision? Fever?"
    - "Has he had hives?"
    - "Has he had insect bites?"
  - Frequency: "Has this ever happened before? When?"

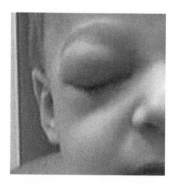

Figure 12-16 Swollen, erythematous right eye in a 3-year-old boy. (Courtesy Dr. Brett Taylor, Dalhousie University, Halifax, Nova Scotia.)

- **Palliative factors:** "Does anything reduce the swelling? If so, what?"
  - NSAIDs
  - Acetaminophen
  - Application of ice
- **Provocative factors:** "Does anything make the swelling worse? If so, what?"
- **PMH/PSH:** Sinusitis, dental infection, dental surgery, recent penetrating trauma, or facial fractures
- **MEDS:** Antibiotics, antipyretics, or immunosuppressants

Physical Examination

- **Vitals:** Evaluate HR and heart rhythm, BP, RR (depth, effort, and pattern), and temperature.
- **General:** Assess the patient's general appearance, work of breathing, and circulation to the skin (see Table 12-3).
- **Skin:** Inspect the skin and nails, noting any flushing or acute eruption (e.g., urticaria).
- **HEENT:** Ensure that the neck is supple (see Figure 12-13). Inspect the eye, noting erythema and whether the child is able to open it. Palpate the periorbital tissues, noting warmth and any tenderness. Gently retract the eyelid, and inspect the conjunctiva. Note any proptosis (protrusion of the eye). Using a brightly colored object, observe ocular mobility (in children with orbital cellulitis, the pain is exacerbated by eye movement). Check the pupillary responses to light. Inspect the nasal mucosa for discharge, and palpate the maxillary sinuses (frontal sinuses do not form until about age 6 years). Inspect the oropharynx, noting any erythema, petechiae, or vesicles on the palate. Note the size of the tonsils and the presence of any exudate. Examine for cervical lymphadenopathy.
- **Resp:** Assess chest expansion for symmetry. Auscultate the lungs, noting breath sounds and adventitious sounds.
- **CVS:** Check capillary refill. Palpate peripheral pulses, noting contour, volume, and rhythm. Auscultate the heart, listening for extra heart sounds or murmurs.
- **Neuro:** Most of the neurologic examination can be performed by simply observing the child play (motor function, cranial nerves).

Pearl

- It is vital to distinguish periorbital from orbital cellulitis. Periorbital cellulitis is associated with swelling, erythema, and warmth with normal ocular mobility and vision. Orbital cellulitis may appear similar, but there may be change in vision, proptosis, pain with eye movement, and systemic symptoms such as fever.

SEVERE INTERMITTENT ABDOMINAL PAIN: HISTORY AND PHYSICAL EXAMINATION

> **INSTRUCTIONS TO CANDIDATE: A 2-year-old girl is brought in by her parents because she is having episodes of screaming, in association with a "sore belly." Between episodes she is playing with her toys. When she has another episode of screaming, the triage nurse asks you to come and assess this patient.**

DD$_X$: VITAMINS C

- **Vascular:** Henoch-Schönlein purpura
- **Infectious:** UTI, pneumonia
- **Traumatic:** Occult trauma (abuse)
- **Metabolic:** Diabetic ketoacidosis (DKA)
- **Idiopathic/iatrogenic:** Intussusception, incarcerated hernia, ovarian torsion, appendicitis, pancreatitis, and stool impaction
- **Substance abuse and psychiatric:** Toxic ingestion
- **Congenital/genetic:** Meckel diverticulum, malrotation with volvulus, and sickle cell crisis

History

- Ask the parents the following questions:
  - **Character:** "Can you tell me about these screaming episodes? How long do they last? How is she between episodes?"
  - **Location:** "Where is the pain in her belly?"
  - **Onset:** "When did this start? How did it come on (sudden versus gradual)?"
  - **Radiation:** "Does it hurt anywhere else?"
  - **Duration:** "How long has this been going on?"
  - **Events associated:**
    - "Has she had a fever or recent infection?"
    - "Has she been vomiting (bilious versus nonbilious)?"
    - "How is her appetite? Any recent weight loss or gain?"
    - "Have you noticed any change in stools (diarrhea, steatorrhea, constipation, melena, or hematochezia)?"
    - "Have you noticed any change in urine (hematuria, dysuria)?"
    - "Is it possible that she ingested any medications or poisons?"
  - **Frequency:** "Has this ever happened before? How many episodes has she had (how often do they occur)?"
  - **Palliative factors:** "Does anything seem to make the pain better? If so, what?"
  - **Provocative factors:** "Does anything seem to make the pain worse? If so, what?"
- **PMH/PSH:** Previous surgery, sickle cell anemia, and diabetes mellitus
- **MEDS**
- **Allergies**
- **SH:** Living arrangements, recent changes at home
- **FH:** Sickle cell anemia, diabetes mellitus

Physical Examination

- **Vitals:** Evaluate HR and heart rhythm, BP, RR (depth, effort, and pattern), and temperature.
- **General:** Assess the patient's general appearance, work of breathing, and circulation to the skin. Check whether the findings of the initial assessment are correlated with the underlying physiologic state (see Table 12-3). Observe any apparent distress, anxiety/crying/screaming (duration), position of comfort, and interaction with her parents; observe behavior between episodes of apparent discomfort.
- **Skin:** Inspect the skin and nails, noting any acute eruption (e.g., purpura).
- **HEENT:** Ensure that the neck is supple (see Figure 12-13). Inspect the conjunctiva and oropharynx, noting any erythema, petechiae, or vesicles on the palate. Examine for cervical lymphadenopathy.
- **Resp:** Inspect for thoracic deformity. Assess chest expansion for symmetry. Auscultate the lungs, noting breath sounds and adventitious sounds.
- **CVS:** Check capillary refill. Palpate peripheral pulses, noting contour, volume, and rhythm. Auscultate the heart, listening for extra heart sounds or murmurs.
- **Abdomen:** Inspect the abdomen. Auscultate for bowel sounds. Percuss lightly in all four quadrants. Perform light and deep palpation, and identify any masses or areas of tenderness. Check for rebound tenderness. Examine the liver and spleen. Check diaper area for any blood or perianal lesions.

Evidence

- When emergency physicians and residents perform the clinical examination in children with abdominal pain, the reliability of their findings is fair at best, in comparison with those of surgeons.[7]

SAMPLE CHECKLISTS

New Peanut Allergy: Counsel

INSTRUCTIONS TO CANDIDATE: A 4-year-old girl is under observation in the emergency department after experiencing an anaphylactic reaction to peanut butter. Counsel the girl's mother about peanut allergy.

Key Points	Satisfactorily Completed
Introduces self to the parent	❏
Determines how the parent wishes to be addressed	❏
Washes hands	❏
Develops a rapport with the parent	❏
States that nut allergy (peanuts, tree nuts) is relatively common (may affect up to 1% of the population)	❏
States that nut allergy is often lifelong	❏
States that peanut allergy can be life-threatening	❏
States that the patient will be referred to an allergist for further evaluation	❏
Counsels the parent on strategies for allergen avoidance:	
• Checking all food labels for the presence of peanuts in the ingredients	❏
• Avoiding high-risk situations such as buffets, ice cream parlors, and unlabeled candy or desserts	❏
Counsels the parent to avoid tree nuts such as walnuts, cashews, and pistachios because cross-reactivity is common	❏
States that symptoms of allergy may develop minutes to hours after the allergen is ingested	❏
Describes early symptoms associated with food-related anaphylaxis:	
• Itching and tingling in the mouth	❏
• Itching at the back of the throat	❏
• Sensation of tightening in the airways	❏
• Abdominal pain, nausea or vomiting	❏
• Flushed appearance	❏
• Hives	❏
• Swelling of the lips and tongue	❏
Advises parent to contact Food Allergy and Anaphylaxis Network (www.foodallergy.org) for more educational materials	❏
Advises the parent that in case of exposure to peanuts and early symptoms and signs of a reaction:	
• Administer injectable epinephrine (intramuscularly in thigh)	❏
• Administer liquid oral diphenhydramine, 1 mg/kg	❏
• Transport patient to an emergency facility	❏
Informs the parent about the importance of educating the child's school or day care personnel about avoidance of nuts and providing them with a written emergency plan	❏
Ensures that the parent understands the emergency instructions (in case of exposure)	❏

Continued

Key Points	Satisfactorily Completed
Provides an opportunity for the parent to ask questions	❏
Provides written instructions for avoiding allergen exposure and an emergency plan in case of reaction	❏
Ensures that the parent has the appropriate prescription for injectable epinephrine	❏
Makes appropriate closing remarks	❏

Nonaccidental Trauma

INSTRUCTIONS TO CANDIDATE: An 8-month-old girl is brought to the emergency department by her grandmother because she is not as active as usual. She cries whenever her grandmother tries to change her diaper and seems to be in pain. Interpret the radiograph (Figure 12-17). What are your responsibilities in this case?

Key Points	Satisfactorily Completed
Checks the name and date on the x-ray film	❏
Comments on the type of view and adequacy of film	❏
Names spiral fracture of the femoral shaft	❏
Looks for other fractures or abnormalities	❏
Comments on need for skeletal survey to detect other acute or healing injuries	❏
Responsibilities in this case:	
• Examine the child	❏
• Ensure adequate pain control	❏
• Treat the fracture	❏
• Obtain an appropriate history from the child's grandmother about potential mechanism of injury	❏
• Ascertain the social history, including information about the child's caregivers	❏
• Explain the finding on the radiograph	❏
• Inform the grandmother of the requirement to report the child's injury	❏
• Contact Child Protection Services to investigate possible abuse	❏
• Consult the orthopedics service	❏

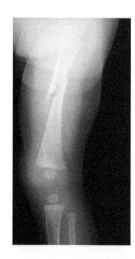

Figure 12-17 Anteroposterior x-ray of left femur. (From Hobbs CJ, Wynne JM. *Physical Signs of Child Abuse.* 2nd ed. London: Saunders; 2001 [p. 107].)

REFERENCES

1. Steiner MJ, DeWalt DA, Byerley JS. Is this child dehydrated? *JAMA*. 2004;291:2746-2754.
2. Stevens MW, Gorelick MH, Schultz T. Interrater agreement in the clinical evaluation of acute pediatric asthma. *J Asthma*. 2003;40:311-315.
3. Ebell MH, Smith MA, Barry HC, et al. The rational clinical examination. Does this patient have strep throat? *JAMA*. 2000;284:2912-2918.
4. McIsaac WJ, Goel V, To T, et al. The validity of a sore throat score in family practice. *CMAJ*. 2000;163:811-815.
5. Margolis P, Gadomski A. The rational clinical examination. Does this infant have pneumonia? *JAMA*. 1998;279:308-313.
6. World Health Organization. *Country Landscape Information System (NLIS): country profile indicators: interpretation guide (online report)*. <http://www.who.int/nutrition/nlis_interpretation_guide.pdf>; Accessed 29.11.10.
7. Yen K, Karpas A, Pinkerton HJ, et al. Interexaminer reliability in physical examination of pediatric patients with abdominal pain. *Arch Pediatr Adolesc Med*. 2005;159:373-376.

CHAPTER 13

Geriatrics

Edited by Katalin Koller, MD, FRCPC, and Paige Moorhouse, MD, MPH, FRCPC

ESSENTIAL SKILLS

APPROACH TO GERIATRIC PATIENTS

The geriatric history includes all aspects of the systems-based histories discussed in Chapters 1 through 11 and 14, with a focus on higher level end points (cognition, mobility, and function) and appropriate use of a collateral historian.

History Taking
- Using the **ChLORIDE FPP** method, you may approach the history of a presenting complaint in the same way as outlined in previous chapters. However, many medical problems in elderly patients manifest in an "atypical" manner in comparison with "classic" descriptions. When an older person is frail, clinical illness manifests first with a failure of cognition, mobility, or function. For example, elderly persons with a serious systemic infection may not mount a fever but often present with delirium, falls, or decreased ability to carry on daily tasks of living. It is particularly important to ascertain the patient's baseline values in each of these areas, so that you may understand the timeline and degree of change associated with acute illness presentations.
- Your ability to take a detailed history is sometimes hindered by the patient's impairments of cognition, speech, or hearing. In the case of suspected cognitive impairment from any cause, you should always indicate that you would like further history from a collateral historian (someone who sees the patient on a regular basis, such as a relative or caregiver). You may wish to speak slowly, ask one question at

a time, and speak loudly, as necessary. Attempt to correct any sensory impairment the patient may have (ask the patient to wear glasses or hearing aid; use hearing amplifier) and allow the patient adequate time to respond to questions. Ensure that the room has good lighting (e.g., some elderly persons adapt by lip reading). Sometimes you may have to resort to communicating through pen and paper. Consider using an interpreter or language-appropriate cognitive test in the setting of language barriers.

Past Medical History/Past Surgical History
- Current medical problems for which the patient is being treated or investigated
- Past medical problems
- Previous hospitalizations
- Previous surgeries

Medications
- Establish a complete list of all current medications and dosing schedules, including prescription, over-the-counter (OTC), and herbal medications. Ensure that the list has been corroborated by a valid source, such as a pharmacy-generated list.
- Ask whether any changes have been made to the medication schedule recently or whether new medications have been added.
- Ask the patient whether he or she takes the medications regularly.
- Ask the patient whether he or she has any concerns about their medications and whether he or she has experienced any side effects.
- In elderly persons, medication use, particularly polypharmacy, is a significant source of iatrogenic health problems. Nonpharmacologic options should be sought as first-line management and always as adjunctive therapy in any medication regimen. Be conscientious about drug-drug interactions. Adjust renally excreted drugs according to the patient's creatinine clearance level. Do not prescribe a drug to manage a side effect of another drug.
- Consider consulting a resource such as the Beers criteria[1] for specific recommendations on medication use in elderly patients. Such resources may help guide decision making with regard to the appropriateness of medications for geriatric patients.

Social History
- Ask the patient the following questions:
  - "What type of home do you have (apartment versus house)? Are there stairs?"
  - "Do you live alone? If not, with whom do you live? Are you taking care of anyone (e.g., spouse)? Is someone taking care of you (e.g., are you dependent or semidependent on a caregiver)?"
  - "Do you have any financial concerns?" (Many elderly persons live on a fixed income. This may affect their ability to get to medical appointments, hire appropriate help, or fill prescriptions.)
  - "What is your primary means of transportation (e.g., driving, caregiver, public transit)?"
  - "Do you smoke cigarettes? Do you drink alcohol (quantify)? Do you use recreational or street drugs?"
  - "Do you currently work outside the home? What is/was your occupation? What is the highest level of education you have received?"
  - "Do you have a Power of Attorney appointed for finances or medical decision making, or both, if you are unable to make these decisions yourself? Do you have an advance directive? Does this include your wishes in the event of a cardiorespiratory arrest? Do you have a substitute decision maker?"
- See pp. 383-384 for specific discussion on advance care directives. In elderly patients, it is particularly important to establish their definition or perception of an acceptable quality of life.

Basic Activities of Daily Living

- Establish the patient's baseline values (when he or she was last well) and current level of function in each area, in view of the patient's self-reported activities, as well as collateral information if you are concerned about the patient's cognitive function.
- Grooming, bathing: Ask for collateral information to determine whether the patient requires cueing to complete these tasks.
- Dressing: Ask for collateral information to determine whether the patient wears the same clothing repetitively or needs cueing to change soiled clothing. Also, check whether the patient is wearing weather-appropriate clothing.
- Ask about the patient's toileting abilities and continence.
- Ask about the patient's ability to feed himself or herself.
- Ambulating: Ask about the patient's ability to transfer from bed or chair to toilet and ability to mobilize outside the home. Ask whether the patient is using any gait aids to ambulate and, if so, when.

Instrumental Activities of Daily Living

- Establish the patient's baseline values (when they were last well) and current level of function in each area; consider the patient's self-reported activities and, if you are concerned about the patient's cognitive function, collateral information:
  - Cooking and cleaning
  - Using a telephone
  - Managing medications
  - Managing finances
  - Shopping
  - Transportation (e.g., driving a car, using public transportation)

Immunization History

- Specifically address whether the patient has received tetanus, influenza, and pneumococcal vaccines.

Symptom Screen

- Sensory impairment: Decreased vision, decreased hearing
- Incontinence: Urinary, fecal
- Malnutrition: Weight loss, dietary habits
- Memory disturbance: Folstein Mini-Mental State Examination (MMSE)
- Depression: Mood, satisfaction with life
- Social isolation: Spending time with family or friends, activities outside the home, recreation, and hobbies

Review of Systems

- Perform a detailed review of systems as outlined in the Introduction (pp. xv-xviii) to this book.

FOLSTEIN MINI-MENTAL STATE EXAMINATION

- The Folstein MMSE tests orientation, registration, attention, recall, comprehension, language, and constructional ability. It takes 10 to 15 minutes to administer. It is a well-studied and useful tool (median positive likelihood ratio [+LR] 6.3, range 3.4 to 47; median negative likelihood ratio [−LR] 0.19, range 0.06 to 0.37).[2] However, scores are affected by age, education level, and language function (i.e., productive aphasia), and it does not test frontal lobe function, beyond the additional clock drawing.
- Prompted answers do not count.
- The test has a total score of 30. Traditional cutoff scores include 21 to 24 for mild dementia, 10 to 20 for moderate dementia, and 0 to 9 for severe dementia. Because the scores are affected by age, education level, and language function, the traditional cutoff scores should not be considered diagnostic rather, they should be used to guide clinical judgment.

Orientation Questions
- "What is the year, season, day of week, date, and month?" (5 points).
- "What is the country, province/state, city, hospital, and floor?" (5 points).

Registration Questions
- Name three objects (e.g., "ball," "car," and "man"), and ask the patient to repeat the three items. Score one point for each item answered correctly (3 points).
- If necessary, repeat the items until the patient learns them. Record the number of trials necessary to achieve this.
- Instruct the patient that you will ask about these three items again later.

Attention Questions
- Ask either of the following (5 points):
  - After ensuring that the patient can spell "world" forward, ask him or her to spell it backward. Score 1 point for each correct letter.
  - Ask the patient to recite the months in reverse order (i.e., December, November, October…)

Memory Question
- Ask the patient to name the three items you asked him or her to remember from the registration part of the examination. Score 1 point for each item recalled correctly (3 points). You cannot test memory if the patient failed to register the items in the first place.

Language Questions
- Show the patient two objects, and ask the patient to name them (e.g., pencil, watch). One point is given for each correctly named item (2 points).
- Ask the patient to repeat the following statement: "No ifs, ands, or buts" (1 point).
- Tell the patient, "Take this piece of paper in your right hand, fold it in half, and put it on the floor." Score 1 point for each stage of the command correctly executed (3 points). Give the three commands, slowly and clearly, but all at once before the patient completes the tasks.
- Ask the patient to read a written command ("Close your eyes") and to do what it says (1 point).
- Ask the patient to write a complete sentence (1 point).

Visual-Spatial Functioning Question
- Ask the patient to copy the design below (two overlapping pentagons. Give 1 point for a correctly completed copy; the intersection of the pentagons must form a four-sided figure (1 point).

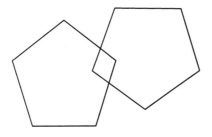

WEAKNESS: HISTORY

> **INSTRUCTIONS TO CANDIDATE:** An 88-year-old woman presents via ambulance from her home with a complaint of "weakness." Obtain a detailed history, exploring possible causes.

DD$_X$: VITAMINS C

The differential diagnosis for such a nonspecific complaint in the geriatric age group is broad and may reflect medications, metabolic derangement, systemic illness, infection, neurologic disease, or something else.

- **V**ascular: Transient ischemic attack (TIA), stroke, and temporal arteritis
- **I**nfectious: Pneumonia, urinary tract infection (UTI), postpolio syndrome
- **T**raumatic: Subdural hemorrhage
- **A**utoimmune/allergic: Myasthenia gravis, Guillain-Barré syndrome
- **M**etabolic: Hypoxia, hyponatremia/hypernatremia, hypoglycemia, hypocalcemia/hypercalcemia, hypomagnesemia, hypokalemia/hyperkalemia, hypoadrenalism, hypothyroidism, and anemia
- **I**diopathic/iatrogenic: Adverse medication effects, orthostatic hypotension
- **N**eoplastic: Constitutional symptoms caused by neoplasm, such as cachexia and asthenia; paraneoplastic syndrome (e.g., Eaton-Lambert syndrome); spinal cord compression
- **S**ubstance abuse and psychiatric: Drug intoxication or withdrawal

History

- Ask the patient the following questions:
  - **Character:** "Describe what you mean by weakness: muscular weakness? Fatigue? Presyncope?"
  - **Location:** "Is the weakness localized? If so, what part of your body is weak?"
  - **Onset:** "How did the weakness come on (sudden versus gradual)?"
  - **Radiation:** "Is the weakness spreading (ascending versus descending)?"
  - **Intensity:** "How severe is the weakness? Are you able to walk? Can you accomplish activities of daily living (feeding yourself, cooking, toileting, dressing)?"
  - **Duration:** "How long has this weakness been going on?"
  - **Events associated:**
    - "Has the weakness caused you to fall?" Elicit a history of falls, if present (see pp. 371-372).
    - "Do you have any difficulty swallowing, chewing, talking, or breathing?"
    - "Have you noticed any changes in bowel or bladder habit? Have you had nausea or vomiting?"
    - Bleeding: "Have you had blood in your urine or stool, black stool, bloody vomit, bloody sputum, or vaginal bleeding?"
    - Constitutional symptoms: "Have you had fever, chills, night sweats, weight loss, or anorexia?"
  - **Frequency:** "Has this ever happened to you before? When? How often (constant versus intermittent)?"
  - **Palliative factors:** "Does anything seem to help? If so, what?"
  - **Provocative factors:** "Does anything seem to make it worse? If so, what?"
- **Review of systems (ROS):** The ROS may help you further delineate the cause of this confusing symptom by looking at the whole picture.
- **Past medical history (PMH)/past surgical history (PSH):** Diabetes, malignancy, vascular disease, falls, or previous surgery
- **Medications (MEDS):** Anticholinergic medications, diuretics, sedatives, insulin, diabetic medications (hypoglycemia), recent medication changes, or new medications
- **Social history (SH):** Smoking, use of alcohol (EtOH), use of street drugs, occupation, and recreational activities
- **Family history (FH):** Malignancy, neurovascular disease

FALL: HISTORY

> **INSTRUCTIONS TO CANDIDATE:** A 79-year-old man presents to the emergency department via ambulance after falling at home. Obtain a detailed history, exploring possible causes.

DD$_X$: VITAMINS C
- **V**ascular: TIA, stroke, drop attack (sudden leg weakness without loss of consciousness), syncope, aortic stenosis, and chronic subdural hemorrhage
- **I**nfectious: Pneumonia, UTI, other diseases
- **T**raumatic: Chronic subdural hemorrhage
- **M**etabolic: Hypoglycemia, electrolyte disturbance, and diabetic neuropathy (impaired sensation/proprioception), dehydration (hypotension, orthostatic changes)
- **I**diopathic/iatrogenic: Deconditioning, Parkinson disease, adverse effects of medications, seizure disorder, and normal-pressure hydrocephalus (ataxia)
- **N**eoplastic: Central nervous system (CNS) tumor
- **S**ubstance abuse and psychiatric: Intoxication, drug withdrawal

Age-Related Factors Contributing to Instability
- Decreased proprioception and peripheral sensation
- Orthostatic hypotension
- Deconditioning
- Osteoarthritis
- Sensory impairment: vision, hearing
- Cognitive decline, depression
- Nocturia (e.g., congestive heart failure, diuretic therapy, prostatism) that leads to bathroom trips in the dark
- Polypharmacy: orthostatic hypotension or excessive sedation

History
- Ask the patient the following questions:
  - **Character:** "Describe what happened to you today. Were you alone? (A witness may offer valuable collateral history.) Are 'falls' a problem for you? How did you fall?"
    - Trip or slip and fall
    - Orthostatic symptoms (stood up, felt weak, and fell)
    - Loss of consciousness leading to a fall
    - Drop attack (sudden leg weakness without loss of consciousness)
    - Vertigo or ataxia leading to a fall
    - Palpitations or shortness of breath before a fall
  - **Location:** "Where did you fall?"
  - **Onset:** "Did you have any warning of the impending fall?"
  - **Intensity:** "How bad was your fall? Did you lose consciousness? Could you get up by yourself afterward? Are you able to walk? Are you injured? Are you having pain?" (Delineate the character, location, and intensity of any identified pain.)
  - **Duration:** "When did you fall? How long was it before you were able to call for help?"
  - **Events associated:**
    - "Do you live alone?"
    - "If you required help getting back on your feet, how did you get help?"
    - "Did you strike your head? Did you lose consciousness after you fell?"
    - "Were you aware of any seizure activity (suggested by tongue bleeding or loss of bowel or bladder function, or by collateral history of witnessed seizure-like activity)?"
    - Environmental factors: "Do you have unstable furniture, poor lighting, uneven stairs, throw rugs, pets, or loose wires or cords (e.g., home O$_2$)?"
    - "Do you use any walking aids (e.g., cane, walker)?"
    - "How able are you to accomplish activities of daily living (feed yourself, cook, toileting, bathe, dress yourself)?"

Table 13-1	Usefulness of the Clinical Examination for Estimating Risk of Falls in Elderly Patients	
Clinical Feature	**+LR (95% CI)**	**−LR (95% CI)**
At least one fall in the last year*	2.8 (2.1–3.8)	—
History of dementia[†]	**17 (1.9–149)**	0.99 (0.97–1.0)
History of Parkinson disease[†]	**5.0 (1.5–16)**	0.98 (0.97–1.0)
Taking a benzodiazepine, phenothiazine, or antidepressant[†]	**27 (3.6–207)**	0.88 (0.82–0.95)
Unable to perform standing heel to toe for 10 seconds without foot movement or manual support (tandem stand)[†]	2.0 (1.7–2.4)	0.74 (0.67–0.82)
Palmomental reflex[†]	2.8 (1.8–4.4)	0.77 (0.67–0.89)

*Data from Chu LW, Chi I, Chiu AY. Incidence and predictors of falls in the Chinese elderly. *Ann Acad Med Singapore.* 2005;34:60-72.

[†]Data from Ganz DA, Bao Y, Shekelle PG, et al. Will my patient fall? *JAMA.* 2007;297:77-86.

CI, Confidence interval; −LR, negative likelihood ratio; +LR, positive likelihood ratio.

Boldface represents findings associated with positive likelihood ratios ≥ 5 or with negative likelihood ratios ≤ 0.2. These are said to be moderate- to high-impact items.

- Frequency: "Has this ever happened to you before? When? How often?"
- Palliative factors: "Does anything seem to help? If so, what (e.g., walking aids)?"
- Provocative factors: "Does anything seem to make it worse? If so, what (e.g., environmental factors such as poor lighting)?"
- **PMH/PSH:** Diabetes, cerebrovascular disease, arrhythmia, ischemic heart disease, valvular disease, Parkinson disease, osteoarthritis of lower extremities, visual deficits, chronic pain, or previous surgery
- **MEDS:** Anticholinergic medications, diuretics, sedatives, insulin, diabetic medications (hypoglycemia), recent medication changes, or new medications
- **SH:** Smoking, use of EtOH, use of street drugs, occupation, and recreational activities
- **FH:** Malignancy, neurovascular disease

Evidence

- For persons aged 65 years and older, the annual risk of falling at least once is 27%. Visual impairment, impairment of gait or balance, and cognitive impairment each seem to increase risk to some extent (Table 13-1). Contrary to popular belief, orthostatic hypotension does not appear to increase risk.[3]

Pearls

- Falls are a major cause of morbidity in elderly persons. The rate of 1-year survival after hospitalization for a fall with hip fractures in this age group is approximately 50%.
- A fall is often an indication of underlying frailty, and you should identify risk factors for future falls so that preventive measures can be instituted (Figure 13-1).

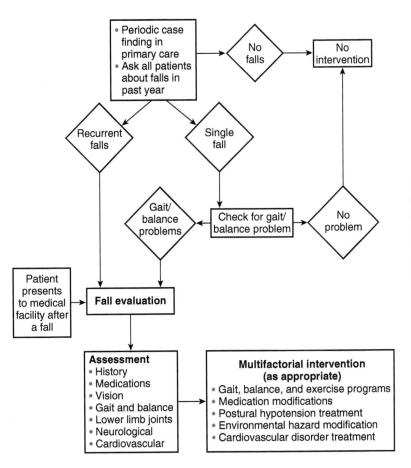

Figure 13-1 Algorithm for assessment and management of falls in elderly persons. (From American Geriatrics Society, British Geriatrics Society, and American Academy of Orthopaedic Surgeons Panel on Falls Prevention. Guideline for the prevention of falls in older persons. Physical examination and health assessment. *J Am Geriatr Soc.* 2001;49:666.)

CONFUSION: DIFFERENTIATE AMONG DELIRIUM, DEMENTIA, AND DEPRESSION

> **INSTRUCTIONS TO CANDIDATE: A 72-year-old man is brought to the hospital by his wife because of his increasing confusion and troubles with memory. She states that he has been found wandering outside, and she is very concerned for his safety. Differentiate among delirium, dementia, and depression (Table 13-2).**

- **Delirium** is acute cognitive dysfunction secondary to underlying medical illness. It was previously referred to as "organic brain syndrome." It is characterized by fluctuating consciousness; reduced ability to focus, maintain, or shift attention; and distractibility.
- **Dementia** is a progressive deterioration of cognitive function that occurs without impairment of consciousness and is severe enough to affect daily life (i.e., there is associated functional impairment). It affects memory, language, orientation judgment, and mood. As it progresses, it can further affect other global brain functions such as praxis, swallowing, and gait.
- **Depression** in elderly persons may cause a dementia-like syndrome (pseudodementia). Major symptoms associated with depression (SIGE CAPS: sleeplessness, loss of interest, guilt, decreased energy, inability to concentrate, loss of appetite, psychomotor retardation, and suicidal ideation) are discussed on pp. 285 and 295. Guilt and negative mood are less commonly self-identified features in older adults, whereas irritability, low energy, poor sleep, and somatic difficulties are more common. Decreased concentration and psychomotor retardation may cause depression to be mistaken for dementia. In general, first onset of depression in an older adult should

prompt suspicion of underlying dementia and necessitates periodic assessment of cognition.

Collateral History

- Obtain collateral history from the wife first (to corroborate the history obtained from the patient and to delineate her specific concerns that precipitated this medical visit). You may ask the patient about his cognitive concerns in general before you begin your objective testing of his cognition.
    - "Have you noticed any memory loss? Does your husband have any difficulty recalling recent events or conversations?"
    - "Does your husband have trouble remembering people's names?"
    - "Does he often have difficulty finding the words he wants to say in conversation?"
    - "Does he ever get lost or forget where he is going?"
    - "Does he seem aware of the date and day of the week?"
    - "When did you first notice these troubles?"
    - "How have these symptoms changed or progressed during the past weeks and months (rapid, gradual, stepwise, or static)?"
    - "How do these problems affect his daily function, namely, reading, writing, using the telephone, and managing money and medications?"
    - Wife's safety concerns: "Does your husband ever wander or get lost? Does he go outside without appropriate clothing (e.g., going outside in winter without coat and shoes)? Has he ever left the stove on or the water running? Do you have concerns about his driving? Does he ever get lost while driving or on foot? Do you have any other safety concerns?"
    - Mood changes: "Has your husband been at all irritable? Have you noticed withdrawal from previous interests?"
    - "How are you managing as your husband's caregiver? Do you feel overwhelmed? Do you need more help at home? Do you ever feel threatened?"
    - Associated symptoms (early onset of these symptoms with cognitive concerns is suggestive of a non-Alzheimer type of dementia):
        - Incontinence
        - Frequent falls
        - Dysphagia
        - Socially inappropriate or disruptive behavior
        - Visual or auditory hallucinations
- **ROS:** The ROS may help you to further delineate the contribution of organic disease to the entity of "confusion."
- **PMH/PSH:** Hypertension, stroke, TIA, depression or anxiety disorder, malignancy, falls, head trauma, or previous surgery
- **MEDS:** Complete list of medications (prescription, OTC, herbals) and dosing schedules, recent medication changes, or new medications
- **SH:** Smoking, use of EtOH, use of street drugs, educational level, occupation, and recreational activities
- **FH:** Dementia, depression or anxiety disorder, or cerebrovascular disease

History from the Patient

- Administer the Folstein MMSE to assess orientation, registration, attention, recall, comprehension, language, and constructional ability. Because the scores are affected by age, education level, and language function, the traditional cutoff scores should not be considered diagnostic; rather, they should be used to guide clinical judgment.
- Perform the Memory Impairment Screen. Give the patient four items to remember (animal, city, vegetable, and musical instrument). After 2 to 3 minutes, ask the patient to name the four items (score 1 point for each item). If the patient cannot recall the items, he may be reminded of the category with which the item is associated (e.g., "The first item is an animal"; score 1 point for each item). The total score is calculated

as [2 × (free recall)] + cued recall (score ranges from 0 to 8). A score of 4 or lower indicates significant memory impairment.[4]
- Administer a brief depression-screening questionnaire such as the **Geriatric Depression Scale (very short form).** The questions are listed as follows; the answer in parentheses is suggestive of depression, and 1 point is scored for each suggestive answer. A score >2 is considered an indication of depression.
  - Are you basically satisfied with your life? (No)
  - Do you often get bored? (Yes)
  - Do you often feel helpless? (Yes)
  - Do you prefer to stay at home rather than going out and doing new things? (Yes)
  - Do you feel pretty worthless the way you are now? (Yes)
- Perform a thorough mental status examination as outlined on p. 287.

Evidence

- The **Memory Impairment Screen** takes only 4 minutes to administer and is very useful (+LR 33, and 95% CI 15 to 72; −LR 0.08, and 95% CI 0.02 to 0.3).[5]
- The importance of collateral history should not be underestimated: At least one study on the subjective complaint of memory loss from a collateral historian had a +LR of 6.5 (95% CI 4.4 to 9.6) for dementia and a −LR of 0.1 (95% CI 0.07 to 0.14).[6]

Table 13-2 Differentiating Among Delirium, Dementia, and Depression

Characteristic	Delirium	Dementia	Depression
Onset	Hours to days (acute)	Often months to years (insidious), although dementia after a stroke may start acutely	Weeks to months
Duration	Variable	Remainder of life	Short
Mood	Labile	Fluctuating	Consistent
Disabilities	New disabilities appear (acute)	Limited insight by patient into deficits	Recognized by patient
Answers	May be incoherent (acute)	Are not correct (but may be close to correct, concealing the deficit)	Poor effort "I don't know"
Folstein MMSE findings	Acute fluctuations Frequent inability to participate in examination	Stable with downward trajectory over time	Fluctuating performance
Progression	Symptoms usually resolve with treatment	Symptoms may improve with treatment for some time, but progression is inevitable	Symptoms resolve with treatment

MMSE, Mini-Mental State Examination.

DECREASED HEARING: HISTORY AND PHYSICAL EXAMINATION

> **INSTRUCTIONS TO CANDIDATE:** An 80-year-old man presents to your office with concern about decreased hearing in his right ear. Obtain a focused history, and perform a focused physical examination.

DD$_X$: VITAMINS C
- Infectious: Otitis media
- Traumatic: Foreign body obstructing external canal, ossicular disruption, and noise trauma (loss of hair cells from organ of Corti)
- Autoimmune/allergic: Multiple sclerosis
- Idiopathic/iatrogenic: Obstruction of external canal by cerumen, otosclerosis, ototoxic medications (e.g., aminoglycosides, furosemide, acetylsalicylic acid), Paget disease, and presbycusis
- Neoplastic: Tumor obstructing external canal, cerebellopontine angle tumor
- Substance abuse and psychiatric: Pseudo-deafness (depression)
- Congenital/genetic: Hereditary deafness (unlikely in this age group)

Definition
- **Presbycusis** is sensorineural hearing loss associated with advanced age (decreased ability to perceive or discriminate sound). Although it affects the majority of persons aged >65 years, only a fraction of these have a functional deficit.

History
- Ask the patient the following questions:
    - **Character:** "Other than decreased hearing, have you noticed anything else? Tinnitus? Hyperacusis? Do you have difficulty localizing sound in noisy environments? In what situations have you noticed the hearing loss?"
    - **Location:** "Is the hearing loss in the right ear only?"
    - **Onset:** "When and how did the loss start?"
    - **Radiation:** "Are there any problems with hearing in the other ear?"
    - **Intensity:** "How severe is the hearing loss?"
    - **Duration:** "How long has the hearing impairment been going on?"
    - **Events associated:**
        - "Do you have any pain in your ears? Headache?"
        - "Do you have any discharge from your ears?"
        - "Do you have any difficulties with speech?"
    - **Frequency:** "How often does your decreased hearing pose a problem for you (constant versus intermittent)?"
    - **Palliative factors:** "Does anything seem to make your hearing better? If so, what (e.g., quiet surroundings, hearing aid)?"
    - **Provocative factors:** "Does anything seem to make your hearing worse? If so, what (e.g., background noise)?"
- **PMH/PSH:** Previous surgery, malignancy, multiple sclerosis, or otitis media
- **MEDS:** Ototoxic medications such as aminoglycosides
- **SH:** Smoking, use of EtOH, use of street drugs, occupational and recreational activities
- **FH:** Deafness, multiple sclerosis, Paget disease

Physical Examination
- **Vital signs (Vitals):** Evaluate heart rate, respiratory rate, blood pressure, and temperature.
    - Fever may be associated with otitis media, inner ear infection, or CNS infection
- **General:** Cachexia may be indicative of malignancy or systemic illness.
- **Skin:** Check for café-au-lait spots and neurofibromas.

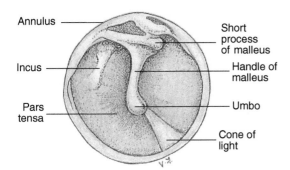

Annulus

Short process of malleus

Incus

Handle of malleus

Pars tensa

Umbo

Cone of light

Figure 13-2 Tympanic membrane. (From Wilson SF, Gidden JF. *Health assessment for nursing practice.* 2nd ed. St. Louis: Mosby; 2001 [p. 289].)

- **Head, eyes, ears, nose, and throat (HEENT):**
  - **Inspection:** Assess the external ear (auricle, tragus) and auditory canal.
  - **Otoscopy:** Examine the normal ear first. Grasp the auricle, and pull it upward, backward, and slightly away from the head. Gently insert the speculum of the otoscope into the ear canal (hold otoscope between thumb and fingers, and brace your hand against the patient's face). Examine the tympanic membrane, and identify landmarks (Figure 13-2). Observe any abnormalities such as discharge, erythema, swelling, or loss of landmarks.
  - **Auditory acuity** should be assessed in a quiet room. Occlude one ear, and ask the patient to speak out loudly. Whisper softly into the other ear, using words or numbers of equally accented syllables. Use a normal voice or a shout, depending on the degree of hearing loss.
  - **Weber's test** (lateralization): Place a vibrating tuning fork (512 Hz or 1024 Hz) firmly on top of the patient's head. Ask the patient whether he hears it in one or both ears. Normally the sound is heard midline. In conductive hearing loss, sound is heard laterally in the impaired ear. In sensorineural hearing loss, the sound is heard laterally in the normal ear.
  - **Rinne's test** (comparing air conduction with bone conduction): Place a vibrating tuning fork (512 Hz or 1024 Hz) on the patient's head over the mastoid bone, behind the ear, level with the external auditory canal. When the patient can no longer hear the sound, place the tuning fork close to the ear canal (with the "U" of the fork facing forward), and ask whether the sound is now audible. In conductive hearing loss, sound is best transmitted by bone conduction.
- **Neurologic system:** Test the motor and sensory aspects of cranial nerve V, as well as the corneal reflex. Test the muscles of facial expression (cranial nerve VII). Observe balance, gait, and speech. Perform tests of coordination (rapid alternating movements, finger-nose testing) and fine motor control (picking up a dime from a table top). Inspect the extraocular movements, and characterize any nystagmus (by the direction of the fast phase).

ADVANCED SKILLS

ABUSE AND NEGLECT: HISTORY

> **INSTRUCTIONS TO CANDIDATE: A 75-year-old woman is brought to your office by her daughter for a checkup. This patient has been dependent on her family for her care since having a stroke last year. Before you see the patient, the nurse tells you that she noted several bruises and decubitus ulcers. Obtain a detailed history, focusing on risk factors for abuse and neglect.**

Definition and Risk Factors
- Abuse of elderly persons is a spectrum that encompasses physical abuse, sexual abuse, emotional or psychologic abuse, neglect, abandonment, and financial or material exploitation. Neglect accounts for the majority of cases of abuse of elderly persons. Such abuse remains underreported by its victims. The vulnerability, both physical and often cognitive, of this population and the risk of social isolation hinder disclosure.
- Abuse and neglect are more likely to take place when the older person is physically, cognitively, or functionally impaired or dependent. Other risk factors include female gender, advanced age, incontinence, and aggressive behavior.
- Caregiver-related risk factors for abuse of elderly persons include alcohol or drug abuse, mental illness, financial or psychosocial stress related to caregiving, lack of caregiving skills, and longer duration as primary caregiver. Social isolation, shared living, and lack of support (resources, family support) further increase the risk.

History
- A thorough history with emphasis on risk factors and direct screening is the most important tool for detecting abuse and neglect.
- The history should be taken from the caregiver alone and from the patient alone, separately.

Patient History
- Ask the patient the following questions:
  - "What brings you here today?" Obtain an appropriate history pertaining to her presenting concerns.
  - Ask for a list of medications. "Do you take your medications yourself, or does your caregiver give them to you? Do you take them regularly? Do you ever have trouble getting your medications when you need them?"
  - "Who lives with you? How are things going at home? Do you feel safe where you live?"
  - "Can you get around inside and outside the house? Do you need help with tasks at home? Do you dress yourself, feed yourself, cook, go to the bathroom on your own, and take a bath or shower on your own? Are you continent?"
  - "Who helps you with the things you cannot do yourself? Do you ever have trouble getting the help you need?"
  - "Are you alone during the day? How often? Do you mind being alone?"
  - "Do you get outside the home? Do you spend time with friends? What do you do for recreation?"
  - "Do you ever have disagreements with your caregiver? How are disagreements handled? What happens?"
  - "Who handles your financial affairs? If a caregiver, do you have any concerns about how he or she is handling your money?"
  - "I notice that you have some bruises; how did that happen?"
  - "Has anyone ever hit, punched, or kicked you? If so, who?"
  - "Has anyone ever invaded your personal space? Has anyone ever touched you sexually in an unwanted way?"

- "Have you ever been locked up or tied down against your will?"
- "Are you ever threatened or yelled at?"
- Note any tension or fearfulness between the patient and her caregiver. Observe the behavior of the patient in your office (e.g., reluctance to make eye contact).
- Perform a mental status examination, and note any signs of anxiety, depression, or cognitive decline.
- For patients who are unable to communicate with you (because of aphasia or cognitive decline, for example), you must rely on the caregiver's history, a collateral history, results of the mental status examination, and findings of the physical examination.

Caregiver History
- Avoid creating a confrontational situation with the caregiver. The history should be obtained in a nonjudgmental manner. Remember that being the caregiver of a dependent adult is often difficult and challenging. Demonstrating sympathy to the caregiver may help you create an alliance with them and facilitate information gathering.
- Direct questions about the initial history to the reasons for the visit today:
  - "Have you noticed any changes in your mother lately? How is she doing?"
  - "Tell me about your mother's routine medications and daily care." Poor knowledge of these essentials may herald neglect.
  - "With what activities do you help her (e.g., feeding, cooking, dressing, bathing)?"
  - "What community resources are you currently using (e.g., respite care)?"
  - "Are you working outside the home? What do you do for recreation?" Social isolation is a risk factor for abuse and neglect.
  - "Describe the current living arrangements. How have things been going at home?"
  - "Have there been any recent stressful events? Are there any financial strains with these living arrangements?"
  - "I noticed that your mother has some bruises and skin breakdown or ulcers. Can you tell me how this happened?"
- Throughout the interview, be alert to clues indicating depression, anxiety, substance abuse, hostility, or indifference.
- Failure of the caregiver to accompany the patient or provide essential belongings, such as glasses, hearing aid, or walking aid, is a red flag.

Red Flags
- Evidence of tension or indifference between the patient and caregiver
- Implausible or vague explanations of mechanism of injury
- Inconsistency in the history of injury given by the patient and caregiver
- Unexplained injuries
- Evidence of old injuries not previously documented
- Patient's lacking glasses, hearing aid, or walking aid
- Caregiver's inability to give details of the patient's routine medications and daily activities
- Potential neglect: Soiled clothing, long toenails, and unkempt hair despite available supports
- Patient's inability to make eye contact or appearing nervous or hesitant to speak
- Caregiver's appearing unwilling to allow the patient to speak

Pearls
- Like violence toward intimate partners, abuse of elderly persons tends to increase in frequency and to escalate in intensity. Abuse and neglect exacerbate underlying medical problems, and elderly persons who are abused appear to have a greater risk of dying than do those who are not abused.
- In some jurisdictions, it is mandatory to report suspected abuse of an elderly person.

SAMPLE CHECKLIST

Urinary Incontinence: History

> **INSTRUCTIONS TO CANDIDATE:** A 76-year-old woman presents to her family doctor with a history of urinary "accidents." This problem limits her activities outside of the home. Obtain a detailed history, exploring possible causes.

Key Points	Satisfactorily Completed
Introduces self to the patient	❏
Determines how the patient wishes to be addressed	❏
Explains the purpose of the encounter	❏
Asks for a description of the problem:	
• Does it occur with coughing, laughing, sneezing, or lifting?	❏
• Is there any urinary urgency?	❏
• Is there a sense of incomplete emptying? Does the urge to void continue even after urinary flow stops?	❏
Asks when the incontinence started	❏
Asks when this poses the greatest difficulty (e.g., overnight)	❏
Asks about quantity of leakage	❏
Asks about continent voids	❏
Inquires about mobility (e.g., difficulty getting to the toilet)	❏
Asks how she deals with the problem:	
• Does she wear an incontinence pad or diaper?	❏
• How often does she have to change it?	❏
Asks what strategies have been tried thus far to manage the problem	❏
Asks how this affects her daily activities:	
• Is she able to participate in activities outside the home, such as grocery shopping?	❏
• Is someone available to help her?	❏
Asks whether the problem is getting better, getting worse, or staying the same	❏
Asks how frequently it poses difficulties (e.g., every day?)	❏
Asks whether she has any abdominal or flank pain	❏
Inquires about constipation (stool impaction can cause incontinence in elderly persons)	❏
Asks about irritative symptoms:	
• Dysuria	❏
• Urgency	❏
• Frequency	❏
Asks about obstructive symptoms:	
• Hesitancy	❏
• Increased force needed for urination	❏
• Sense of incomplete emptying	❏
Asks about hematuria (blood in the urine)	❏
Asks about palliative and provocative factors	❏
Asks about normal pattern of fluid intake	❏
Asks about past medical problems and past surgery	

Key Points	Satisfactorily Completed
• Genitourinary trauma: childbirth	❏
• Genitourinary or pelvic surgery	❏
• Diabetes	❏
• Congestive heart failure	❏
• Neurologic disorders and conditions that decrease mobility	❏
Documents medications:	
• Asks for a complete list of medications, including dosages (prescription, OTC, and herbal medicines)	❏
• Clarifies any recent changes to medication regimen (e.g., addition of diuretics)	❏
Makes appropriate closing remarks	❏

Pearl

• Potentially reversible causes of urinary incontinence can be sought with the mnemonic **DRIP:**

Drugs, **d**elirium

Restricted mobility, **r**etention (overflow incontinence)

Infection, **i**mpaction (stool)

Polydipsia

REFERENCES

1. Fick DM, Cooper JW, Wade WE, et al. Updating the Beers criteria for potentially inappropriate medication use in older adults: results of a US consensus panel of experts. *Arch Intern Med.* 2003;163:2716-2724.
2. Holsinger T, Deveau J, Boustani M, et al. Does this patient have dementia? *JAMA.* 2007;297: 2391-2404.
3. Ganz DA, Bao Y, Shekelle PG, et al. Will my patient fall? *JAMA.* 2007;297:77-86.
4. Buschke H, Kuslansky G, Katz M, et al. Screening for dementia with the memory impairment screen. *Neurology.* 1999;52:231-238.
5. Kuslansky G, Buschke H, Katz M, et al. Screening for Alzheimer disease: the memory impairment screen versus the conventional three word memory test. *J Am Geriatr Soc.* 2002;50:1086-1091.
6. Carr DB, Gray S, Baty J, et al. The value of informant versus individual's complaints of memory impairment in early dementia. *Neurology.* 2000;55:1724-1726.

CHAPTER 14

Ethics

ESSENTIAL SKILLS

END-OF-LIFE CARE

> **INSTRUCTIONS TO CANDIDATE: A 68-year-old woman is brought to the emergency department by her husband because of worsening shortness of breath. She has cyanosis, is tachypneic, and is having difficulty speaking in complete sentences. She is known to have end-stage chronic obstructive pulmonary disease. In the past year, she has been admitted to the hospital three times, and her functional abilities have continued to decline despite optimal medical management. She does not have an advance care directive. When asked by the attending physician about intubation and resuscitation, she says, "Let me die." Talk to the patient and her family about her wishes.**

Advance Care Planning

- Unfortunately, this patient does not have an advance care directive. Like informed consent, advance care planning is a process rather than an event. Using this process, capable patients make decisions with regard to their future health care (in the event that they should become unable to express their wishes). This may take the form of a written document called an *advance care directive* that outlines specific wishes, usually with regard to resuscitative measures, or appoints a substitute decision maker to carry out these wishes, or both. In this process, patients may identify the standard of living or quality of life that would be acceptable for them. Alternatively, the patient may simply make family members and friends aware of his or her wishes with the expectation that they would make decisions consistent with these expressed wishes.
- An advance care directive takes effect only when the patient is not able to make his or her own decision.
- Advance care planning should be reevaluated on an ongoing basis as the patient's disease changes.

End-of-Life Care
- High-quality end-of-life care is often recognized as lacking in modern medical care.
- Singer and MacDonald[1] identified three main elements in quality end-of-life care:
  - Control of pain and other symptoms (e.g., breathlessness, nausea, fatigue)
  - Use of life-sustaining treatment
  - Support of dying patients and their families

In the Course of a Compassionate Conversation, the Candidate Should:
- Ask the patient about resuscitative measures (intubation, noninvasive positive pressure ventilation, defibrillation, cardiopulmonary resuscitation [CPR]).
- Ask the patient about the process through which she came to this decision and whether she has discussed it with her family.
- Provide information about the likelihood of success and the potential risks or harms of attempting resuscitation.
- Ascertain that the patient understands her disease process and the proposed treatment.
- Ascertain that the patient understands the consequences of her decision (i.e., death).
- Ascertain that the decision is consistent with the patient's values (i.e., not based on delusions, depression, or other pathologic state).
- Ask the patient's husband about their previous discussions regarding resuscitation.
- Agree to respect the patient's request (if applicable).
- Reinforce the fact that withholding resuscitative measures does not imply withdrawal or withholding of all treatment.
- Describe a plan for treatment in light of the discussion (may include admission or transfer to a quieter area of the department, symptom management, and comfort care).
- Offer to answer any questions or address the patient's concerns.
- Ask what else can be done to help (e.g., access to phone to contact other family members, access to spiritual care or social worker).
- State that the patient can change her mind.

FUTILITY AND WITHDRAWAL OF CARE

> **INSTRUCTIONS TO CANDIDATE:** A 47-year-old man presented to the emergency department via ambulance, intubated, ventilated, and comatose. Paramedics were called to the scene after he had a "seizure" at home. On arrival he was "decerebrate" (i.e., rigid extension). He had previously been in good health. His pupils are now fixed and dilated. A computed tomographic scan shows a major intracerebral hemorrhage. The consulting neurosurgeon says that the chances of meaningful recovery or even survival are negligible. His wife arrives and would like to be updated on his condition.

Medical Futility
- Medical futility is a controversial concept that refers to situations in which medical treatment is not likely to benefit the patient. In situations such as these, futile treatments need not be offered at all and may be refused if demanded by family members. This idea has not been universally accepted and has not been tested conclusively within the court system. As such, institutional variation is to be expected. There are two types of medical futility:
  - *Quantitative futility:* When the treatment is physiologically incapable of achieving the goals of care (i.e., essentially useless)
  - *Qualitative futility:* When the gain produced by an intervention (quality) is exceptionally poor (e.g., the patient remains in a permanent state of unconsciousness)
- In catastrophic situations in which the prognosis for recovery or survival is bleak, timely communication with the family is essential. They should be apprised of the prognosis and what it means for their loved one in terms of treatments and outcomes. The attending physician should assure the family that everything will be done to ensure the patient's comfort, but no further life-sustaining treatment will be offered.

Withdrawal of Life-Prolonging Treatment

- There is no ethical or legal distinction between withholding and withdrawing life-prolonging treatment that has already been started.
- It is appropriate to withdraw a life-sustaining measure when it is no longer of benefit to the patient or at the request of a capable patient or substitute decision maker.

In the Course of a Compassionate Conversation, the Candidate Should:

- Assure the wife of the certainty of her husband's diagnosis and prognosis.
- Ask whether the patient has made an advance care directive or a living will.
- Ascertain whether the wife is the substitute decision maker.
- Ensure that the wife understands that the role of the substitute decision maker is to make a decision that would be consistent with the patient's prior stated wishes.
- Offer to facilitate a family meeting.
- Ask about discussions regarding the previously expressed wishes of the patient.
- State that life-prolonging medical care should be withdrawn.
- Reinforce the fact that withholding further life-prolonging measures does not imply withdrawal or withholding of all treatments.
- Offer to answer any questions or address her concerns.
- Describe a plan for treatment in reference to the discussion (discontinuation of ventilation with or without extubation, symptom management and comfort care, transfer to a quieter area of the department, availability of spiritual care, or other support).
- Ask what else can be done to help (e.g., access to phone to contact other family members, access to spiritual care or social worker).
- Mention that the patient *may* be a candidate for tissue donation (organ donation can be considered only when brain death is confirmed).
- Ask about any previous discussions with her husband about tissue or organ donation.

INFORMED CONSENT

> **INSTRUCTIONS TO CANDIDATE: A 61-year-old woman presents to her family physician for the results of a recent screening mammogram. You inform her that something suspicious has been detected, and you are recommending a biopsy. She had a biopsy 3 years ago, the results of which were negative. She was disturbed by the scar from that procedure. Discuss the proposed procedure for the purposes of "informed consent" (or refusal).**

Process of Informed Consent

- The need for informed consent arises from a fundamental societal tenet that the human body be protected from violation by another person, and from the ethical duty to involve patients in their health care decisions. Within the law, medical treatment, intervention, or investigation without consent can be interpreted as assault, battery, or both.
- Informed consent is a *process*, not a form; completing a consent form does not by itself imply that "informed consent" was obtained. Consent is a two-part process that involves disclosure of information and the patient's subsequent decision (to consent or to refuse the procedure).
- Using understandable language, you should disclose the nature of the procedure and its purpose, including how the outcome will alter further management plans. This discussion should also include the possible benefits and the severity and likelihood of risks (according to the standard of what a patient would want to know under the circumstances, within reason). The patient should be offered possible alternatives to the procedure (possible benefits and the severity and likelihood of risks), including the possibility of doing nothing.

- You should present an opportunity for the patient to ask questions and express concerns. Seek confirmation that the patient understands the procedure, its risks, and its benefits before she makes the decision.
- The patient's decision must be voluntary and not coerced. The patient may elect to take further time to consider her options or have discussions with her family or friends.
- The setting may also be of importance. For example, it would not be appropriate to seek informed consent for nonemergency surgery in the hallway outside the operating room. It is arguable that this setting is coercive in itself.
- A mnemonic for essentials of informed consent is **Dduv** (pronounced "dove"):
  - **Decision-making capacity**
  - **Disclosure**
  - **Understanding**
  - **Voluntariness**

Capacity

- Although the terms are often used interchangeably, capacity and competency are not equivalent. *Competency* tends to be stable over time and is often a legal determination. *Capacity* is applied to particular decisions (e.g., where to live or whether to undertake chemotherapy) and may fluctuate over time and across domains (e.g., finances, personal care, health care). The treating physician and the health care team determine a patient's capacity in the health care setting. This is not to be confused with involuntary admission to hospital for risk of harm to self or others; such patients may still retain the capacity to refuse medical treatment.
- If a patient has been deemed capable of making a particular decision, it must be respected whether it is in accordance with your recommendations or not. Refusal to comply with treatment recommendations is not evidence of incapacity, nor is difficulty in making the decision.
- A patient's capacity is determined according to the following criteria:
  - Ability to understand the medical problem, the proposed treatment, and possible alternatives
  - Ability to appreciate the consequences of undergoing the proposed treatment
  - Ability to appreciate the consequences of refusing the proposed treatment
  - Ability to make the decision within a stable set of values (not based on delusions or depression)

In the Course of a Compassionate Conversation, the Candidate Should:

- Explain the nature of the procedure, its purpose, risks, and benefits.
- Offer alternatives to the procedure, including the possibility of doing nothing and the consequences.
- Ask whether the patient has any concerns about the procedure.
- Confirm whether the patient understands the information, including the consequences of refusing the procedure.
- Ask whether the patient needs more time or information to make the decision.
- Allow the patient to make a voluntary decision.
- Explore reasons for refusing to consent (if applicable).

DECISION-MAKING CAPACITY AND REFUSAL OF CARE

> **INSTRUCTIONS TO CANDIDATE:** A 56-year-old man with a complicated in-hospital course of recovery from pancreatitis is having upper gastrointestinal bleeding. As the intensive care unit staff person on call, you have been asked to see this patient. His hemoglobin level is 56 g/L, but he is currently refusing blood products because of religious convictions. He is now having chest pain. You note acute ischemic changes on his electrocardiogram, but he continues to refuse blood products. His wife pleads with you in the hallway to "do something to help him." Discuss the situation with the patient and his wife, and ascertain his wishes.

Substitute Decision Making

- A substitute decision maker is one who makes decisions on behalf of a patient who is not capable of doing so. These decisions should reflect what the patient would want in a particular circumstance as much as possible, rather than the wishes of the decision maker for the patient.
- Ideally, the substitute decision maker would be appointed by a patient who is still capable and who has informed the decision maker about his or her wishes in particular situations.
- In the absence of an appointed decision maker, the task falls to the spouse, child, parent, sibling, another relative, or a public guardian. The substitute decision maker should be someone who knows the patient well, because decisions should still be based on the *patient's* beliefs and values, rather than the wishes of the decision maker for the patient. The laws about identifying substitute decision makers vary from province to province and from state to state.
- A parent's religious beliefs do not include the right to deny life-prolonging treatment, including blood transfusions, for a child. In the case of such patients, the child would be made a ward of the court, and all necessary treatments would be provided in accordance with the principles of nonmaleficence and beneficence.

Process of Informed Consent

- Consent is a two-part process that involves disclosure of information and the patient's subsequent decision (to consent to or refuse the procedure).
- Using understandable language, you should disclose the nature of the procedure and its purpose, including how the outcome will alter further management plans. This discussion should also include the possible benefits and the severity and likelihood of risks (according to the standard of what a patient would want to know under the circumstances, within reason). The patient should be offered possible alternatives to the procedure (with explanations of possible benefits and the severity and likelihood of risks), including the possibility of doing nothing.
- You should present an opportunity for the patient to ask questions and express concerns. Seek confirmation that the patient understands the procedure and its risks and benefits before he makes the decision.
- The patient's decision must be voluntary and not coerced.

Capacity

- A patient's capacity is determined according to the following criteria:
  - Ability to understand the medical problem, the proposed treatment, and possible alternatives
  - Ability to appreciate the consequences of undergoing the proposed treatment
  - Ability to appreciate the consequences of refusing the proposed treatment
  - Ability to make the decision within a stable set of values (not based on delusions or depression)

In the Course of a Compassionate Conversation, the Candidate Should:
- Explain the seriousness of the patient's condition and that because of ongoing bleeding and acute myocardial ischemia, having no transfusion will likely lead to death.
- Ask whether the patient has discussed his wishes with his wife.
- Ascertain the reason for refusing blood products (e.g., Jehovah's Witness teachings).
- Ensure that the patient is not depressed, suicidal, or delusional.
- Ascertain that the patient understands the seriousness of the consequences of refusing blood products (i.e., death).
- Allow the patient to make a voluntary decision.
- Offer to facilitate the patient's discussion with his wife.
- Explain that the patient retains capacity to make informed decisions about health care.
- State that the patient's wishes will be respected.
- Address any additional concerns raised by the patient and his wife.
- Ask the patient whether he desires other life-sustaining treatments (intubation, defibrillation, CPR).
- State that the patient can change his mind.

CONFIDENTIALITY, CONSENT, AND THE MATURE MINOR

> **INSTRUCTIONS TO CANDIDATE: A 14-year-old girl presents to the emergency department with right lower quadrant pain and "spotting." On investigation, she is found to have an ectopic pregnancy and requires surgery urgently. She understands the importance of having the surgery. She came to the hospital with a friend but would like to see her parents. She does not want them to find out what kind of operation she is having because they do not know she is sexually active. Discuss these concerns with her.**

Confidentiality
- Confidentiality is a fundamental underlying premise of the physician-patient relationship. Trust is necessary to maintain the therapeutic relationship and to ensure that patients feel secure in being forthcoming with their symptoms and concerns. Withholding information may prove detrimental to the patient's care.
- The autonomous patient has the right to decide when to disclose information to others (if there is no risk of harm).
- Specific information should be disclosed in the following cases:
  - Suspicion of child abuse
  - Reportable diseases (a matter of public health)
  - Public safety risk such as unsafe drivers
  - Imminent serious risk of harm to an identifiable individual

Process of Informed Consent
- Consent is a two-part process that involves disclosure of information and the patient's decision (to consent to or refuse the procedure).
- Using understandable language, you should disclose the nature of the procedure and its purpose, including how the outcome will alter further management plans. This discussion should also include the possible benefits and the severity and likelihood of risks (according to the standard of what a patient would want to know under the circumstances, within reason). The patient should be offered possible alternatives to the procedure (possible benefits and the severity and likelihood of risks), including the possibility of doing nothing.
- You should present an opportunity for the patient to ask questions and express concerns. Seek confirmation that the patient understands the procedure and its risks and benefits before making the decision.
- The patient's decision must be voluntary and not coerced.

Mature Minor

- A mature minor is a child who meets criteria for capacity and is able to participate in informed consent. Provincial laws generally do not specify an age below which a child is presumed incapable.
- A patient's capacity is determined according to the following criteria:
  - Ability to understand the medical problem, the proposed treatment, and possible alternatives
  - Ability to appreciate the consequences of undergoing the proposed treatment
  - Ability to appreciate the consequences of refusing the proposed treatment
  - Ability to make the decision within a stable set of values (not based on delusions or depression)

In the Course of a Compassionate Conversation, the Candidate Should:

- Explain the nature of the surgery and its purpose, risks, and benefits.
- Offer alternatives to the surgery, including the possibility of doing nothing and the consequences.
- Ask whether the patient has any concerns, questions, or comments.
- Confirm whether the patient understands the information, including the consequences of refusing the surgery.
- Ask whether the patient needs more time or information to make the decision.
- Allow the patient to make a voluntary decision.
- Assure the patient that her confidentiality will be respected.
- Inform the patient that her parents' inquiries will be redirected to her (i.e., you will not lie to them about the nature of her surgery).
- Address the nature of the patient's relationship with her parents.
- Encourage her to consider being honest with her parents.
- Offer to facilitate and be present for a discussion with her parents.
- Offer local support services to her, such as crisis team or social work.

BRAIN DEATH AND ORGAN DONATION

> **INSTRUCTIONS TO CANDIDATE: An 18-year-old woman is in the intensive care unit for 36 hours. She was intubated for acute decline in level of consciousness. Although previously healthy, she is now known to have extensive thrombosis of her cavernous sinus. Her family has expressed concern to the nursing staff about the idea of organ donation and worry that the doctors are interested only in her organs. You have confirmed that she now meets the criteria for brain death. Approach the family, and discuss her current condition.**

Brain Death

- Brain death is the complete and irreversible cessation of all brain function.
- The brain-dead patient is comatose and apneic and does not have brainstem reflexes.
- At the time of brain death declaration, the patient is considered medically and legally dead, even though, with the assistance of a ventilator and critical care, vital signs may still be present.
- Brain death is an ethically challenging concept for some people. Some cultural and religious groups may not be able to accept death until the cessation of all vital functions.
- Brain death can usually be determined at the bedside. Electroencephalography is not required in order to determine brain death; in fact, it may yield unreliable readings. Clinical criteria for the declaration of brain death (in a patient aged >2 months)[2] are as follows:
  - Lack of reversible causes of cerebral unresponsiveness, such as hypothermia and depressant or sedative medications. This may require a period of observation.
  - Absence of brainstem reflexes, including oculovestibular (cold caloric), oculocephalic (doll's eye), pupillary, corneal, gag, and respiratory (apnea testing) reflexes. Apnea

testing includes disconnecting the ventilator for approximately 10 minutes to allow the partial pressure of arterial CO_2 to increase to 60 mm Hg (pH <7.28). Absence of respiratory effort at this point confirms apnea (absence of respiratory reflexes).

- Absence of motor responses in the cranial nerve distribution to stimuli applied anywhere on the body. Spinal reflexes may remain intact.

Organ Donation

- Organ retrieval cannot be performed unless the patient is no longer alive.
- Declaration of brain death for the purposes of organ retrieval should be declared by two separate physicians not involved in the care of potential organ recipients. Furthermore, physicians who participate in the declaration of brain death should not participate in the transplantation procedures.
- Most institutions have dedicated teams of personnel for organ donation and retrieval.
- Laws about organ and tissue donation may vary from province to province, state to state, and institution to institution. Ensure that you are aware of the laws in your region and the policies of your institution.

In the Course of a Compassionate Conversation, the Candidate Should:

- Assure the patient's parents that everything possible has been done in the investigation and treatment of their daughter's condition.
- Explain the meaning of "brain death" (e.g., complete and irreversible cessation of brain function, including the brainstem).
- Assure her parents of the certainty of the diagnosis (i.e., clinical criteria have been satisfied and verified by two separate physicians).
- Assure her parents of the certainty of the prognosis (i.e., brain damage is complete and irreversible; there is no chance of recovery).
- State clearly that their daughter is dead now (i.e., brain death is a legal definition of death).
- State that ventilatory support and other critical care measures should now be stopped.
- Give the family an opportunity to ask questions.
- Address any concerns raised by the patient's parents.
- Ask about previous discussions with the patient about organ donation and whether she had an organ donation card.
- Explain that their daughter is now a candidate for organ donation.
- Ask the family's views regarding donation of the patient's organs.
- Address their concerns if possible (e.g., organ donation does not affect burial).
- If the family expresses interest in learning more about the option of organ and tissue donation, offer the option of discussing it further with the organ donor personnel at your institution.

REFERENCES

1. Singer PA, MacDonald N. Quality end-of-life care. In: Singer PA, ed. *Bioethics at the Bedside: A Clinician's Guide.* Ottawa, ON: Canadian Medical Association; 1999: 117-124.
2. Lazar NM, Shemie S, Webster GC, Dickens BM. Bioethics for clinicians: 24. Brain death. *CMAJ.* 2001;164(6):833-836.

Sample In-Depth OSCE Case

Graham Bullock, MD, FRCPC (used with permission)

> **INSTRUCTIONS TO CANDIDATE:** You are a clinical clerk working in the emergency department. Mark Bartholomew presents to the emergency department with a 2-day history of "jaundice." During the next 10 minutes, obtain a detailed history of the onset and nature of his symptoms, exploring possible causes. Examine the liver. Describe the examination and your findings to the examiner. Communicate your impressions to the patient.

PATIENT SCRIPT: MARK BARTHOLOMEW

DEMOGRAPHICS

Age: 24 years
Sex: male
Marital status: single
Educational background: university student majoring in computer science

CHIEF CONCERN

"I think I have jaundice."

PATIENT BEHAVIOR, AFFECT, AND MANNERISMS

The patient is a young man ("woman" could be substituted) of average build. He is wearing an examining gown and shorts. He appears a little anxious but is otherwise in no distress and is cooperative. No makeup is required.

During examination, on deep palpation of the epigastric area and right upper quadrant (RUQ), he complains of mild discomfort. He demonstrates no guarding or evidence of peritoneal irritation.

HISTORY OF CURRENT ILLNESS

He has been feeling essentially well until approximately 7 days ago, when he experienced the onset of nonspecific symptoms, including nausea, chills, and loose stools. These symptoms continued for several days but have now largely abated and left him with a general feeling of fatigue, muscle aches, and vague abdominal discomfort. He has been sleeping much more than usual—up to 10 hours per night—and has had to skip classes. Today his roommate told him that she thought he looked yellow and should get to a doctor. He had not yet sought medical attention for this illness.

PAST MEDICAL/SURGICAL HISTORY

No events of significance are noted. He has not had hepatitis testing or hepatitis vaccinations to date. He has had no previous blood transfusions, no previous hospitalizations, and no surgery.

MEDICATIONS

- **Prescription medications:** None.
- **Over-the-counter (OTC) medications:** Caffeine tablets, taken on a regular basis when studying; acetaminophen and ibuprofen, taken occasionally but not recently and never to excess.

ALLERGIES

None known.

RELEVANT SOCIAL HISTORY

- Mr. Bartholomew is a third-year university student studying computer science. He is not aware of any exposures to infectious hepatitis. He has no past employment or history suggestive of exposure to hepatotoxic drugs.
- He is currently dating and has no fixed partner. Although he has had several different sexual partners in the past year, he uses condoms "religiously." He has no children.
- He does not smoke. He drinks a "case" of beer (24 beers) per week, mostly on the weekends.
- He has dabbled with amphetamines and "wake-ups" to help him study for examinations. He denies intravenous drug use but has smoked marijuana and tried cocaine nasally in the remote past.
- He enjoys skiing and extreme sports. He took part in a cross-country adventure race in the southern United States (Nevada) 4 weeks ago. He drank filtered water on that trip and is not aware of any other participants who are sick. He did not have any immunizations before this trip.

RELEVANT FAMILY HISTORY

- Father, aged 58 years, has high blood pressure and angina.
- Mother, aged 52 years, is "pretty healthy."
- Brother, aged 28 years, is not aware of any health problems.
- There is no known family predisposition to cancers or liver disease.

REVIEW OF SYSTEMS

- **General:** The patient had chills last week and a poor appetite this week; no documented fever; and no weight change.
- **Head, eyes, ears, nose, and throat (HEENT):** No abnormal findings are noted.
- **Respiratory (Resp):** No abnormal findings are noted.
- **Cardiovascular system (CVS):** No abnormal findings are noted.
- **Gastrointestinal (GI):** Vague dull, constant upper abdominal pain has been present for the past week. The pain does not radiate. No exacerbating or relieving features are noted. The patient had several loose, nonbloody stools last week. Now bowel movements are about normal, with no color change. The patient had some diarrhea while in the southern United States for a few days that resolved spontaneously.
- **Genitourinary system (GU):** Urine is slightly darker than normal. Otherwise, findings are negative.
- **Skin:** Possible jaundice is documented. Otherwise, findings are negative.

PHYSICAL EXAMINATION

- The patient appears anxious but is otherwise in no distress.
- He should not have any visible surgical scars.
- He is able to cooperate with the history taking and physical examination.
- During examination, on deep palpation of the epigastric area and RUQ, he complains of mild discomfort. He demonstrates no guarding or evidence of peritoneal irritation.

EXAMINER'S CHECKLIST: JAUNDICE

Please indicate which items were satisfactorily completed.

General/Introductory

❑	1. Introduces self to the patient	
❑	2. Determines how patient wishes to be addressed	
❑	3. Washes hands	
❑	4. Establishes the purpose of the encounter	
❑	5. Establishes presenting concern in the patient's own words	
❑	6. Uses open-ended questions to obtain story	

Presenting Concern: Jaundice and Associated Symptoms

❑	7. Establishes onset	Noticed by roommate today; otherwise not sure
❑	8. Preceding symptoms	Yes, unwell for 1 week
❑	9. Fever/chills	Chills earlier this week
❑	10. Nausea/vomiting	Nausea with reduced appetite, no vomiting
❑	11. Abdominal pain	Yes
❑	12. Onset of abdominal pain	Not sure; about 1 week ago
❑	13. Nature of abdominal pain	Dull, ache
❑	14. Severity of pain	Mild
❑	15. Location of pain	Upper abdomen
❑	16. Aggravating or alleviating factors for pain	None
❑	17. Nature of stools: diarrhea?	Yes, last week
❑	18. Color of stools	Normal, brown

Review of Systems: Other Relevant Features

❑	19. Skin rash	No
❑	20. Myalgias	Yes, mild and generalized
❑	21. Urine color	No change

Relevant Social History

❑	22. Alcohol consumption	Yes
❑	23. Quantifies recent alcohol consumption	24 Beers per week
❑	24. Intravenous drug use	No
❑	25. Sexual contacts: number of partners and frequency	Several different sexual partners in past year
❑	26. Sexual practices: barrier precautions	Uses condoms
❑	27. Recent travel	Yes, southern United States
❑	28. Possible exposure to contaminated water	Yes, recent trip

Past Medical History

❑	29. Previous hepatitis	No
❑	30. History of biliary/gallbladder disease	No
❑	31. Previous vaccinations against hepatitis	No
❑	32. Prescription medications	None
❑	33. OTC medications: specifically acetaminophen	Occasional acetaminophen, ibuprofen; regular use of caffeine tablets when studying

Physical Examination

❑	34. Drapes the patient appropriately	
❑	35. Inspects for rash and discoloration of the skin and sclerae	Faint jaundice?
❑	36. Percusses liver span from above	
❑	37. Percusses liver span from below	
❑	38. Palpates for liver edge, beginning in the right lower quadrant	Not enlarged
❑	39. Palpates liver for tenderness, including Murphy's sign	
❑	40. Palpates RUQ/liver edge for mass, including gallbladder	None

Closure

❑	41. Makes appropriate closing remarks	

Note: Page numbers followed by b, f, or t indicate boxes, figures, and tables, respectively.

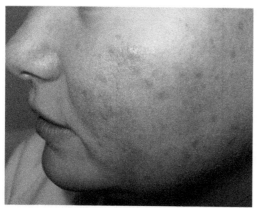

Figure 7-6 Acne rosacea. Note prominent background erythema and inflammatory papules of similar size and shape in the absence of comedones. Note subtle telangiectasias (small, threadlike blood vessels) account for the erythema but are not clearly visible in this image. (Courtesy of Dr. Peter Green.)

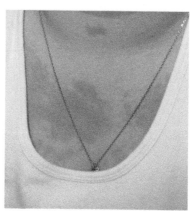

Figure 7-7 Note prominent flushing response on chest in a patient with rosacea. (Courtesy of Dr. Peter Green.)

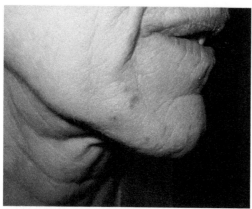

Figure 7-8 Acne excoriée. Patient presented with "acne unresponsive to treatment." Note absence of any primary acne excoriée; only excoriations are present. (Courtesy of Dr. Peter Green.)

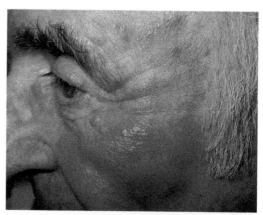

Figure 7-9 Steroid acne. An acneiform eruption confined to cheeks and temples, where moderate-potency topical steroids had been applied over a number of years. Again, note the presence of telangiectasias and absence of comedones. Rosacea could have a similar appearance; thus the history was instrumental in making the appropriate diagnosis. (Courtesy of Dr. Peter Green.)

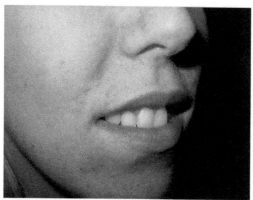

Figure 7-10 Perioral dermatitis: a subtle collection of monomorphic red papules in a perioral distribution. Note sparing of vermillion line of the lip and lack of comedones. (Courtesy of Dr. Peter Green.)

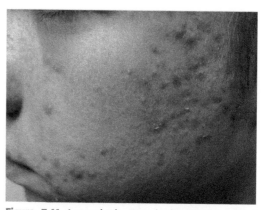

Figure 7-11 Acne vulgaris. Note simultaneous presence of open comedones (blackheads), papules, pustules, small nodules, and subtle scarring. The patient was treated successfully with oral isotretinoin. (Courtesy of Dr. Peter Green.)

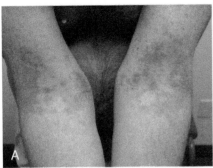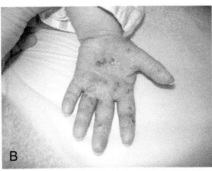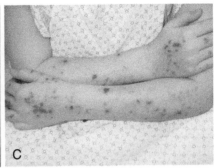

Figure 7-12 Manifestations of atopic dermatitis. **A,** Typical flexural location for atopic dermatitis; ill-defined, red, lichenified plaques with no vesicles or evidence of secondary infection. **B,** Eczema herpeticum: that is, secondary infection of underlying atopic dermatitis with herpes simplex type 1. Note hemorrhagic vesicles and pustules, which were painful. **C,** Atopic dermatitis that is secondarily infected with *S. aureus.* Note significant crusts and erosions. (Courtesy of Dr. Peter Green.)

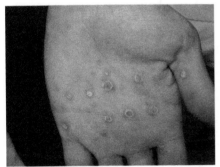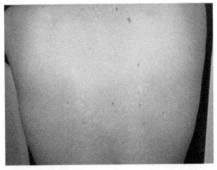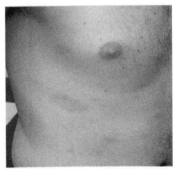

Figure 7-13 Secondary syphilis involving palm. (Courtesy of Dr. Peter Green.)

Figure 7-14 Pityriasis versicolor with predominance of hypopigmentation and subtle scale. (Courtesy of Dr. Peter Green.)

Figure 7-15 Herald patch of pityriasis rosea; note adjacent smaller, oval, and scaly plaques. (Courtesy of Dr. Peter Green.)

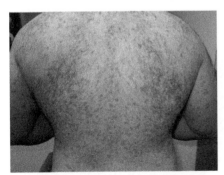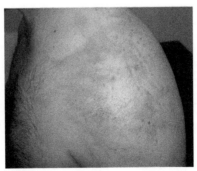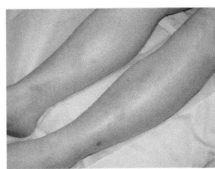

Figure 7-16 Guttate psoriasis on trunk following streptococcal pharyngitis. (Courtesy of Dr. Peter Green.)

Figure 7-17 Urticaria. (Courtesy of Dr. Peter Green.)

Figure 7-18 Ill-defined red nodules on shins of a patient with erythema nodosum and associated asymptomatic pulmonary sarcoid. (Courtesy of Dr. Peter Green.)

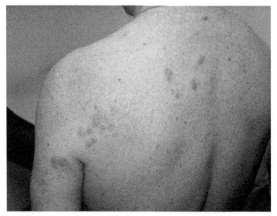

Figure 7-19 Dermatomal pattern of herpes zoster on trunk; note clusters of vesicles. (Courtesy of Dr. Peter Green.)

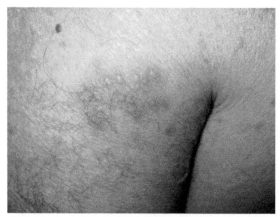

Figure 7-20 Close-up of herpes zoster, demonstrating vesicles on an erythematous base. (Courtesy of Dr. Peter Green.)

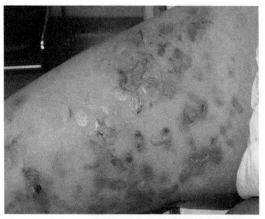

Figure 7-21 Tense bullae adjacent to ruptured bullae on lower extremity in a man with bullous pemphigoid. (Courtesy of Dr. Peter Green.)

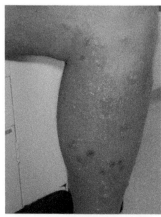

Figure 7-22 Linear vesicles and bullae on an urticarial, erythematous base of poison ivy allergic contact dermatitis. (Courtesy of Dr. Peter Green.)

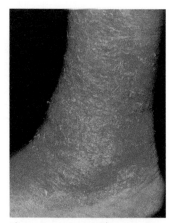

Figure 7-23 Venous stasis ulcer. (From Habif TP. *A color guide to diagnosis and therapy: clinical dermatology,* ed 4, St. Louis, 1996, Mosby, p 72.)

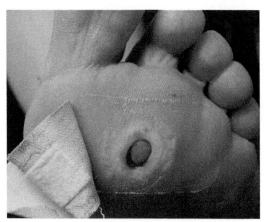

Figure 7-24 Mal perforans ulcer (diabetic). (Courtesy of Dr. Peter Green.)

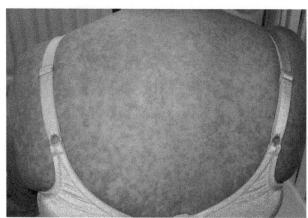

Figure 7-25 Drug exanthem after ingestion of amoxicillin. (Courtesy of Dr. Peter Green.)

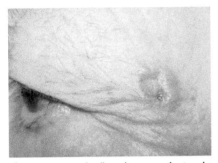

Figure 7-26 Basal cell carcinoma on the temple. (Courtesy of Dr. Peter Green.)

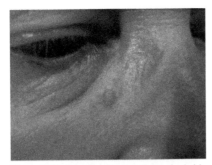

Figure 7-27 Seborrheic keratosis, irritated, mimicking a squamous cell carcinoma. Note waxy, stuck-on appearance. (Courtesy of Dr. Peter Green.)

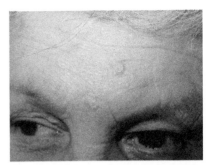

Figure 7-28 Sebaceous gland hyperplasia on the forehead: a soft yellow papule with central umbilication. (Courtesy of Dr. Peter Green.)

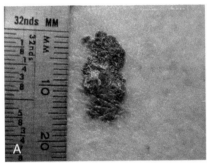
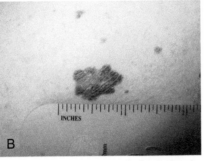

Figure 7-29 A, Malignant melanoma on the scapula. **B,** Malignant melanoma on the lower extremity. Note multiple colors in the lesion, including pink, tan, brown, and black. (Courtesy of Dr. Peter Green.)

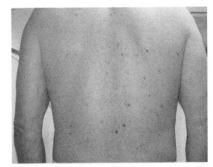

Figure 7-30 Dysplastic or atypical nevi on the back. (Courtesy of Dr. Peter Green.)

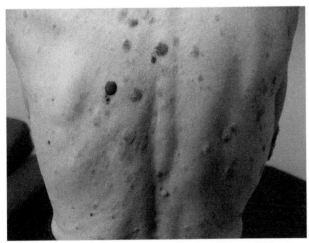

Figure 7-31 Multiple seborrheic keratoses on the back. (Courtesy of Dr. Peter Green.)

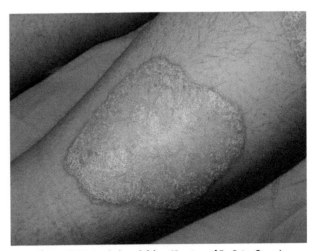

Figure 7-32 Psoriasis on left leg. (Courtesy of Dr. Peter Green.)